Practical Sample Size Determination for Medical and Health Researchers

This book provides a clear, comprehensive guide to sample size determination across medical and health-related disciplines, including epidemiology, clinical trials, rehabilitation sciences, and reliability studies. Beginning with essential topics – such as estimating means and proportions or comparing two groups – it progresses to advanced applications including one- and two-way ANOVA, ANCOVA, repeated-measures ANOVA, multiple outcomes, correlation analysis, linear and logistic regression, intraclass correlation coefficients, Kappa statistics, Cronbach's alpha, and more. Each topic is illustrated with real-world, fully worked numerical examples and supported by practical reference tables for commonly used values.

The ability to generalise findings from a sample to a reference population is one of the most compelling goals for researchers, yet achieving this requires an adequate sample size in practice. Determining the right sample size is also one of the most challenging steps in study design and proposal development, as it demands a careful balance between feasibility, resource constraints, and statistical rigour. Many novice or non-methodologist researchers fall into common pitfalls: relying on arbitrary, predetermined, or conventional sample sizes so they can collect data first and manipulate other factors later; modelling their studies on previous research without recognising key differences – overlooking the fact that sample size is influenced by numerous dynamic factors; or adjusting software inputs and default values without fully understanding the underlying concepts and specialised terminology simply to obtain a preconceived sample size. These missteps can compromise both the validity and interpretability of results.

Drawing on more than 40 years of teaching and research experience in biostatistics, sampling, and study design, the author – an associate professor and seasoned expert in sample size determination – provides readers with both the theoretical foundation and the practical tools needed to design statistically sound studies with confidence. The author has published several books, including *Practical Biostatistics for Medical and Health Sciences* (2024) and *A Tale of Research: A Novice Exploring the World of Scientific Research* (2020), the latter written in the style of theatrical plays.

Practical Sample Size Determination for Medical and Health Researchers

Seyed Hassan Saneii

CRC Press
Taylor & Francis Group
Boca Raton London New York

CRC Press is an imprint of the
Taylor & Francis Group, an **informa** business
A CHAPMAN & HALL BOOK

Designed cover image: Seyed Hassan Saneii

First edition published 2027
by CRC Press
2385 NW Executive Center Drive, Suite 320, Boca Raton FL 33431

and by CRC Press
4 Park Square, Milton Park, Abingdon, Oxon, OX14 4RN

CRC Press is an imprint of Taylor & Francis Group, LLC

ISBN: 978-1-041-26278-7 (hbk)
ISBN: 978-1-041-26281-7 (pbk)
ISBN: 978-1-003-74978-3 (ebk)

DOI: 10.1201/9781003749783

Typeset in Palatino
by Deanta Global Publishing Services, Chennai, India

Contents

Introduction

In today's rapidly evolving world, research serves as the cornerstone of advancements in biological, medical, and health sciences. At the heart of meaningful discoveries lies the critical process of sampling and sample size determination. The ability to generalise findings from a sample to a larger population is essential, yet it demands meticulous planning and scientifically robust methodologies. Among the most challenging aspects of research is determining the appropriate sample size, which requires a delicate balance between feasibility, resource efficiency, and statistical rigour.

In my 40 years of teaching and research, I have observed several common yet flawed practices in sample size determination:

1. **Manipulating Factors to Fit Desired Outcomes**: Researchers often fix the number of individuals they can examine and then manipulate factors influencing sample size to match their preferred outcome using statistical formulas or software. This approach, lacking justified reasoning, is fundamentally flawed.
2. **Overreliance on Default Values in Software**: While sample size calculation software is based on scientifically valid methods, many researchers, unfamiliar with specialised terminology, rely on default values or tweak inputs to achieve their predetermined sample size. Such practices undermine the integrity of the research process.
3. **Bypassing Methodological Consultation**: It is not uncommon for researchers to base their sample size on similar studies, thereby bypassing necessary methodological consultation. This approach neglects the fact that sample size is influenced by numerous dynamic factors, including significance level, statistical power, trait variability, dropout rate, sampling method, and the type of statistical test (one-tailed or two-tailed tests). These factors can vary over time, across locations, and between study populations, necessitating a tailored calculation for each specific research context.

This book is designed to guide students and researchers through the complexities of sampling and sample size determination. It offers practical tools, numerical examples, and step-by-step guidance to ensure scientifically robust results. Whether you are a novice researcher or an experienced scientist, this book will equip you with the knowledge and confidence to make informed decisions about sample size and sampling methods.

Structured into 12 comprehensive chapters, the book begins with "Fundamentals: Core Principles, Terminology, and Definitions" (Chapter 1), laying a solid foundation for understanding sampling concepts. Chapters 2 and 3 explore non-probability sampling methods and probability sampling techniques, enriched with real-world examples and visual aids. Chapter 4, "Key Factors in Determining Sample Size", explores the critical elements that influence sample size, such as significance level, statistical power, and variability. Subsequent chapters address specialised applications, including "Population Size Estimation Techniques" (Chapter 5), "Sample Size for Estimating and Comparing Means and Totals" (Chapter 6), "Sample Size Determination for Proportions" (Chapter 7), "Sample Size Estimation for Epidemiological Studies" (Chapter 8), "Sample Size for ANOVA Family" (Chapter 9), "Sample Size for Correlation and Regression Analysis" (Chapter 10), "Sample Size Estimation for Survival Studies" (Chapter 11), and "Sample Size Estimation for Reliability Studies" (Chapter 12).

With its practical approach and comprehensive coverage, this book is an indispensable resource for researchers striving for excellence in their work. It is my hope that this guide will empower you to conduct impactful research, ensuring that your findings are both scientifically valid and applicable to the broader population.

1

Fundamentals: Core Principles, Terminology, and Definitions

1.1 Introduction

The primary objectives of research are to identify general relationships between specific events and the evidence that supports them, as well as to generalise findings from a sample to an entire population. Studying every individual within a population is often impractical and, in many cases, impossible. Additionally, in large populations, target values may change before the study can be completed. Therefore, research is frequently conducted on a smaller scale using sampling techniques, which rely on careful observation of selected units within the population.

Most scientific research employs sampling methods to enable generalisation from a sample to the broader population. For example, in clinical research, patients in a study are considered a sample representing the larger population of all comparable patients. A clear understanding of specialised terminology related to sampling is essential for selecting appropriate sampling techniques and accurately calculating sample sizes. Key terms and concepts relevant to sampling will be defined before exploring these topics in greater detail.

1.2 Terminology

1.2.1 Population

In everyday language, the term "population" typically refers to a collection of people living in a defined area, such as a country. In statistics, however, the concept is broader. A population is defined as the target group for a given study, to which the research findings are intended to apply and generalise. The elements, or units, within this group must share at least one common characteristic, which constitutes the target population. These units do not have to be human; they can include objects, animals, patients, children in

DOI: 10.1201/9781003749783-1

schools, medical units, manufactured products, and so on. Accordingly, the number of units may be either finite or potentially infinite.

TIP

In statistics, a population refers to the target group under study, which may consist of humans, objects, or any clearly defined entities. Defining the population precisely ensures that the study's findings are both applicable and relevant, thereby enhancing the validity and reliability of the research.

The more characteristics shared by members of a population, the more specific – or "closed" – the population becomes. For example, the population of women athletes aged 30–40 is more narrowly defined than the broader population of all women athletes, which, in turn, is more specific than the general population of women. In most research studies, the population size – the total number of subjects in the population – is typically large. Collecting data from every member of such a population usually requires substantial time, financial resources, facilities, logistical support, and transportation.

Furthermore, factors such as sample loss, variations in participants' behaviour and mobility, and limited access to certain population members – due to travel, occupational commitments, or other constraints – complicate the data collection process. For these reasons, in medical research, only a small volume of a patient's blood (a few cubic centimetres) may be analysed to determine its composition and characteristics.

Given these challenges, it is often impractical to study every member of a population. Consequently, sampling becomes a logical and necessary strategy. This is particularly relevant in social, epidemiological, and scientific research, making sampling a common and widely accepted practice. For instance, only a portion of a population may be surveyed to determine the community's attitudes towards a specific television programme or social initiative.

1.2.2 Census

When the population is small, or when researchers possess adequate resources, logistics, budget, and facilities, it may be possible to study the entire target population through a **census**. In this approach, the attribute of interest is measured for every member of the population, providing complete certainty about the collected data. In rare cases, all subjects within the target population can be examined, resulting in what is known as complete enumeration or a census.

However, in most situations, conducting a census is impractical due to the large size of the population or because financial and logistical constraints hinder the collection of data from every member. In some cases, researchers can make a census possible by redefining the population, such as by limiting its size or geographical extent (Frey, 2021).

1.2.3 Sample

In statistics, a *sample* is a subset of a given population that is randomly selected and measured to represent that population. By studying a smaller number of subjects rather than including every member of the target population, researchers can measure variables and obtain the necessary information in less time, at lower cost, and with fewer resources. Such a sample provides insights into the original population, often referred to as the *parent population, reference population,* or *target population.* In other words, the sample should accurately reflect the characteristics of the main population.

To draw valid conclusions about the entire population from which the sample is taken, the sample must be selected in a way that allows each subgroup within the population to be adequately represented. For example, if a class consists of 50 students and we wish to select eight of them, each student's name could be written on a small piece of paper, placed in a container, and thoroughly mixed before drawing eight names at random. Alternatively, each student could be assigned a number from 1 to 50, and eight numbers could then be selected at random from a table of random numbers. The students corresponding to the selected numbers would form the sample.

In this example, every student has an equal probability of being chosen. However, if only students from the front row were selected, the resulting sample would not accurately represent the entire class. The characteristics of front-row students – such as vision difficulties or higher levels of enthusiasm – might differ from those of students seated elsewhere. Therefore, the sample selection process must be based on chance and randomness, ensuring that each member of the population has an equal and appropriate opportunity to be chosen. This approach is known as *random sampling.*

TIP

Sampling is a vital research technique that enables researchers to make inferences about a larger population without examining every individual. By selecting a representative subset, researchers can conserve time and resources while still gaining meaningful insights – making sampling an efficient and practical approach across various fields of study.

The primary advantage of sampling is that the results obtained can be generalised to the population from which the sample was drawn. This feature is essential for producing the most accurate estimate of the population parameter under investigation. For instance, if research comparing men and women indicates that men have higher blood cholesterol levels than women, we would expect similar results in the reference population. Such interpretations are valid only when the sample is representative and the sample size is sufficiently large to support reliable and robust conclusions.

1.2.4 Sampling Unit

Any reference population consists of a group of subjects or units from which a sample is drawn. Each unit within the reference population that may be selected is referred to as a *sampling unit*. In other words, it is the basic element drawn from the population, the unit for which data are collected, and the unit for which information is processed. The terms *population unit* (also known as *population element*) and *sampling unit* are often used interchangeably. Depending on the research question, the population under study, and the sampling technique employed, the characteristics and definition of a sampling unit may vary.

In accordance with the sampling technique, the sampling unit must be clearly defined to ensure that each intended unit has an appropriate chance of being selected. In simple, one-stage sampling designs, the sampling units are the same as the elements of the population. However, in more complex sampling techniques, different levels of sampling units must be defined.

For instance, there are two approaches that may be used to collect data on the distribution of citizens' ages and genders in a city:

- **First Approach:** Create a comprehensive list of all residents in the city and select a representative sample from this list. In this case, the sampling units and population units are equivalent.
- **Second Approach:** Select a number of census blocks within the city, then choose families from those blocks, and finally select individual members from the chosen families. In this three-stage sampling plan, census blocks, families, and individual family members are selected step by step, with each level drawn from the units chosen in the previous stage.

In the second sampling design, the terms *primary sampling unit* (*PSU*), *secondary sampling unit* (*SSU*), and *enumerating sampling unit* (*ESU*) are used to refer to these successive stages.

It is important to note that, ideally, sampling units should be independent of one another; however, this separation is not always feasible. Alternative designs – such as area, circular, household, or block sampling – can sometimes reduce costs, travel time, and the overall duration of data collection. These sampling patterns are frequently employed in agricultural, environmental, and animal research.

1.2.5 Observation Unit

The observation unit, or data collection unit, refers to a member or a combination of members of the population from whom information must be collected. Although the unit of observation and the unit of analysis are often the same, this is not always the case. For example, a researcher may collect information about an entire family (the observation unit) through interviews with the head of the family (the analysis unit).

When the unit of observation and the unit of analysis are identical, the research process is somewhat simplified. However, when the observation units and the analysis units differ, additional expertise is required to collect accurate data on the analysis units. In such cases, the researcher must have the necessary knowledge and initiative to act effectively without first directly assessing the observation units.

1.2.6 Parameter

In statistics, a parameter is any numerical quantity or feature of a population that summarises or describes a particular aspect of that population, such as the mean or standard deviation (Kotz et al., 2005). It serves as a measure of the population as a whole, taking into account all individual data points. It is crucial to first identify the population because a parameter always corresponds to a specific population (Salkind, 2006, 2010).

A parameter is to a population what a statistic is to a sample (Lavrakas, 2008). A parameter is a fixed, unknown numerical value, whereas a statistic is a known number that varies depending on the subset of the population.

TIP

A parameter summarises the key characteristics of a population, describing it as a whole using measures such as the mean or standard deviation. In contrast, a statistic is a value calculated from a subset of the population, and it can vary from sample to sample. While a parameter represents a fixed – often unknown – numerical value for the population, a statistic serves the same role for a sample.

The parameter has a fixed value because it applies to every member of the population. For example, consider the mean height of students in a university with a population of 15,000 students. This value would remain consistent even if different researchers measured each student's height individually. Although the exact value of the parameter may be unknown, it is nonetheless fixed.

Additionally, different statistical notations are employed to distinguish between sample statistics and population parameters.

1.2.7 Statistic

The singular noun *statistic* (without the ending 's') has three definitions: (1) an observed number or event; (2) a mathematical operation (and the resulting number) performed on sample data; and (3) an operation (and the resulting number) derived from a sampling distribution (Salkind, 2010). The term *statistics* (with an 's') typically refers to the field of mathematics that scientists and others use to analyse data from empirical studies.

For instance, descriptive statistics include measures such as the mean $\left(\frac{\Sigma X}{n}\right)$, median, standard deviation, and the 95th percentile, each defined by its own formula. In addition to the formula itself, the resulting numerical value may also be referred to as a *statistic* (Salkind, 2006).

An alternative definition of a statistic is a numerical value derived from the observed values of a random variable (or variables) in a sample. The term "random" pertains to both the variable's value and its statistic. A *statistic* serves as a numerical summary of a particular variable (or variables) in the population and is used to estimate a parameter (Lavrakas, 2008).

In the context of parameters, if researchers each take random samples from a student population and calculate the mean height, their calculated means will differ due to the randomness of the sample selections.

1.2.8 Estimation

The objective of estimation is to approximate the values of unknown quantities using available data. These unknown quantities, referred to as parameters, may include well-known population metrics such as the population mean (μ), population proportion (p), population variance (σ^2), and population median (ν). In some cases, the parameters are components of more complex statistical models, such as the coefficients (β_0, β_1, ...) in a linear regression model (Levy, 2005).

1.2.9 Sampling Frame

A survey can either be a census of the entire population being studied or conducted using a sample from the target population. A sampling frame, which identifies and characterises every element of the target population, is essential for both census and sample surveys. For a census, the frame consists of a complete list of all known units in the population, where each unit must be surveyed. For a sample survey, the frame includes the target population units from which the sample is drawn (Lavrakas, 2008).

TIP

The sampling frame is a complete list of all elements within a population from which a sample is drawn. An accurate and well-defined sampling frame is essential to ensure that the sample properly represents the population. It should be comprehensive and up-to-date to minimise bias in the selection process. Additionally, the sampling frame must include all relevant elements while excluding any irrelevant ones. A deep understanding of the sampling frame is crucial for maintaining the validity and reliability of the sample results.

In single-stage sampling, the sampling frame is essentially a list of the previously identified members of the population being studied. For example, if a simple random sample of students residing in a dormitory is chosen, the list of names maintained by the dormitory office or on a computer serves as the sampling frame.

Ideally, the sampling frame should include every element of the population, although this is not always achievable. Preparing the frame requires a clear specification of both the sampling unit and the population. The quality of the sample – and, to some extent, the survey itself – depends on the quality of the sampling frame. All members of the target population must be accessible and have an equal chance of being selected in the sample.

A crucial step in designing a survey is to provide a sampling frame that is of high quality and suitable for both the population being studied and the data collection method. The units within the frame must be mutually exclusive, and the frame should consist of an exhaustive list (Indrayan & Holt, 2016). When developing a sampling frame, two key aspects should be considered: (1) it must cover the entire population under study, and (2) it should be appropriate for the method of data collection (Lavrakas, 2008). Therefore, it is essential to minimise potential flaws in the sampling frame, including missing units, duplicate units, multi-unit assemblies with the same name, and empty units.

1.2.10 Sampling Design

A sampling design outlines the procedure for selecting study participants from a specific population. It refers to the techniques used to acquire the sample and serves as a roadmap for choosing survey participants. This design describes the methods the researcher employs to select each component of the sample. The objectives of a sampling design – such as increasing sample representativeness, reducing systematic bias, and minimising sampling error – ensure that the chosen sample allows for generalisation of findings to the entire target population. Additionally, the sampling design determines the sample size, i.e., the number of elements to be included in the sample. Therefore, a robust and well-structured sampling design must be established prior to data collection.

TIP

A well-structured sampling design is essential for conducting effective research. It serves as a roadmap for participant selection, focusing on key objectives: enhancing representativeness, minimising bias, and reducing sampling errors.

A properly designed sampling strategy ensures that findings can be accurately generalised to the entire target population, thereby increasing the study's validity.

Sampling designs may utilise either probability (random) or non-probability (non-random) techniques. Among the various sampling design procedures, the researcher must select methods that are reliable and appropriate for the study. It is important to note that a sampling design provides detailed information regarding the sampling method, sample size calculation, and estimation of population parameters for a specific study. The sampling design should align with the study's objectives, taking the following key points into account:

- **Define the Study Population:** The researcher must clearly specify and understand the study population, which includes the subjects under examination. The population may be finite (with a known number of elements) or infinite (with an unknown number of elements).
- **Provide a Sampling Frame:** A sampling frame, sometimes referred to as a "source list", is a comprehensive and accurate list of all items in the population from which the sample will be drawn. This list should be reliable and representative of the population.
- **Consider the Sampling Unit:** Before selecting a sample, the researcher must assess the sampling unit. A sampling unit can be social (e.g., a family, club, or school), geographical (e.g., a state,

district, or village), structural (e.g., a house or apartment), or individual (e.g., a person such as Sourena, Sara, or Aren).

- **Estimate Sample Size:** The sample size is the number of items drawn from the population to form the sample. Determining the appropriate sample size can be challenging. The sample should be sufficient – not too large or too small – to meet the criteria for confidence level, study power (Type I and Type II errors), and representativeness (dispersion). When calculating sample size, it is crucial to consider the study's objectives, parameters of interest, and budgetary constraints. This book provides several formulas and equations for calculating an adequate sample size.
- **Budgetary Considerations:** Budgetary constraints influence both the sample size and the choice of sampling technique, potentially necessitating the use of non-probability sampling.
- **Sampling Procedure:** The researcher must decide on the type of sample and the methods for collecting sample items.
- **Determine the Estimation Method:** The researcher must select appropriate methods for estimating population parameters.

A well-designed sampling strategy should possess the following characteristics:

- **Representativeness:** The sample should accurately reflect the characteristics of the population. If the true characteristics of the population are known, this can be achieved. The design should be straightforward, adequate, appropriate, and practical, allowing each stage to be executed precisely according to the protocol.
- **Minimisation of Sampling Errors:** The design should aim to reduce sampling errors. Practical considerations must be made to address defects arising from the study process and non-responsiveness of sample units. An advanced approach to minimising sampling errors is essential.
- **Cost-Effectiveness:** The design should collect the most important information at the lowest possible cost. Utilising previously available information whenever feasible can help avoid unnecessary expenses.
- **Control of Systematic Bias:** The design must effectively manage systematic bias, which refers to the inherent tendency of a process to favour certain subjects or disproportionately affect data in one direction.
- **Generalisability of Results:** The sampling design should allow the findings from the sample to be confidently applied to the broader population.

- **Chance of Selection:** Each unit in the population must have a known, non-zero probability of selection. In other words, a random sampling technique based on probabilities should be employed to accurately calculate standard errors.

1.2.11 Population and Sampling Frame Interaction

The target population and the sampling frame interact closely and should correspond with one another. Unfortunately, researchers often pay insufficient attention to this correspondence, which is crucial when constructing a sampling frame.

In a one-stage sampling design, the list of population members and the sampling frame are identical. However, in practice, researchers frequently define the study population based on existing sampling frames, which is conceptually incorrect. Therefore, the sampling frame should be defined based on the population being studied, rather than vice versa.

Once the study population has been identified and characterised, the next step is to identify and specify the sampling units for that population. Following this, researchers should seek potential sampling frames. This process involves analysing and assessing available frames to determine which one best represents the target population and is most suitable for the research objectives.

One reason the sampling frame may not encompass all members of the population is that the list of population units may not be updated regularly or in a timely manner. To ensure an up-to-date sampling frame, a portion of the research budget should be allocated for its development. For example, obtaining a list of patients referred for a clinical trial may require visiting hospital statistics offices or accessing hospital computer records, which demands both time and resources. Importantly, such a list, consisting of patients who have undergone surgery at the hospital, cannot be used as a sampling frame unless it has received approval from the hospital management.

Figure 1.1 illustrates the relationship among the sampling frame, target population, and sampling population (Lohr, 2021, p. 4).

1.2.12 Independent Information

Independent information refers to observations and data collected either concurrently with or prior to the survey from other external and independent sources. The purpose of collecting such information is to enhance the study's validity and improve its realism; however, its collection is not among the primary objectives of the research project. Independent information can serve multiple functions, including classifying the population, determining the appropriate sample size, identifying key variables, and developing questionnaires and response options.

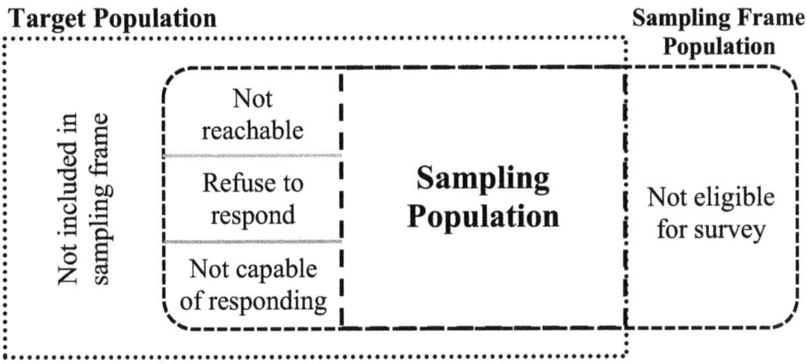

FIGURE 1.1
The relationship between the sampling frame, target population, and sampling population.

1.2.13 Sampling Variation

The primary objective of sampling is to estimate population parameters, such as the mean or proportion, using data collected from a sample (Scheaffer et al., 2011). However, these estimates are rarely identical to the true population values. The differences that are expected to occur across all potential samples, or the differences between individual sample estimates and the true population parameters, are referred to as **sampling variations**.

TIP

Sampling variation refers to the differences that occur when multiple samples are drawn from the same population. Factors such as sample size and sampling techniques can significantly influence this variation, affecting the accuracy of estimates.

Recognising and accounting for these variations is essential for improving the reliability and validity of research findings.

Sampling variation arises from the inherent differences that may appear in the results when multiple samples are drawn from the same population. These variations can occur due to factors such as sample size, sampling technique, errors during the sampling process, and other factors that influence the sample's representativeness. As a result, two or more samples drawn from the same population, even if they share nearly identical population characteristics, are likely to yield different results.

To illustrate this concept, let's assume that Sarah, John, and Sourena each decide to estimate the average number of part-time hours worked per week by college students. While their estimates may vary, none would be considered incorrect, as these differences reflect natural sampling variation. The sources of sampling variations can be summarised as follows:

1. **Sampling Design (Sampling Process and Sample Size):** Variations in sampling design can arise depending on the sampling technique employed and its alignment with the study objectives. Probability sampling methods provide an unbiased representation of the population, whereas non-probability sampling methods may introduce biases and limit the generalisability of findings. While sampling variations cannot be entirely eliminated, they can be minimised through appropriate sampling techniques. Additionally, sample size significantly affects sampling variation: larger sample sizes increase the precision of population parameter estimates and reduce variability, whereas smaller sample sizes tend to increase variability and diminish the representativeness of results.
2. **Population Characteristics:** The characteristics of the population under study can influence sampling variation. Careful consideration of these traits is essential to ensure that the sample adequately represents key demographic, socioeconomic, and other relevant factors. Neglecting population characteristics may result in a biased or unrepresentative sample, leading to differences in findings. Furthermore, highly heterogeneous populations tend to produce greater variability in results compared to more homogeneous populations.

1.2.14 Error of Estimation

Assume we want to estimate μ by taking a sample and calculating M. How accurate is this estimate? Since our estimation is based on a sample, there is a discrepancy between M and μ ($M - \mu$), known as the **error of estimation**. This error varies depending on the specific sample drawn. The sample means tend to cluster around μ but typically fall slightly to the right or left of μ, where μ represents the centre of the sampling distribution of the mean. The distance by which they deviate from μ represents the estimation error, denoted as ($M - \mu$). In general, the **error of estimation** is defined as the difference between a point estimate derived from the sample and the corresponding population parameter being estimated, expressed as ($M - \mu$) (Cumming, 2013).

1.2.15 Difference between "Sampling Variations" and "Error of Estimation"

Sampling variation and error of estimation are two related but distinct concepts in statistics. While they are interconnected, they are not interchangeable terms.

Sampling variation refers to the natural variability that occurs when different samples are drawn from the same population. These variations can arise due to several factors, including the sampling technique employed, sample size, errors during the sampling process, and the inherent characteristics of the population being studied. Sampling variation is a fundamental concept in statistics because it affects the accuracy and precision of estimates and the inferences made from sample data.

In contrast, the error of estimation refers to the difference between a sample statistic (such as the sample mean or proportion) and the corresponding population parameter (such as the true mean or proportion). This error arises because the sample represents only a subset of the population and may not perfectly reflect the characteristics of the population as a whole. The error of estimation quantifies how well the sample statistic approximates the population parameter.

This error can occur due to multiple factors, including sampling variation, measurement error, and bias. Although sampling variation contributes to the error of estimation, it is not the only factor. Other sources, such as measurement error and systematic bias, can also influence the magnitude of the estimation error.

In summary, sampling variation refers to the natural variability that arises when different samples are taken from the same population, whereas the error of estimation represents the difference between the true population parameter and the corresponding estimate derived from a sample. While sampling variation contributes to the error of estimation, it is not its sole cause. Sampling variation is an inherent part of the sampling process and cannot be completely eliminated, whereas the error of estimation can be reduced by increasing the sample size and employing more accurate measurement and data collection techniques.

1.2.16 Measurement Error

Measurement is the process of assigning symbols, usually numbers, to objects based on a defined standard. This process involves both the establishment of a rule and the assignment of values according to that rule. The symbols assigned represent the characteristics or attributes of the object being measured. Any deviation between the assigned symbol and the "true" value that should be attributed to the object is considered a *measurement error* (Lavrakas, 2008). Furthermore, measurement error can be defined as the variation in repeated measurements of the same quantity on the same item (Salkind, 2006).

Construct validity refers to the degree of precision with which a concept or variable is measured. Just as misclassification applies to qualitative data, measurement error pertains to quantitative data. This means that when categorical variables are measured with error, they become misclassified (Levy, 2005).

TIP

Measurement error can significantly impact research outcomes. It occurs when a discrepancy exists between the true value and the measured value of a variable. This error may arise from various sources, including poor survey design, instrument limitations, or human error. Minimising measurement error is essential for ensuring the accuracy and reliability of research results.

Measurement errors can arise from several factors, including poor survey design, sampling variability, inherent biological variation, and laboratory or analytical errors. Measurement error is generally categorised into two types: systematic error and random error (Salkind, 2006).

1.2.17 Difference between "Measurement Error" and "Error of Estimation"

Measurement error and error of estimation, while related concepts, originate from different sources and influence statistical studies in distinct ways. Although both terms refer to deviations from the true value, their meanings differ within the context of research. In summary, measurement error pertains to the accuracy of individual measurements (i.e., the measured data), whereas error of estimation relates to the accuracy of statistical estimates (i.e., estimated values, statistical estimations, and analyses) derived from those measurements. Each concept is described in more detail below:

- **Error of Estimation:** The error of estimation refers to the difference between the true value of a population parameter and its estimated value based on a sample. In regression analysis, the difference between an observed value and its predicted value is often referred to as a residual. This error arises because a sample represents only a subset of the population and may not fully capture the characteristics of the entire population.

  Various factors, including measurement error, model misspecification, random variation, and sampling error, can contribute to estimation errors. For example, if one estimates the average height of a population using a sample, the error introduced by using only a portion of the population will affect the accuracy of the estimate. This error can be reduced by increasing the sample size or employing more precise estimation techniques. Statistical tools such as confidence intervals and margins of error are commonly used to quantify estimation errors.

- **Measurement Error:** Measurement error refers to the difference between the true value of a variable, as determined by an instrument or measurement technique, and its observed (measured) value. Such errors can lead to inaccuracies in data, resulting in systematic or random deviations from the true values and ultimately affecting the validity and reliability of study findings.

  Measurement error can be classified into two main categories: random error and systematic error. Random errors are unpredictable and occur by chance, whereas systematic errors are consistent and predictable, often stemming from flaws in measurement instruments or procedures. Numerous factors can cause measurement error, including instrument calibration problems, environmental conditions, observer bias, human error, respondent bias, and other systematic biases. These sources of error should be minimised through appropriate study design, proper calibration, and rigorous data collection procedures. For example, using a slightly bent ruler to measure the length of a table may produce inaccurate results due to imperfections in the measuring instrument.

  Estimation errors are inherent in statistical modelling and can be evaluated using various methods, including the mean squared error (MSE) and the residual sum of squares (RSS). However, if measurement error is not properly accounted for in statistical analysis, it can lead to biased estimates and incorrect inferences. Therefore, distinguishing between these two types of error and implementing appropriate procedures to minimise their effects is critical for improving the accuracy, validity, and reliability of statistical analyses.

1.2.18 Random Error

The term "random error" refers to any unpredictable variation that occurs in the measurement of a variable. It acknowledges that any survey measure obtained repeatedly may deviate – by some small amount – from other measurements simply due to imprecision in the measurement process. Consequently, when compared to the true value of the measure for a specific respondent, the observed value may sometimes be higher and at other times lower.

This difference between the observed and true values is commonly represented by "e" in the formula $X = T + e$ (Lavrakas, 2008). Such errors are inherent and unpredictable, occurring when repeated measurements of the same characteristic are taken under identical conditions, excluding bias or human error (Indrayan & Holt, 2016).

For example, consider a patient whose weight is measured in a hospital. If two different nurses weigh the patient, they might record slightly different values. Even if the same nurse takes two measurements in quick succession, variations in eye position while reading the scale could lead to discrepancies. Because these variations lack a consistent pattern, the recorded weight may be either higher or lower than the true value.

In principle, the total amount of random error across a series of measurements on the same variable should sum to zero. Therefore, random error exerts minimal influence on the average measurement value. The mean of the observed values should, in theory, equal the true value when derived from multiple similar measurements of the same variable. This means that random error has minimal impact on the average measurement value. This type of error is often referred to as "noise", and by definition, it is not considered a component of bias (Lavrakas, 2008; Salkind, 2006).

Statistical inference fundamentally relies on the concept of random error. Statistical tests are used to determine the degree of confidence that can be placed in an inference by assessing the magnitude of random error. Every sample statistic is associated with a corresponding random error, which is typically expressed as its **standard error**. Researchers can partially control the magnitude of random error by increasing the sample size or employing a more precise sampling design (Lavrakas, 2008).

1.2.19 Systematic Error

Systematic error refers to a bias that arises when a data collection or analysis process consistently yields results that differ from the true value of the quantity being estimated. Unlike random error, systematic error is not reduced by increasing the sample size; doing so only produces more precise but still biased estimates of the desired value (Levy, 2005).

Systematic errors result from bias in measurement or estimation techniques, leading to consistent overestimation or underestimation of key parameters. Effective survey research methodologies seek to minimise systematic error through probability-based sampling procedures and careful survey design. In survey research, two major sources of systematic error are sample selection bias and response bias (Lavrakas, 2008).

For example, if a patient-weighing scale consistently shows readings that are five pounds above the actual weight, this indicates a calibration issue with the scale. Through proper experimental design and planning, systematic errors can often be reduced or even eliminated. The term "bias" is commonly used to describe this type of error (Salkind, 2006).

1.2.20 Bias

Bias in statistics is defined as the "deviation of results or inferences from the truth, or processes leading to such deviation". In other words, it represents the extent to which a population parameter differs from the expected value of its estimate (Levy, 2005). Thus, bias depends on both the parameter and the statistic. When a statistic is used as an estimator of a parameter, its bias (the difference between the statistic and the true parameter value) becomes particularly important (Kotz et al., 2005).

Bias can be interpreted as "wrong", with the added nuance of being "wrong due to a systematic error". Therefore, a biased estimate is considered incorrect within statistical and scientific contexts. In epidemiology, the term *bias* is often used to describe distortions in measures of association between exposure and outcome, such as the rate ratio, relative risk, attributable risk, and odds ratio (Boslaugh, 2007).

Identifying the nature and extent of bias in survey measures remains one of the most challenging tasks for survey researchers. Quantifying and minimising bias are ongoing concerns in survey research. In some cases, the bias is so small that it may be disregarded; in others, it is unavoidable and can significantly distort survey results (Lavrakas, 2008).

The term "bias" specifically refers to systematic errors that reduce the validity of estimates, whereas random errors primarily reduce the precision of those estimates. Unlike random error, bias cannot be eliminated or reduced by increasing sample size. Bias may arise at various stages of the research process, including literature review, study design, implementation, data collection, analysis, interpretation of results, and publication (Levy, 2005).

1.2.21 Systematic Error and Bias

The concept of systematic error is closely related to the broader statistical notion of bias. To illustrate this relationship more concretely, consider a situation in which a researcher seeks to estimate the population mean of a continuously measured variable – such as the amount of funding that should be allocated to a particular policy. After selecting a random sample of participants and collecting their opinions, the researcher calculates the sample mean and variance.

If a systematic error exists in the sampling procedure – such as when the sample overrepresents or underrepresents certain segments of the population – or if the survey questions are worded in a way that distorts respondents' true opinions, the resulting sample mean will not accurately represent the population mean. In such cases, even if the researcher were to draw repeatedly and survey multiple random samples, the sample means would, on average, fail to coincide with the true population mean. This example demonstrates that bias can arise from systematic errors in the measurement or estimation of key parameters (Lavrakas, 2008).

1.2.22 Sampling Error and Fluctuations

Any sample drawn from a population will almost certainly differ from another, as the second sample may include some or all new participants. Consequently, the findings derived from one sample may not fully align with those obtained from another. This variability is referred to as sampling fluctuation or sampling error, which constitutes one of the primary sources of statistical uncertainty. The term denotes the difference between sample estimates and the true population values. Thus, sampling errors can be expressed as the difference $(x - \mu)$ in the case of the mean and $(p - \pi)$ in the case of a proportion. Therefore, a sampling error represents a variation resulting from the process of sampling itself, rather than an "error" in the conventional sense. Because estimates vary from one sample to another, sampling error will also fluctuate accordingly (Indrayan & Holt, 2016).

Sampling errors can be evaluated statistically. The variability among all possible samples is quantified through measures of sampling error (Chakwana & Violence, 2005). For a specific sampling design and sample size, the magnitude of sampling error can be determined. The standard error of a particular statistic (e.g., mean or proportion) is typically defined as the square root of its variance (Chakwana & Violence, 2005). Since these errors occur randomly and are equally likely to deviate in either direction, they are compensatory in nature, meaning that their expected value is zero (Kothari, 2004).

The magnitude of sampling error primarily depends on the sampling method, sample size, and the variability within the population (Indrayan & Holt, 2016).

1. **Sample Size:** Sampling error decreases as the sample size increases (Kothari, 2004). When a sample is chosen randomly, the probability of substantial sampling error diminishes with larger sample sizes. Including a greater number of subjects in the sample ensures that the findings from one sample are less likely to differ significantly from those of another sample of the same size, as both samples provide a more accurate representation of the population. This relationship does not hold for smaller samples, which are more prone to variability (Indrayan & Holt, 2016).
2. **Method of Sampling:** It is essential to select subjects in a manner that adequately represents the diversity of the population and ensures that repeated sampling produces consistent results. Employing a representative sampling technique is critical for the validity of the study.
3. **Variability among Subjects in the Population:** Sampling error is lower in a homogeneous population (Kothari, 2004). Conversely, if the characteristics of the population vary widely, the resulting

samples are likely to exhibit substantial variability, increasing the potential for sampling error (Indrayan & Holt, 2016).

1.2.23 Non-sampling Errors

Non-sampling errors arise from mistakes made during data collection and processing. These errors can include failing to identify or interview the appropriate participants, misunderstandings between the interviewer and respondent regarding the questions, and errors in data entry (Chakwana & Violence, 2005). Non-sampling errors often present a greater challenge than sampling errors, as they cannot be mitigated merely by increasing the sample size (Cuddeback et al., 2004).

TIP

While sampling errors primarily affect the reliability of a study, non-sampling errors directly reduce the validity of the results. When substantial non-sampling errors are present, the study may fail to accurately address the original research question.

Non-sampling errors do not imply that sampling was not employed; rather, they refer to human errors arising from various sources, including conceptual mistakes, sample-selection biases, data-collection errors, analytical shortcomings, and misinterpretation of results. In contrast to sampling errors, which are natural and random, non-sampling errors are systematic and can compromise the validity of study conclusions. While sampling errors primarily affect the reliability of a study, non-sampling errors directly compromise the validity of the results. When substantial non-sampling errors are present, the study may fail to adequately address the original research question.

In addition to bias, other factors contributing to non-sampling errors include:

1. Unclear questions and ineffective communication,
2. Non-response and inaccurate responses,
3. Errors in data entry and coding,
4. Improper statistical methodology or techniques, including inadequate analyses that fail to account for all confounding factors,
5. Incorrect interpretation of computer output based on incomplete or flawed analyses.

These biases that lead to non-sampling errors represent significant concerns in many research studies. Non-sampling errors can be minimised through improved methodology, enhanced training, thoughtful research design, and other preventive techniques. Close engagement with respondents may also be necessary to elicit accurate and reliable responses.

A large sample that contains non-sampling errors tends to exacerbate bias rather than reduce it, creating a false sense of confidence in the results. Non-sampling errors are often subtle and may remain undetected until new evidence emerges that contradicts earlier, incorrect conclusions derived from such errors (Indrayan & Holt, 2016). These errors – arising from inadequate study design, poor reporting, flawed judgement, inaccurate recording, non-response, and similar issues – are genuine sources of error. They are exogenous in nature, and efforts to control them are essential at every stage of the research process.

1.2.24 Probability versus Non-probability Sampling

Researchers rarely have the opportunity to observe every member of a target population – the group to which they wish to generalise their study results – because of limitations in time and resources. Instead, a subset of that population must be selected. To do so, researchers may employ either probability sampling or non-probability sampling techniques.

In *non-probability sampling*, participant selection is non-random and typically based on availability or researcher judgement. Common non-probability sampling methods include snowball sampling, quota sampling, convenience sampling, and purposive sampling. Because it is impossible to determine how closely a non-probability sample represents the target population, findings derived from such samples cannot be generalised to the entire population. This limitation arises because not all members of the population have an equal chance of being selected, which increases the potential for bias.

In contrast, probability sampling involves selecting participants from the target population through random selection techniques, producing findings that are generalisable to the population – provided that other sources of bias are absent. In probability sampling, every member of the target population has a non-zero probability of being included in the sample, and the probability of selecting any individual can be explicitly calculated (Boslaugh, 2007).

References

Boslaugh, S. (2007). *Encyclopedia of epidemiology*. Sage Publications.

Chakwana, C., & Violence, D. (2005). *Malawi demographic and health survey 2004*. National Statistical Office (NSO)[Malawi], and ORC Macro.

Cuddeback, G., Wilson, E., Orme, J. G., & Combs-Orme, T. (2004). Detecting and statistically correcting sample selection bias. *Journal of Social Service Research, 30*(3), 19–33.

Cumming, G. (2013). *Understanding the new statistics: Effect sizes, confidence intervals, and meta-analysis.* Routledge.

Frey, B. B. (2021). *The SAGE encyclopedia of research design.* Sage Publications.

Indrayan, A., & Holt, M. P. (2016). *Concise encyclopedia of biostatistics for medical professionals.* Chapman and Hall and CRC Press.

Kothari, C. (2004). *Research methodology: Methods and techniques.* New Age International.

Kotz, S., Balakrishnan, N., Read, C. B., Vidakovic, B., & Johnson, N. L. (2005). *Encyclopedia of statistical sciences* (Vol. 1). John Wiley & Sons.

Lavrakas, P. J. (2008). *Encyclopedia of survey research methods.* Sage Publications.

Levy, P. S. (2005). *Encyclopedia of biostatistics* (ArmitageP. & T. Colton, Eds., 2nd ed.). Wiley.

Lohr, S. L. (2021). *Sampling: Design and analysis.* Chapman and Hall and CRC Press.

Salkind, N. J. (2006). *Encyclopedia of measurement and statistics.* Sage Publications.

Salkind, N. J. (2010). *Encyclopedia of research design* (Vol. 1). Sage Publications.

Scheaffer, R. L., Mendenhall III, W., Ott, R. L., & Gerow, K. G. (2011). *Elementary survey sampling.* Cengage Learning.

2

Exploring Non-probability Sampling Methods

2.1 Introduction

A scientifically selected sample is necessary for conducting population-based research. The population of interest may include the entire population – such as all individuals residing in a country's urban areas – or a specific subpopulation. Obtaining a representative sample of the target population is fundamental to ensuring the validity of such studies, whereas an inappropriate or biased sample can compromise the accuracy of the findings (Boslaugh, 2007). The sampling technique refers to the methodological process of selecting a sample from the target population. Depending on the method of sample selection, sample surveys are generally classified into two main categories: *probability sampling* (also known as random sampling) and *non-probability sampling* (also referred to as non-random sampling) (Indrayan & Holt, 2016).

2.2 The Necessity of Non-probability Sampling

Although probability sampling has greater potential for generalisability and is more effective in capturing the characteristics and events of the reference population, it is generally considered to yield samples that are more representative than those obtained through non-probability sampling. Consequently, most researchers and statisticians prefer probability-based methods over non-probability (non-random) sampling techniques. However, probability sampling is not always feasible due to limitations in time, resources, or accessibility. In such cases, researchers may employ non-probability sampling methods to select participants and obtain the necessary data.

DOI: 10.1201/9781003749783-2

TIP

In epidemiological and medical research, particularly when involving human participants, researchers often select sampling units and individuals from volunteers or readily accessible populations for surveys and intervention studies. However, random (probability) sampling is not always practical or feasible due to time constraints, financial limitations, or other logistical and ethical considerations.

In epidemiological and medical research involving human participants, researchers frequently draw samples from volunteers or readily accessible individuals for surveys and intervention studies. The practical challenges of implementing random sampling – such as limited budgets, strict timelines, ethical considerations, or difficulty identifying a complete sampling frame – often necessitate the use of non-probability sampling.

Similarly, in behavioural and social research, especially when it comes to human participants, investigators commonly recruit participants from easily accessible or volunteer populations when forming survey samples or designing intervention studies. Random (probability) sampling is frequently impractical due to financial, temporal, logistical, or other practical constraints.

Concrete examples further illustrate this necessity. In studies evaluating the effectiveness of two therapeutic interventions for addiction, probability sampling may be unfeasible because addiction is frequently stigmatised as immoral or even criminal. As a result, the population of individuals with addiction and the corresponding sampling frame are often unknown. In such cases, researchers must employ non-probability sampling methods, recruiting participants who are willing to participate, readily available, or mandated to undergo treatment.

2.3 Practical Considerations and Limitations

To approximate the benefits of random sampling, researchers may still employ probability-based procedures within the study design – for example, by randomly assigning participants to experimental and control groups. Likewise, when investigating opinions of television viewers, researchers may use non-probability approaches – such as surveying individuals passing through a specific location or gathered at a particular venue – because the overall population of viewers and the sampling frame for the programme's audience are unknown.

However, results obtained from non-probability samples cannot be readily generalised to the reference population. Broader inferences can only be supported through repeated studies across diverse contexts and conditions.

2.4 Types of Non-probability Sampling

In non-probability sampling, there is no guaranteed or equal chance that any individual or unit from the reference population will be included in the sample. Instead, samples are typically determined by participants' accessibility, availability, and willingness, as well as the judgment and expertise of the researcher. In some cases, sampling decisions may also be informed by prior experience or knowledge of the researcher and the research instrument. These factors introduce potential selection bias, as sample composition is influenced by characteristics beyond random chance and cannot be assumed to represent the population reliably.

TIP

Conducting research on taboo behaviours within a society – such as smoking among school students, the consumption of restricted foods in certain cultures, suicide across cultural contexts, sexual relationships between close relatives, academic dishonesty, abortion in specific cultures, and the use of illegal drugs or the misuse of prescription medications – can be highly challenging. This difficulty is particularly evident when employing random (probability) sampling methods, as obtaining a comprehensive and representative sample of the target population is often not feasible. In such cases, non-probability sampling methods may be more appropriate and practical.

Thus, non-probability sampling is based on a technique in which, first, not all members of the target population have a chance of being selected for the sample, and many have no chance at all. Second, if individuals do have a chance of being chosen, it is not proportional to their frequency in the population. Third, the probability of selection is neither predetermined nor calculable. Consequently, statistical significance tests cannot be applied to evaluate the sample, and the observed results from the sample cannot be generalised to the entire reference population; they can only be described.

Non-probability sampling, on the other hand, is generally less expensive and easier to implement than probability sampling. In such sampling, the population may not be fully specified, and researchers have no concrete methods to assess statistical properties of estimators, such as reliability, validity, or unbiasedness, because the selection probability of each element is unknown ("Encyclopedia of Biostatistics", 2005; Levy & Lemeshow, 2013).

Despite these limitations, the results of this type of sampling cannot be generalised to the entire population from which the sample was drawn, but they may still be useful in certain situations the sample was taken (Indrayan & Holt, 2016). They are frequently used, particularly in surveys of public opinion and market research, because probability sampling is often time-consuming, costly, and not always feasible (Levy & Lemeshow, 2013).

In some specific cases, neither a representative nor a random sample is required. Non-random sampling is often employed to define a group of volunteers for phase I clinical trials. Although non-random samples limit generalisability, they can still be valuable when the primary purpose is to assess the tolerability of a treatment regimen, as in phase I trials. This approach provides a practical way to collect a purposive or targeted sample. Such approaches are collectively referred to as non-random sampling methods (Indrayan & Holt, 2016).

Researchers also use non-probability sampling to identify members of a population pool when it is not possible to define the population needed for probability sampling (Boslaugh, 2007). The four main categories of non-probability sampling – purposive, quota, convenience, and snowball sampling – are discussed further in this chapter. Figure 2.1 illustrates the various types of non-random/non-probability sampling.

2.4.1 Convenience or Haphazard Sampling

One type of non-probability sampling is convenience sampling, in which participants are selected as "convenient" sources of data for researchers (Boslaugh, 2007). As the name suggests, a convenience sample is chosen based on ease of access. For example, it may include anyone the researcher can readily contact who is available and willing to participate. Volunteers are a common example of a convenience sample (Agresti et al., 2020). This sampling method is often employed when a large number of participants representing the study's target demographic are unavailable (Indrayan & Holt, 2016). In essence, a convenience sample consists of a portion/subset of the population selected primarily because the researcher can easily access or contact its members (Lavrakas, 2008). Convenience sampling is also referred to as *haphazard sampling* (Indrayan & Holt, 2016).

Because participants are not selected randomly, convenience samples can be highly biased. Consequently, findings from such samples cannot be generalised to the broader population; however, they can still provide useful insights in certain circumstances (Indrayan & Holt, 2016). While convenience

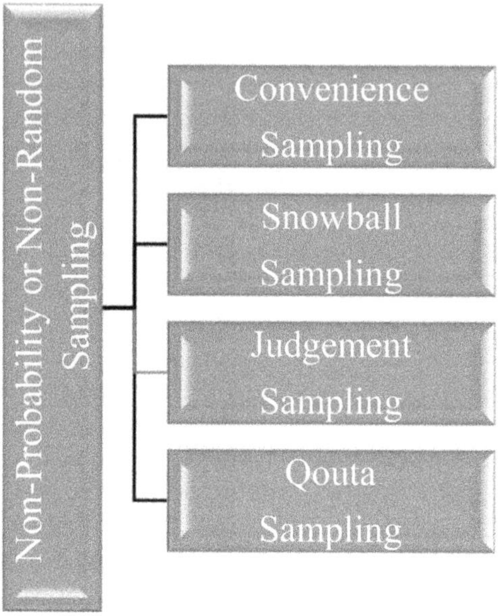

FIGURE 2.1
Different types of non-probability sampling.

samples are not considered scientifically rigorous, they may be valuable to researchers and practitioners who are aware of their limitations. For instance, they can offer a preliminary or quick exploration of a hypothesis that may later be tested using probability sampling methods (Boslaugh, 2007). The primary criterion for convenience sampling is the ease of obtaining the sample rather than achieving representativeness. This ease can relate to factors such as the cost of locating participants, their geographic distribution, and the practicality of collecting interview data (Boslaugh, 2007). In many cases, convenience samples are not a waste of resources, particularly when the research aims to examine attitudes, causes, or characteristics of relatively unknown phenomena (Indrayan & Holt, 2016).

Convenience sampling techniques may involve recruiting participants through friends and acquaintances, administering surveys via social media or online platforms, or approaching individuals in crowded public locations such as shopping malls and streets. One of the most common applications of convenience sampling is the use of student volunteers as study participants. Another example includes selecting participants from a clinic, classroom, or organisation that is easily accessible to the researcher. More specific instances might involve choosing the first five students in a class or the top five names on a patient list.

Figure 2.2 presents a schematic representation of convenience sampling, illustrating how samples are selected non-randomly according to colour proportions.

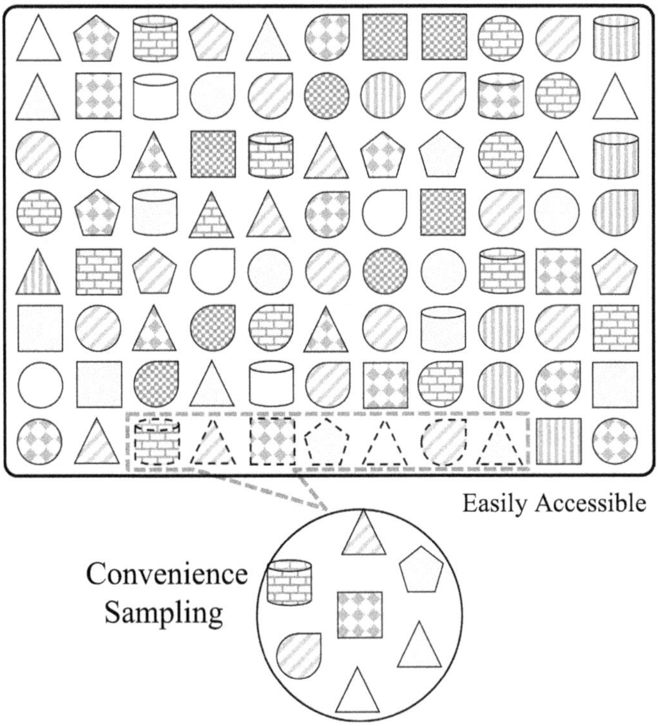

FIGURE 2.2
Presentation of convenience sampling.

2.4.2 Snowball Sampling

Snowball sampling is a limited multistage sampling technique in which sample units or participants are selected at the beginning of the process. The primary participants in the first stage then introduce and refer other potential participants (sampling units) in subsequent stages. For interview and sampling purposes, the initial participants provide the names and contact information of individuals they know. In this kind of sampling method, the initial respondents may be selected either randomly or non-randomly, for instance, from a telephone directory. In subsequent stages, additional respondents are recruited through introductions and referrals provided by participants from earlier stages.

This sampling technique creates a chain of eligible individuals in an attempt to reach a closed or hidden population. It is commonly used to identify rare or hard-to-reach populations. Snowball sampling continues to be widely applied in contemporary social, behavioural, biological, medical, health, and epidemiological research. It is also a popular approach for studying social networks in qualitative and sociometric research. Furthermore, by asking programme participants to identify individuals who are similar to them but are not enrolled in the programme, snowball sampling can be employed to establish control groups for programme evaluations ("Encyclopedia of Biostatistics", 2005).

Typical examples of hard-to-reach populations include sex workers and drug users, who are often difficult to identify and may not self-disclose their status. Once a single drug user is identified, the researcher can use that participant's network to locate additional individuals, who may, in turn, refer others. For this reason, snowball sampling is sometimes referred to as *chain referral sampling, chain sampling, network sampling,* or *referral sampling. It is also known as friend-to-friend sampling* (Indrayan & Holt, 2016). Some participants may choose to share their contacts, while others may not.

If each participant identifies at least three new individuals, the sample size could theoretically increase to 81 after four stages. Although it is unrealistic to expect a large sample size using this method, it can still help researchers recruit a reasonably sized sample for empirical studies.

This approach typically involves at least two stages:

(a) selecting an initial sample of respondents who possess a particular characteristic x at the zero stage (s_0), and
(b) obtaining referrals for additional respondents who are likely to exhibit characteristic x in subsequent stages (s_1 through s_k).

The referral process continues, or "snowballs", until a sufficient number of qualified respondents is obtained. If probability-based selection techniques are employed at the zero stage, statistical inferences can be drawn from that stage alone. However, samples obtained at stages s_1 through s_k, or samples combining the zero and snowball stages, are not representative and therefore cannot be used to draw valid statistical conclusions ("Encyclopedia of Biostatistics", 2005).

Despite the fact that this sample is not random, it can still provide valuable insights into the phenomenon under investigation. However, because this method does not rely on random sampling, statistical procedures such as confidence intervals cannot be applied.

Snowball sampling is a relatively inexpensive and straightforward method for reaching individuals you want to investigate, but it rarely yields a sample that is representative of the target population. Since participants tend to recruit others who are similar to themselves, a strong clustering effect may occur, leading to biased estimates. After several recruitment waves, the process may also become repetitive, with the same individuals being referred multiple times. Furthermore, as many participants in such studies may be engaged in illegal or stigmatised activities, special attention must be given to ethical considerations, participant sensitivity, and building sufficient trust to secure their cooperation (Indrayan & Holt, 2016).

Snowball sampling is associated with several well-known disadvantages. The most critical issue is that respondent selection across the stages s_1 through s_k is non-random. This non-randomness can introduce bias and restrict the generalisability of the findings. In studies of sensitive, unusual, or deviant behaviours, the nomination process may also raise confidentiality concerns, discouraging informants from providing honest responses. Moreover, this method assumes that members of the target population are acquainted with one another – an assumption that is often unrealistic and challenging to verify.

To address these limitations, several refinements of snowball sampling have been proposed, including the *random walk* approach for social network analysis, *targeted sampling*, *targeted personal network sampling*, and *respondent-driven sampling* (RDS). These variants are designed to improve representativeness and to estimate the size of hidden populations more accurately.

Despite its drawbacks, snowball sampling remains a widely used method across a variety of research settings. It offers a cost-effective and efficient means of identifying hard-to-reach populations and collecting data quickly. In exploratory research, particularly when the characteristics or parameters of a population are largely unknown, snowball sampling provides a practical first step for designing more systematic sampling strategies ("Encyclopedia of Biostatistics", 2005).

The term *snowball sampling* derives from the analogy of a snowball growing in size as it rolls downhill; similarly, the sample expands as participants recruit additional participants.

Figure 2.3 provides a schematic illustration of snowball sampling, in which samples are selected non-randomly based on proportional colour representation.

Example 2.1: To collect data for a study on the recruitment practices of military security groups, the researcher must interview recent recruits to obtain sample data. He asks each participant, *"Who introduced you to this organisation?"* In the next stage, the researcher approaches the individual identified by the recruit. After completing the necessary forms and conducting the interview, he asks the same question to this new participant. This referral process continues, with the researcher completing forms and interviewing each newly referred individual, until a sufficient sample size is reached.

Example 2.2: Studying the distribution of drug users and the underlying causes of their addiction presents significant challenges. Many individuals conceal their addiction due to its stigmatised and sensitive nature, making it difficult to establish an effective sampling framework. In this context, the snowball sampling method can be advantageous. By initially selecting a random sample of well-known addicts, researchers can inquire about individuals who have influenced their addiction or those who are also struggling with similar issues. This referral process continues until the desired sample size is achieved.

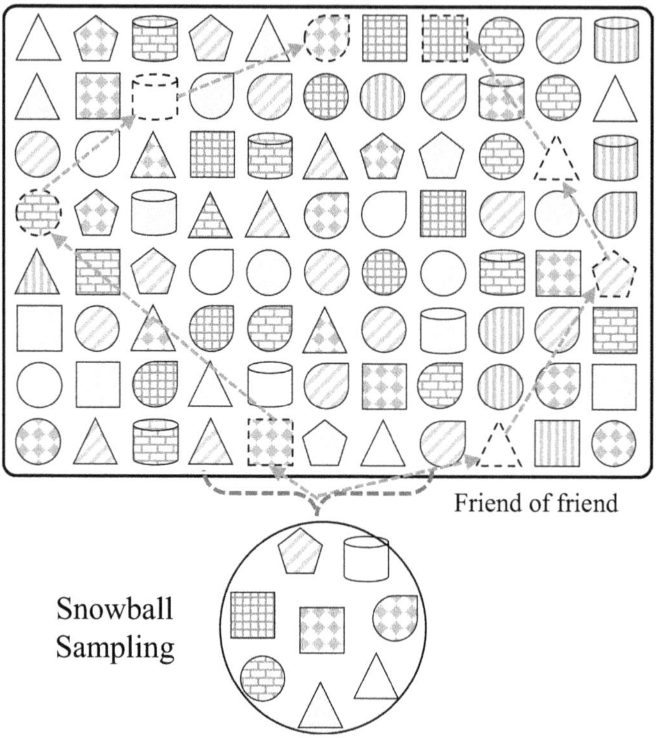

FIGURE 2.3
Presentation of non-probability snowball sampling.

> **Example 2.3:** Similar to research on drug users, studying sex workers poses substantial challenges, making snowball sampling a recommended approach. Between 1967 and 1968, Mrs. Sattareh Farmanfarmaian (1921–2012) employed the snowball sampling method to conduct one of the most notable studies of female sex workers in Tehran.

2.4.3 Purposive Sampling

Purposive Sampling (also known as judgmental sampling, expert sampling, or deliberate sampling) is a non-probability sampling technique in which researchers select participants based on predetermined criteria, specific characteristics relevant to the study's objectives, or the knowledge, experience, and expertise of the researcher (Kotz et al., 2005; Lavrakas, 2008). Unlike probability sampling, in which participants are randomly chosen, purposive sampling relies on the expert judgment of the researcher to identify individuals who are most appropriate for the study.

This type of sampling is generally conducted by selecting a non-random subset of elements from the population that is believed to represent a cross-section of the group under study. The effectiveness of the sample depends heavily on the knowledge, experience, and judgment of the expert making the selections. However, assessing or quantifying these qualities is inherently challenging, making the reliability of the method dependent on the skill and insight of the researcher (Lavrakas, 2008).

Purposive sampling is particularly useful when researchers aim to focus on a specific population or subgroup. Its main goal is to gather data from individuals who meet predefined standards or criteria, ensuring that the sample is relevant to the research questions being addressed (Cozby et al., 2016). Furthermore, specific criteria must be defined to determine which individuals or elements are included in the sample, in accordance with the research questions the study is designed to address (Salkind, 2010).

The term *purposive sampling* broadly refers to any sampling technique in which the probability of selecting a particular unit cannot be calculated ("Encyclopedia of Biostatistics", 2005). To illustrate this, consider a hospital setting where patients are the target population. In a probability sampling approach, each patient could be labelled and selected using random numbers, so that every individual has an equal chance of inclusion (e.g., a simple random sample). In contrast, a purposive sample would be chosen based on the researcher's judgment – such as selecting "this patient", "that female patient", or "this elderly individual". The researcher may believe that applying judgment will result in a sample that is more representative of key variables or better distributed across important characteristics than a purely random approach would provide ("Encyclopedia of Biostatistics", 2005).

Purposive sampling may be useful to a researcher in the following situations: when the target population is rare or difficult to reach; when the researcher wants to ensure that a specific group or population with unique characteristics is included in the study; when the researcher seeks participants with a specific experience or perspective; or when the researcher wants to ensure that the sample comprises individuals with specific experiences or viewpoints that are relevant to the study (Kotz et al., 2005). It is also frequently used in clinical research, where the goal is to enrol a specific patient population with a particular disease or condition (Boslaugh, 2007). For example, a researcher studying the experiences of cancer survivors may use purposive sampling to identify individuals who have recently received their diagnosis, completed their course of treatment, and undergone chemotherapy. If a participant meets the study's eligibility criteria, the investigator may choose to recruit them through online forums or cancer support groups.

Purposive sampling is not a representative sampling technique, since participants are selected by the researcher based on predetermined criteria rather than at random from the population. This can introduce bias into the research and limit the generalisability of the findings (Kotz et al., 2005). Additionally, it has the limitation of providing no statistical insight into the reliability of the resulting estimates, because the probability of selection

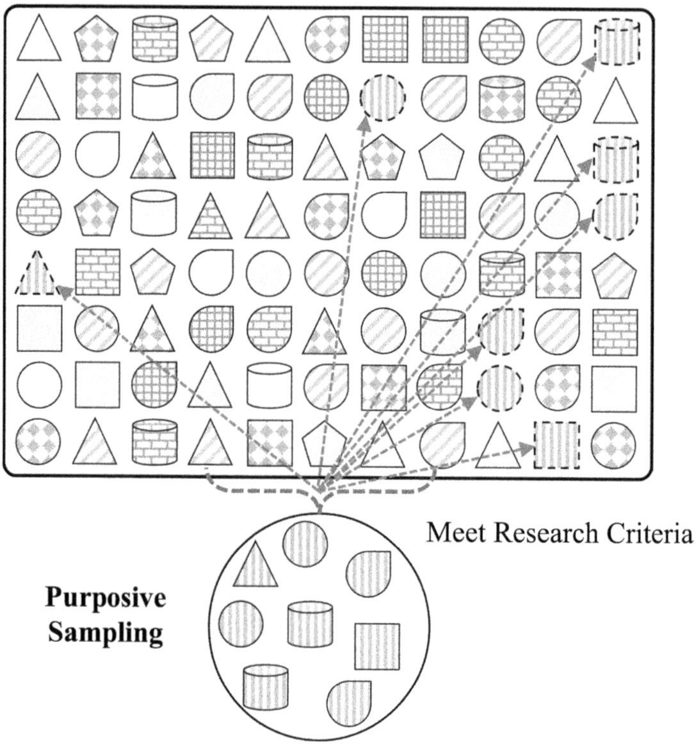

FIGURE 2.4
Presentation of purposive sampling.

for the various sampling units cannot be calculated ("Encyclopedia of Biostatistics", 2005; Levy & Lemeshow, 2013).

Figure 2.4 shows a schematic representation of purposive sampling, in which samples are chosen non-randomly based on colour proportion.

2.4.4 Quota Sampling

Quota sampling is a form of non-probability sampling in which the researcher designs the sampling plan so that the sample structure for specific variables mirrors the structure of the reference population, based on their knowledge of these variables within the population. In this approach, participants are selected according to pre-established quotas for specific demographic or other characteristics, such as age, gender, race, or socioeconomic status ("Encyclopedia of Biostatistics", 2005; Kotz et al., 2005).

To implement quota sampling, the researcher first divides the reference population into categories based on their understanding of the variables of interest (e.g., gender into two classes – men and women; geographical region into four areas – north, south, east, and west; work status; marital status; age groups; etc.). These divisions are often based on multiple variables simultaneously. The researcher then assigns quotas proportional to the frequencies and sizes of each category in the population. This technique is termed "quota sampling" because each sample category has a predetermined quota corresponding to its size in the reference population. Consequently, the structure and composition of the sample reflect those of the population, ensuring that each subgroup is represented in the sample in the same proportion as in the population. By using this approach, the researcher can be confident that every class represented in the sample is represented in the population in the same proportion. Consequently, the structure and composition of the sample reflect those of the population.

TIP

Stratified sampling and quota sampling are regarded as similar techniques, with the primary distinction being that quota sampling involves the non-random selection of final units within each subgroup.

Within each quota, participants may be selected using convenience sampling, purposive sampling, or other non-random strategies. Unlike random sampling, these methods do not require a complete sampling frame for each category ("Encyclopedia of Biostatistics", 2005; Indrayan & Holt, 2016). The sampling process continues using non-random selection methods until the required number of completed interviews for each subgroup is obtained (Lavrakas, 2008).

The probability of obtaining representative estimates is higher in quota sampling than in the other three non-probability sampling techniques (convenience, snowball, and purposive), due to the similarity between the sample and population structures. However, because participants within each category are not selected at random, this technique is classified as a non-probability sampling method. Similar to probability sampling, stratified sampling allows the researcher to preselect the proportions of desired strata in the final sample. From this, it can be concluded that stratified sampling and quota sampling are analogous, such that "the stratified method is to probability sampling as the quota method is to non-probability sampling".

Researchers frequently use quota sampling to ensure that the sample is representative of the overall population and includes a specific number of individuals from different categories or subgroups. This method helps maintain population representativeness ("Encyclopedia of Biostatistics", 2005).

It is particularly useful in situations where obtaining a random sample is difficult or impractical, such as in large, dispersed populations or when

TABLE 2.1

The Distribution of University Students by Gender and Faculty of Study

	Gender		
Faculty	**Female**	**Male**	**Total**
Social sciences	130 (13%)	120 (12%)	250 (25%)
Medicine	150 (15%)	200 (20%)	350 (35%)
Rehabilitation	100 (10%)	50 (5%)	150 (15%)
Health school	150 (15%)	100 (10%)	250 (25%)
University	530 (53%)	470 (47%)	1000

logistical constraints complicate data collection. Quota sampling is commonly applied in market research and opinion polls to obtain a sample that accurately reflects the population's distribution on key variables of interest (Kotz et al., 2005).

Since participants in quota sampling are not chosen at random, the method cannot be considered a random sampling technique. Additionally, this approach may introduce bias, as the researcher selects participants based on predetermined criteria ("Encyclopedia of Biostatistics", 2005; Kotz et al., 2005). Non-random selection reduces the generalisability of results and can compromise the validity of statistical inference methods, including confidence intervals and hypothesis testing (Indrayan & Holt, 2016).

A typical example of quota sampling is a random-digit dialling telephone survey in which 50% of the interviews are conducted with men and 50% with women. Another example involves a researcher seeking to consider the opinions of students in a sample of 200 participants. The university has 1,000 students distributed across five faculties. Basic details about the faculties and the gender composition of students are provided in Table 2.1.

In order to ensure that the quotas correspond accurately to the reference population, the researcher utilises the available information to distribute the number of samples proportionally to the percentages presented in the table.

This distribution is conducted independently for each faculty and gender within the total sample. Specifically, there will be 26 female students from the Faculty of Social Sciences, representing 13% of the total sample, and 10 male students from the Faculty of Rehabilitation Sciences, representing 5% of the total sample. Table 2.2 presents the number of samples in each subgroup.

2.4.4.1 Advantages of Quota Sampling

- **Cost-Efficiency:** This method is relatively inexpensive, as it simplifies the selection process in the final stage and reduces the need for extensive human resources and time.
- **Speed:** For routine and repetitive projects, such as surveys on television programmes, quota sampling can be implemented more rapidly than other sampling methods.

- **Flexibility:** This approach is not constrained by the rigid structures of random sampling, making it more adaptable – particularly when an appropriate sampling frame is unavailable.

TABLE 2.2

The Distribution of Sampled Students by Gender and Faculty of Study

	Gender		
Faculty	**Female**	**Male**	**Total**
Social sciences	26	24	50
Medicine	30	40	70
Rehabilitation	20	10	30
Health school	30	20	50
University	106	94	200

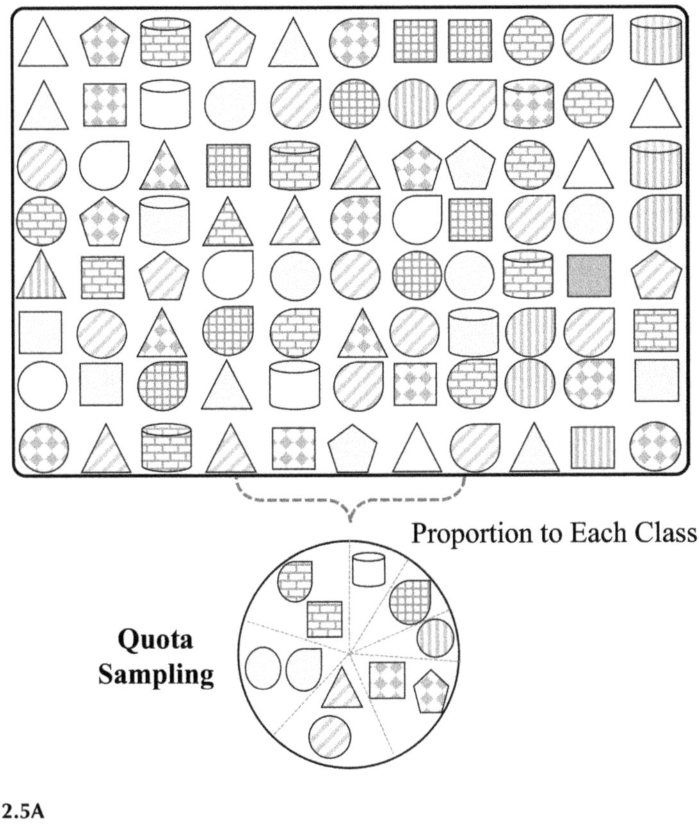

FIGURE 2.5A
Illustration of quota sampling.

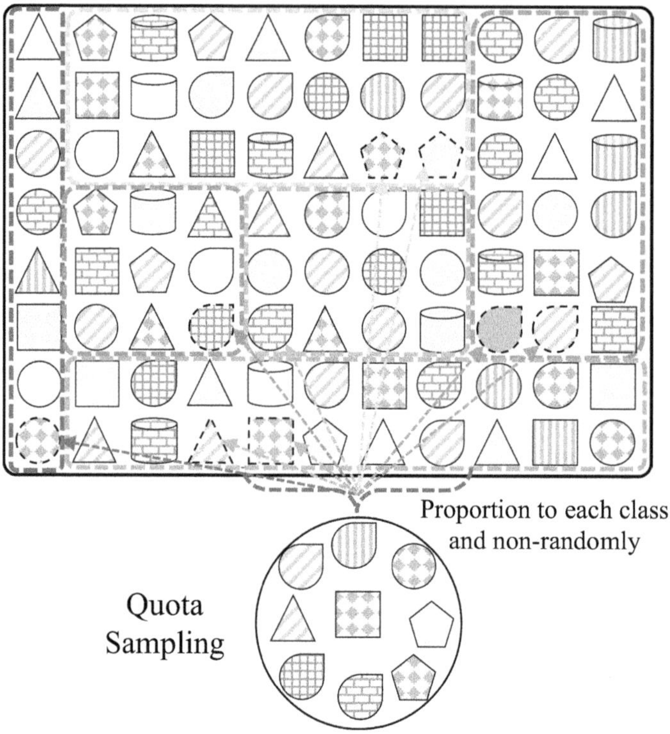

FIGURE 2.5B
Illustration of quota sampling.

2.4.4.2 Disadvantages of Quota Sampling

- **Difficulty in Error Estimation:** Although it is possible to estimate the standard error, accurately calculating the sampling error is not feasible without conducting repeated samples.
- **Potential for Bias:** Interviewers' personal biases and preferences may influence participant selection. Characteristics such as appearance or gender can affect whom interviewers choose to include. Furthermore, variations in participant willingness – some individuals declining to participate while others being overly eager – can lead to systematic bias, potentially skewing the sample and compromising its representativeness.

Figure 2.5a illustrates a schematic representation of quota sampling, in which samples are selected non-randomly based on proportional representation by colour.

Figure 2.5b illustrates a schematic representation of quota sampling, in which samples are selected non-randomly based on proportional representation by stratum size.

References

Agresti, A., Franklin, C. A., & Klingenberg, B. (2020). *The art and science of learning from data*. Pearson.

Boslaugh, S. (2007). *Encyclopedia of epidemiology*. Sage Publications.

Cozby, P. C., Bates, S. C., Krägeloh, C. U., Lacherez, P., & Van Rooy, D. (2016). *Methods in behavioural research*. McGraw-Hill Education.

Indrayan, A., & Holt, M. P. (2016). *Concise encyclopedia of biostatistics for medical professionals*. Chapman and Hall and CRC Press.

Kotz, S., Balakrishnan, N., Read, C. B., Vidakovic, B., & Johnson, N. L. (2005). *Encyclopedia of statistical sciences* (Vol. 1). John Wiley & Sons.

Lavrakas, P. J. (2008). *Encyclopedia of survey research methods*. Sage Publications.

Levy, P. S. (2005). *Encyclopedia of biostatistics* (ArmitageP. & T. Colton, Eds., 2nd ed.). Wiley.

Levy, P. S., & Lemeshow, S. (2013). *Sampling of populations: Methods and applications*. John Wiley & Sons.

Salkind, N. J. (2010). *Encyclopedia of research design* (Vol. 1). Sage Publications.

3

Probability Sampling Techniques

3.1 Introduction

A sample is considered random when the inclusion or exclusion of a particular eligible subject is determined purely by chance and cannot be predicted in advance. However, the probability of inclusion is not necessarily equal for all subjects within the sample. For this reason, it is often more accurate to describe such sampling as probability sampling (Indrayan & Holt, 2016).

Probability sampling is a technique used to select a sample from a defined population, ensuring that every element has a known and non-zero probability of being included. In this method, the sample is selected through a random mechanism, allowing each element of the population to have a specified probability of selection (Levy, 2005).

Because each element has a known probability of selection, probability sampling allows for the assessment of the statistical properties of estimators for population parameters (such as means and proportions) derived from sample data. This approach facilitates unbiased estimation and the construction of estimators with desirable statistical attributes. These attributes can then be generalised to the target population, assuming no additional biases are present (Levy, 2005; Levy & Lemeshow, 2013). For example, it enables the determination of whether the expected value of an estimator, across repeated samples of the same parameter, corresponds to the true value of the parameter being estimated (i.e., unbiasedness).

TIP

The core principle of sampling is that the sample must accurately represent the population from which it is drawn. Achieving representativeness not only reduces the number of observations required but also enables valid and effective generalisation of the findings from the sample to the larger population.

DOI: 10.1201/9781003749783-3

Although random sampling is a widely used method for generating a representative sample, it is not the only available approach. Other techniques that achieve representativeness may also be employed; however, empirical evidence indicates that no method is more effective than random sampling. Moreover, the larger the sample size relative to the population, the greater the likelihood that the sample will be representative, regardless of the sampling method used (Indrayan & Holt, 2016).

3.2 The Logic of Probability Sampling

Consider a hypothetical population in which all members share the same attributes under study. In this case, selecting a single member can represent the entire population. For example, if you are in an elementary school and want to determine the grade level of the pupils, asking just one pupil would be sufficient. This single observation can represent the entire class (the population).

Similarly, when visiting a medical diagnostic laboratory for a blood test, it is not surprising that only a few cubic centimetres (CCs) of blood drawn from one area of the body are sufficient to assess a patient's health. This is because the blood within the body is relatively uniform and homogeneous. However, it is advisable to take multiple blood pressure readings, as blood pressure can vary due to several factors such as nutrition, sleep quality, stress, anxiety, and physical activity. Likewise, an individual's blood glucose levels fluctuate after meals and during fasting periods.

In reality, populations are typically diverse and heterogeneous. Therefore, the number of samples collected must be sufficient to accurately represent the population. This means that the sample should reflect the essential variations that exist within the population. The key principle is that the sample must be representative, comprehensive, and inclusive. Being comprehensive implies that every individual in the population has an equal probability of being selected. To represent the population accurately, the sample should be chosen based on the variability of relevant characteristics across different contexts. Consequently, a larger sample size is required when the variable of interest exhibits substantial variation (heterogeneity), whereas a smaller sample size may be adequate for a more homogeneous population with limited variation.

The objective of most sampling surveys is to estimate specific parameters of certain characteristics of the reference population, such as means, totals, proportions, percentiles, standard deviations, or other distributional features (Levy & Lemeshow, 2013). The fundamental principle of sampling is that the sample must accurately represent the population from which it is drawn. Additional objectives include reducing the number of observations required by the researcher (Machin et al., 2018) and providing a practical means of generalising data from the sample to the population. These principles require that all members of the reference population have a clear and equal probability of selection. In such cases, sampling is based on probability, and the terms *probability sampling* and *random selection* are closely related – both indicating that the likelihood of selecting each member of the population is proportional to their representation within it.

3.3 Types of Probability Sampling

This chapter discusses the principal types of probability sampling methods, including:

- Simple random sampling (SRS),
- Systematic random sampling (SyS),
- Cluster random sampling (CRS),
- Stratified random sampling (StRS),
- Multistage random sampling (MRS),
- Area sampling,
- Probability proportional to size sampling (PPS).

Each type of random sampling will be examined in detail, accompanied by illustrative designs to enhance understanding.

Figure 3.1 presents the various types of probability sampling.

3.3.1 Simple Random Sampling (SRS)

Simple random sampling (SRS) is the most fundamental type of probability sampling and serves as the basis for more advanced sampling methods (Lohr, 2021; Peregrine, 2018). This method is conceptually straightforward: samples are selected entirely at random, such as by flipping a coin or drawing numbers from a hat, which is why it is called *"simple random sampling"*. SRS provides an unbiased representation of a population, making it one of the most widely used techniques for data collection. A random subset of participants can effectively represent the characteristics of the entire population.

The primary objective of SRS is to generate a manageable and balanced subset of individuals that accurately reflects a larger population, particularly when it is impractical to sample the entire group.

The process of conducting an SRS typically involves the following steps:

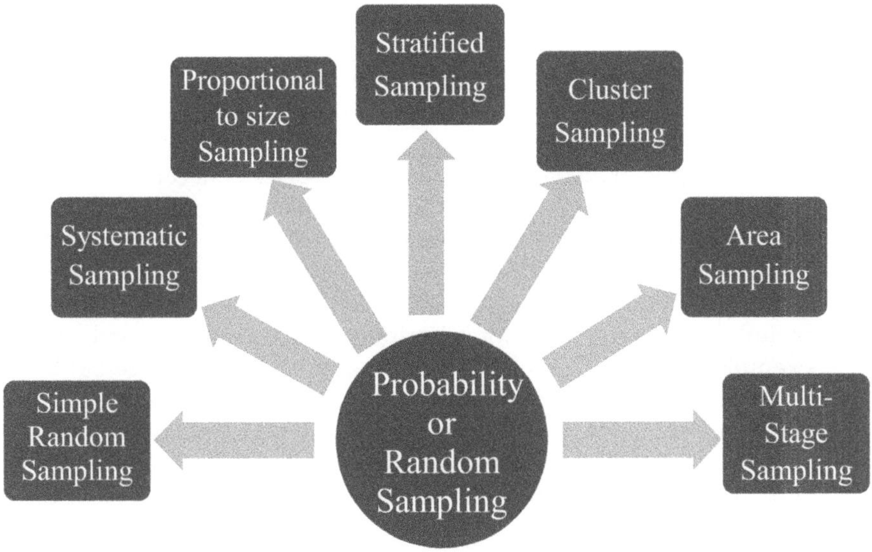

FIGURE 3.1
Various types of probability sampling.

1. **Define the Target Population:** Identify the population to be studied and determine an appropriate sample size. A smaller sample size may reduce representativeness and limit the generalisability of findings.
2. **Establish the Sampling Frame:** Create a comprehensive list of all individuals or units in the population from which the sample will be drawn. Examples include schools, treatment centres, or electoral registers.
3. **Assign Numbers:** Assign each individual or unit in the sampling frame a unique sequential number.
4. **Select Participants:** Use unbiased selection methods – such as lotteries, random number tables, random number generators, or computer algorithms – to select the sample.

TIP

Simple Random Sampling (SRS) is a fundamental probability sampling method that provides an unbiased representation of a population. By selecting participants entirely at random, SRS minimises sampling bias and enhances the generalisability of research findings, making it one of the most widely used techniques for reliable data collection.

SRS can be implemented in two main ways:

- **Without Replacement:** Each unit in the sample is unique; once a unit is selected, it cannot be chosen again (Lohr, 2021). This approach serves as the foundation for many other probability sampling techniques (Kotz et al., 2005). An SRS without replacement can be drawn from a sampling frame using random number tables or computer-based algorithms. Obtaining a comprehensive and accurate sampling frame is crucial for effective implementation (Kotz et al., 2005). Many programming languages and statistical software packages include built-in functions for selecting a simple random sample; for example, the "deal" function in A Programming Language (APL). Similar random selection functions are also available in statistical software such as SPSS – for instance, the Random Numbers function under *Transform* → *Compute* or the Random Sample of Cases procedure – both of which can be used to generate simple random samples.
- **With Replacement:** A unit may appear more than once in the sample. For instance, when drawing 5 balls from an urn containing 20, each ball is returned to the urn before the next draw, maintaining the same population for each selection. In this case, each unit has a $1/N$ probability of being selected, where N is the total population size (Everitt & Howell, 2021, p. 2570).

In contrast, simple random sampling (SRS) without replacement involves selecting units randomly from a population without returning them to the sampling frame. For example, if five balls are drawn from an urn without replacement, the population size decreases with each draw, resulting in five distinct balls after five selections. Consequently, the probability of obtaining a specific sample differs from that in sampling with replacement (Everitt & Howell, 2021, p. 2570).

It is important to note that most statistical procedures – such as the estimation of odds ratios, regression coefficients, and confidence intervals – assume that SRS has been performed. In other words, the development of statistical estimation is fundamentally based on the principles of SRS. Although estimates can be derived from non-SRS sampling methods, they may be biased or inaccurate if the assumptions underlying random sampling are violated (Boslaugh, 2007).

In practice, SRS provides desirable statistical properties, including minimal variance and the smallest possible confidence intervals. Its straightforward design makes it easy to implement using standard statistical software, thereby reducing analytical complexity. However, it is essential to acknowledge that SRS does not always guarantee the most efficient estimates in all research contexts (Boslaugh, 2007).

3.3.1.1 Advantages and Disadvantages of SRS

3.3.1.1.1 Advantages

Simple random sampling (SRS) offers two primary advantages: it minimises bias and enhances the representativeness of the target population. This sampling method is among the least biased because every member of the population has an equal probability of selection. By giving each individual an equal opportunity to be chosen, SRS helps eliminate researcher bias. Although sampling error can never be entirely avoided, this approach strives to be as objective and unbiased as possible. Moreover, SRS ensures that the selected sample accurately reflects the characteristics of the overall population, thereby increasing the likelihood that the results can be generalised to the entire group.

3.3.1.1.2 Disadvantages

Despite its strengths, SRS also has certain disadvantages, including high time and cost requirements, potential sampling errors, and challenges in accessing respondents. Constructing a comprehensive sampling frame (a complete list of the target population) can be expensive, time-consuming, and logistically difficult – particularly for large or dispersed populations. Even when a complete list is available, obtaining accurate contact information for all individuals can pose significant challenges, particularly if the population is large or geographically dispersed. In addition, sampling errors may still occur if the selected sample fails to accurately reflect the population as a whole, which may necessitate restarting the sampling process.

Figure 3.2 illustrates the simple random sampling (SRS) method.

3.3.1.2 Table of Random Numbers

A table of random numbers or digits is a set of numbers (0, 1, 2, 3, 4, 5, 6, 7, 8, 9) arranged randomly in rows and columns, as illustrated by the small sample below. Typically, five-digit numbers are organised in rows and columns to facilitate reading. A complete table usually spans four or more pages. But what distinguishes a table of randomly selected digits from any other listing of numbers? There are two key characteristics of a random digit table. First, every digit from 0 to 9 has an equal probability of appearing in each table entry. Second, the entries are independent of one another. These features ensure that a table of random digits exhibits no discernible pattern, meaning that any digit from 0 to 9 has an equal chance of being selected when a number is chosen at random from the table.

Knowing the entries in some parts of the table does not allow one to predict the entries in other parts. Most statistical textbooks include tables of random numbers. Since 1927, random number tables have been generated using various methods.

Note: In modern practice, tables of random numbers have been almost entirely replaced by computational random number generators. Like random

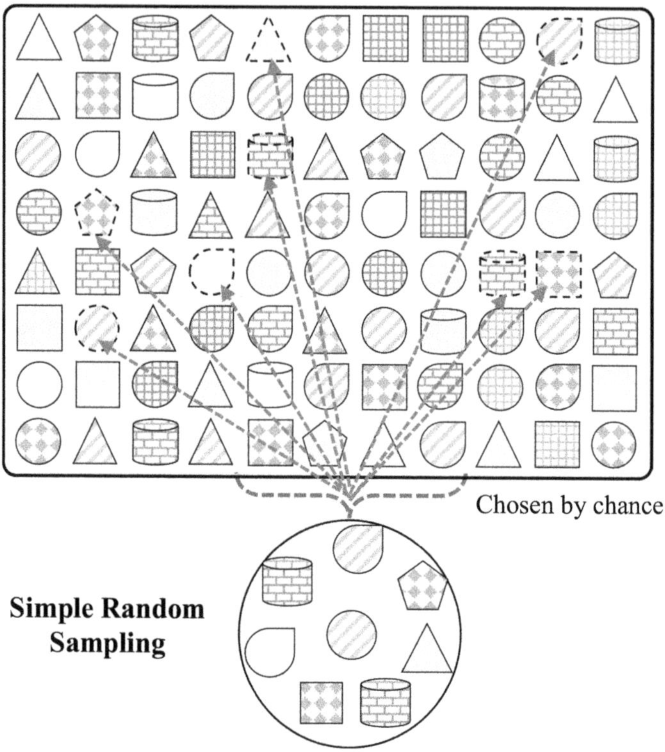

FIGURE 3.2
Schematic presentation of simple random sampling.

number tables, these generators produce random data using different algorithms. Most calculators and software programs, however, cannot generate truly random numbers; they produce numbers using a formula based on a seed, which introduces the possibility of repeated sequences and prevents the numbers from being completely random. Nevertheless, for most research purposes, such pseudo-random numbers are sufficient.

Table 3.1 presents a section of a table containing random digits, as commonly found in statistical textbooks.

3.3.1.3 Using Random Number Tables in Practice

There are various methods for reading numbers from random number tables. One such method is outlined below:

1. Suppose you have examination results for 200 students in your class. Each student is assigned a unique identification number from 1 to 200. For this demonstration, we will randomly select five students.

TABLE 3.1

Part of Table of Random Numbers

61424	20419	86546	00517
90222	27993	04952	66762
50349	71146	97668	86523
85676	10005	08216	25906
02429	19761	*15370*	43882
90519	61988	40164	15815
20631	88967	19660	89624
89990	78733	16447	27932

2. Since the population size is represented by a three-digit number, we will use the first three digits of the numbers in the random number table.
3. Next, we determine a direction for reading the table (downward, in this example, and then to the right). We choose a random starting point on the table without looking. Assume that the starting point corresponds to the number 20419 (the first entry in the second column of Table 3.1).
4. The first three digits of this number are 204. Because 204 exceeds the total number of students (200), it is excluded. We then move to the next number to the right. Recall that valid student numbers must fall within the range 001–200.
5. The first three digits of the next number, 865, are also too large. We continue moving to the right until we find a number whose first three digits are within the valid range. The number 005 meets this condition, as its first three digits are less than or equal to 200.
6. Continuing in this way, we obtain the following valid three-digit numbers from the table: 049 (04952), 100 (10005), 082 (08216), 024 (02429), and 197 (19761). Therefore, the students selected for the random sample are those with identification numbers 49, 100, 82, 24, and 197.

3.3.1.4 Why SRS Implementation Is Difficult and Less Commonly Used

Simple random sampling (SRS) forms the foundation of sampling theory and serves as the benchmark for evaluating other sampling methods. As the most basic form of probability sampling, SRS ensures that every participant has an equal probability of being selected. However, despite its conceptual simplicity, implementing SRS in practice can be challenging, often proving to be costly and impractical.

A major difficulty lies in constructing a realistic sampling frame – the complete list of all elements in the population from which the sample is to be drawn. Developing such a list is frequently constrained by financial and temporal limitations. A comprehensive sampling frame must be established before data collection begins, yet it may be missing, incomplete, or outdated. For instance, as Indrayan and Holt (2016) note, if a study involves multiple hospitals, each institution may maintain its own patient registry, but a consolidated list encompassing all hospitals' patients may not be readily available (Indrayan & Holt, 2016).

Another challenge arises from the nature of random selection process itself. Because each sampling unit has an equal probability of being chosen, selected units may be widely dispersed across large geographic areas. This spatial dispersion can substantially increase the cost and time required for conducting interviews and administering questionnaires. Furthermore, such geographic spread does not necessarily improve the representativeness of the sample. There is no assurance that SRS will adequately capture all relevant subgroups within the target population (Indrayan & Holt, 2016). Random selection can, by chance, lead to overrepresentation of certain subgroups relative to their actual proportions in the population. For example, a sample might include several cases with moderate or severe conditions while excluding those with mild conditions. Similarly, studies primarily involving adults might yield little to no representation of children (Indrayan & Holt, 2016). Additionally, despite its theoretical neutrality, bias can still infiltrate samples obtained through SRS, particularly if the sampling frame is incomplete or inaccurately defined.

Given these challenges, it is understandable why researchers often opt for alternative sampling methods. While SRS possesses strong statistical properties and provides unbiased estimators in theory, it frequently encounters the practical limitations described above and may not fully align with the specific objectives of a given study. These constraints highlight the importance of considering other sampling techniques better suited to real-world research contexts (Boslaugh, 2007).

3.3.2 Systematic Sampling (SyS)

Systematic sampling is easier to implement in the field and serves as a practical alternative to simple random sampling (SRS). It is the sampling technique most similar to SRS in nature, and systematic samples are generally assumed to behave in a similar manner to simple random samples for estimation purposes (Boslaugh, 2007). Systematic sampling involves an easy-to-use and straightforward selection process.

A sampling method is referred to as *systematic random sampling* when the first unit is selected at random from the initial set according to the sampling fraction, and the remaining units are automatically selected based on the same sampling fraction or interval (Indrayan & Holt, 2016). The researcher begins at a random starting point and selects items separated by a fixed interval. Specifically, a random number between 1 and k is first selected from a list or another device defining the target population. Starting with this random number, every kth element is subsequently added to the sample (Boslaugh, 2007).

Assume for the time being that $k = \frac{N}{n}$ is an integer and that a sample of n elements is required from a population list of N elements. Every kth element on the list is then selected to create a systematic sample, where k represents the sampling interval. The first sampled element is usually chosen by selecting a random number, say m, between 1 and k. The $m_{th}, [m+k]_{th}, [m+2k]_{th}, \ldots, and\ [m+(n-1)\}k]_{th}$ elements on the list constitute the selected sample. When a random start is used, every element in the population has the same probability of selection, equal to $\frac{1}{k}$ (Kotz et al., 2005).

TIP

Start with a random point: Always begin your systematic sampling process by choosing a random starting position within the population. This approach ensures that each unit has an equal probability of selection, thereby preserving the representativeness and integrity of your sample.

Let the population consist of N subjects, numbered from 1 through N in any arbitrary order. The sampling fraction for a sample size of n is given by $k = \frac{N}{n}$; although the fraction is technically $\frac{n}{N}$, using $k = \frac{N}{n}$ is more convenient when conducting systematic sampling (Indrayan & Holt, 2016).

In practice, the sampling interval k is rarely an integer. Several approaches can be used to handle non-integer values of k. One common method is to round k to the nearest integer and proceed with the selection as before. Although the final sample size may not exactly match the initially intended size, this discrepancy is usually acceptable. Alternatively, k can be rounded down to the nearest integer. In this approach, a random start is chosen for the entire population, and $(n-1)$ additional elements are selected by repeatedly adding the rounded-down k to the random start one after the other. This process effectively creates a circular list, where the last element is followed by the first.

As an illustration, consider a systematic sample of 25 subjects selected from a target population of 200 subjects. The sampling fraction in this case is 1 out of 8. After the first subject is chosen at random, the others are automatically selected by adding the sampling interval. For example, if number 3 is chosen at random, the subsequent selected numbers would be 11, 19, 27, 35, 43, 51, and 59. This example assumes that subjects follow a predetermined order and that each has a known serial number. When subjects are not arranged sequentially, each must be assigned a serial number prior to sampling.

Now, assume that there are $N = 101$ subjects in the target population and that $n = 8$ of them will be selected using the systematic method. The integer part of the sampling interval, calculated as $k = \frac{101}{8}$, is 12 (Indrayan & Holt, 2016).

When the sampling interval is an integer, the systematic sampling method performs well; however, two types of anomalies may arise in other situations:

- **Exclusion of the Final Units:** It is possible that the last few units in the population will not have a chance to be selected. In the example above, if the first selected number is 12, the last number in the sample will be 96. Consequently, units 97–101 can never be chosen.
- **Sample Size Inflation:** In certain cases, the sample size may exceed the intended number. For instance, if the fourth unit is the first randomly selected unit in this example, the hundredth unit becomes the last selected unit. In this scenario, the sample would include nine units instead of the required eight. This issue is negligible when the sample size n is large, such as greater than 30. One way to address this problem is through circular sampling, in which the starting point is a random number between 1 and N, and every k^{th} unit is selected cyclically. In other words, after reaching the Nth unit, the selection continues from the first unit again until n units are chosen (Indrayan & Holt, 2016, p. 619).

TIP

Monitor for Periodicity: Be alert to periodic patterns within your population. If the sampling interval aligns with a periodic trend, it can produce biased results. Regularly examine your population structure to ensure that sampling remains representative and to avoid skewed outcomes.

Systematic sampling is widely used in industry to ensure quality control. It tends to yield a representative sample of the population when specific items start to malfunction consistently, whereas simple random sampling may over- or under-represent defective items (Frey, 2021).

3.3.2.1 Merits and Demerits of Systematic Sampling

3.3.2.1.1 Merits

- **Ease of Implementation:** Systematic sampling is straightforward to carry out. For example, when patients arrive at a clinic, it is simple to select every eligible i^{th} patient after randomly choosing the first patient for study inclusion. This method also tends to be faster than simple random sampling (SRS), which requires random selection of each individual unit.
- **No Need for a Complete Sampling Frame:** Systematic sampling does not require a complete list of all population units; it only requires knowledge of the total population size. For instance, if a clinic sees $N = 275$ patients per month and a sample of $n = 30$ is to be selected, the sampling interval is $k = 9$. No patient list is necessary; if the first randomly selected patient is the seventh, the subsequent patients included would be the 16th, 25th, and so on, according to the order of arrival.
- **Proportional Representation:** Because selection occurs at evenly spaced intervals, all sections of the population can be represented, potentially producing a more representative sample than SRS. For example, if a clinic operates six days a week, with teenage patients scheduled on Mondays and Thursdays, adult male patients on Tuesdays and Fridays, and adult female patients on Wednesdays and Saturdays, systematic sampling covering all days will automatically ensure proportional representation of each patient group.

3.3.2.1.2 Demerits

- **Risk of Bias due to Periodicity:** Systematic sampling may produce a biased sample if hidden periodicities or trends exist among the population as units are numbered from 1 to N. Systematic sampling performs poorly when the survey variable follows a periodic pattern and the sampling interval coincides with a multiple of this periodicity. For example, consider a list of married couples where husbands are listed first and wives second. Using an even sampling interval could result in a sample consisting entirely of husbands or entirely of wives. In contrast, an odd sampling interval would yield nearly equal proportions of husbands and wives.
- **Avoid Sampling Intervals Matching Periodicity:** When periodicities are present, sampling intervals that are multiples of the periodicity should be avoided. Regular periodic cycles are relatively uncommon in practice. Kotz and colleagues also discussed several methods for improving the precision of systematic sampling in the presence of linear trends (Kotz et al., 2005, p. 8601).

TIP

Maintain Proportional Representation: When sampling from diverse groups, ensure that your systematic approach captures all segments of the population. Adjust your sampling intervals based on the distribution of different groups within the population to achieve proportional representation.

3.3.2.2 Key Points in Systematic Sampling

1. **Use of Systematic Sampling When a Population List Is Absent or Randomly Ordered:** When there is no population list or only a roughly random list, systematic sampling is often employed as an alternative to simple random sampling (SRS). If the population is arranged in a monotonic order, systematic sampling typically produces estimators with smaller variances – although, in some cases, these variances may be inestimable – compared to SRS. Repeating systematic sampling with distinct random starting points allows researchers to estimate the variance of the overall sample by analysing variability across the subsamples (Frey, 2021).
2. **Considerations When the Population Is Periodic:** When the population exhibits periodic order, selecting an appropriate sampling interval is critical for obtaining a representative sample. Systematic sampling can be considered a form of cluster sampling in which each cluster comprises non-contiguous units. For example, suppose the population values, in order, are:

   $$1, 2, 3, 1, 2, 3, 1, 2, 3, 1, 2, 3,$$

   and the sampling interval is 3. In this case, all elements selected in the systematic sample would be identical, illustrating the importance of avoiding sampling intervals that coincide with the population's periodicity (Lohr, 2021).

Systematic sampling must be representative of the population and cover the full range of the population to be effective. A basic example is interviewing individuals in a long queue about their political opinions. To select a sample of size 50 from a queue of 700 people, one would first randomly select a number between 1 and 14, then choose every 14th person thereafter. If the individuals in the queue are arranged in random order, both a simple random sample and a systematic sample will yield similar results.

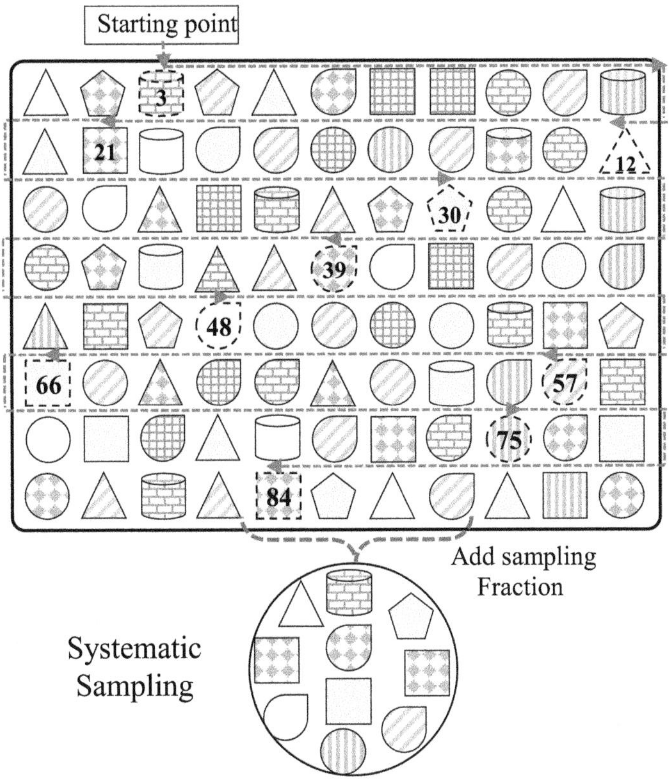

FIGURE 3.3
Schematic presentation of systematic sampling.

However, systematic sampling may yield more representative results than random sampling when individuals with similar political views are grouped together.

Figure 3.3 illustrates the process of selecting a systematic sample from a hypothetical population.

To collect samples using systematic approaches, the following steps should be followed:

1. **Identify the Size of the Parent Population (*N*):** Determine the total number of individuals in the parent population and calculate the sample size (n) to be selected from it.
2. **Determine the Sampling Interval:** Calculate the sampling interval using the formula $k = N / n$ or determine the sampling fraction using n / N. If the sampling interval is not an integer, discard the decimal portion to ensure a sufficiently large sample size (n). Alternatively, use the solutions discussed in the previous section.

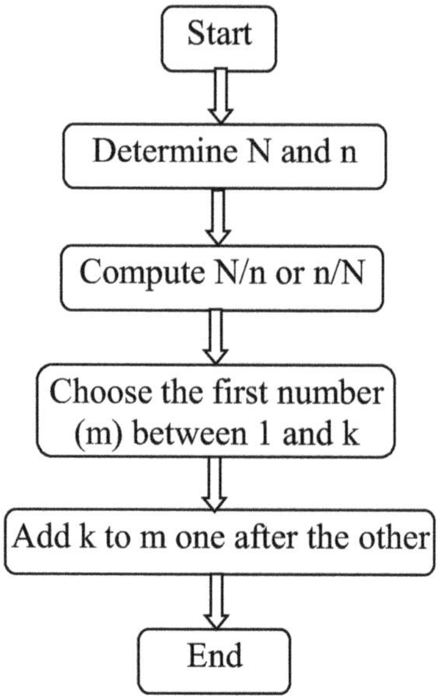

FIGURE 3.4
How to select systematic samples.

3. **Select a Random Starting Point:** Choose a random number (e.g., m) between 1 and k for the first sample.
4. **Select Subsequent Samples:** For the remaining samples, sequentially add k to m until $(n-1)$ additional elements are selected. The members of the sample will be the mth, $[m+k]^{th}$, $[m+2k]^{th}$, ..., and $[m+(n-1)k]^{th}$ elements of the list.

Figure 3.4 provides a visual representation of these steps.

3.3.3 Cluster Sampling

Cluster sampling is a cost-effective probability sampling technique in which groups of units are selected instead of individual units. A *cluster* is defined as a collection of related or similar units, which may include any physically connected grouping such as homes, classrooms, hospital wards, or other spaces (Indrayan & Holt, 2016, p. 108).

As the name suggests, units are selected in groups. When any primary sampling unit in the frame contains more than one observation unit (element), these primary sampling units are referred to as *clusters,* and a sample composed of such units is known as a *"cluster sample"* (Kotz et al., 2005).

Typically, researchers employ pre-existing units as clusters, such as cities or schools. In cluster sampling, a simple random sample of these groups (clusters) is selected, thereby dividing the entire population into smaller subgroups known as clusters. A *one-stage cluster sampling plan* involves sampling every element within each selected cluster (Saneii & Doosti, 2024). In contrast, a *multistage cluster sample* includes only a subset of observation units within each cluster and is also referred to as a *sample with subsamples*. Many applications employ sampling across more than two stages. Each subsample is used sequentially to estimate the total for the unit from which it was selected, thereby producing estimators of totals (Kotz et al., 2005, p. 1020).

TIP

Remember that researchers will always incur costs when making observations. It is not advisable for them to select very large clusters, as this can lead to unnecessary expenditure of time, money, and resources. Consequently, the advantages of clustering may be reduced – or even completely lost.

For instance, a *two-stage cluster sample* involves two stages of random selection, while *three-stage* or *multistage cluster sampling* involves three or more stages of selection. The units chosen during the first stage are termed *primary sampling units* (*PSUs*), those selected in the second stage are *secondary sampling units* (*SSUs*), and the final elements chosen are referred to as *ultimate sampling units* (*USUs*) (Salkind, 2006, p. 151).

Clusters may also be created during the design stage to improve efficiency or convenience. One method for forming cluster samples is *systematic sampling*. Formally, when only one starting value is used, a systematic sample is equivalent to a sample of one cluster. In certain situations, organising the population using auxiliary information can result in more efficient systematic (cluster) samples than stratified samples of the same size (Kotz et al., 2005).

TIP

A common mistake made by researchers using survey data is analysing a cluster sample as if it were a simple random sample (SRS).

3.3.3.1 Relation to Systematic Sampling

Another perspective suggests that systematic sampling is essentially a subset of cluster sampling (Cochran, 1977, p. 207; Lohr, 2021, p. 166). A systematic sample can be viewed as a single cluster unit drawn at random from a population of k cluster units. There are k possible systematic samples of size n when $N = n \times k$. The population is divided into k large sampling units, each comprising n of the original elements. Selecting a randomly located systematic sample thus involves choosing one of these large sampling units at random.

For example, suppose we want a sample of size 3 from a population of 12 elements:

$$1\ 2\ 3\ 4\ 5\ 6\ 7\ 8\ 9\ 10\ 11\ 12.$$

To obtain a systematic sample, randomly choose a number between 1 and 4, draw that element, and then select every fourth element thereafter. Under this scheme, the population contains four primary sampling units (PSUs), which function as clusters even though the elements are not contiguous:

$$(1, 5, 9) \quad (2, 6, 10) \quad (3, 7, 11) \quad (4, 8, 12).$$

Clusters can be selected using various sampling techniques. For instance, a sample of clusters may be selected by simple random sampling or systematic sampling. Clusters may also be grouped into strata to obtain a stratified random sample of clusters (Levy & Lemeshow, 2013, p. 226). After the first stage of sampling, the sampling frame is constructed using only the clusters selected in the sample. Once the sample clusters are identified, the listing of second-stage sampling units is prepared only for these sampled clusters. Similarly, if the sampling involves more than two stages, units at each subsequent stage are listed only for those units chosen in the preceding stage.

Because the listing of clusters or units is often an expensive field operation, listing costs are generally lower for cluster-sampling designs than for other designs (Levy & Lemeshow, 2013, p. 226).

Clusters may be chosen with equal probability or using probability proportional to size (PPS). Under PPS sampling, the probability of selecting a cluster is proportional to its size, meaning that larger clusters have a higher probability of selection than smaller ones. The advantage of this approach is that, when clusters are selected with probability proportional to size, the same number of interviews can be conducted in each sampled cluster, ensuring adequate representation of each sampled unit.

3.3.3.2 Reasons for Using Cluster Sampling

Cluster sampling is widely adopted for three main reasons: its practicality, economic feasibility, and efficiency. Although researchers may initially intend to use individual elements as sampling units, numerous studies have shown that the elements of a population are often poorly listed, making the creation of a comprehensive list costly and time-consuming.

TIP

Cluster sampling offers several advantages, including practicality, cost efficiency, and a reduced need for comprehensive sampling frames. By using larger geographical units as clusters, researchers can minimise travel time and expenses while still obtaining reliable estimates, making it a cost-effective approach for studying dispersed populations.

In many cases, it is impractical to develop a sampling frame that includes every person or household in the population, especially when estimates are required on a per-person basis. Even when a list of individual households can be developed, it is often more economical to use larger geographic entities as sampling units, particularly when the target population is dispersed over a wide area (Cochran, 1977, p. 233; Levy, 2005, p. 1027). Cluster sampling is therefore employed for the following reasons

1. **Challenges in Creating a Sampling Frame:** Compiling a complete list of observation units can be difficult, expensive, or impractical. For example, it is not feasible to include every social media user or every store visitor in a region. While it may be possible to generate a list of individuals in a city using housing data or Wi-Fi purchase records, this process is both costly and time-consuming. In such cases – where a comprehensive and up-to-date sampling frame is unavailable – cluster sampling or the use of regional maps becomes essential. The study area can be divided into manageable units, such as city blocks or defined land segments in rural areas. Thus, cluster sampling is recommended when identifying individual units is challenging or when no reliable list of population elements exists.
2. **Distribution of the Target Population:** The population may be widely dispersed, particularly in remote areas, or it may be naturally grouped into clusters such as households, schools, hospitals, malls, or community centres. Sampling entire clusters is generally more cost-effective than conducting simple random sampling (SRS) of individuals (Lohr, 2021; Saneii & Doosti, 2024). For example, if

the target population consists of nursing homes in a specific region, it is far more economical to sample entire nursing home facilities and interview all residents than to carry out an SRS of individual residents. Interviewing a single individual at a nursing home often requires more resources than sampling all residents within the selected facilities. Likewise, in archaeological surveys, examining all artefacts within a defined region, rather than focusing on isolated sites, demonstrates the efficiency of cluster-based sampling approaches (Lohr, 2021, p. 166).

3. **Cost-Efficiency and Accuracy:** Observing groups of units can yield more precise results (i.e., smaller mean square error for an estimator) for a fixed level of expenditure. The operational costs of this method are relatively low; instead of travelling n times to different units located in n separate locations, researchers need only make a single trip to where all n units are located. This substantially reduces travel expenses between sampling sites. Additionally, constructing the sampling frame is less expensive. For instance, travelling to 40 randomly selected homes across a state is generally costlier than travelling to 10 clusters containing 4 homes each.

Another form of cluster sampling is *area sampling*, also known as *geographical cluster sampling*. When surveying a geographically dispersed population, it is often more cost-effective to group respondents within local areas into clusters rather than employ simple random sampling (Saneii & Doosti, 2024).

3.3.3.3 Merits and Demerits of Cluster Sampling

3.3.3.3.1 Merits

1. **Cost Reduction with Accuracy:** The primary motivation for using cluster sampling is to reduce total costs while maintaining the required level of accuracy. When most of the population's variation occurs within groups rather than between them, the expected random error for a fixed sample size is smaller.
2. **Reduced Need for Sampling Frames:** One key advantage of cluster sampling over simple random sampling (SRS) is that it does not require a complete list of all individual units; only a list of clusters is needed. This approach also allows researchers to increase the sample size, and consequently precision, without a proportional increase in cost. For example, compiling a list of hospitals is much easier than creating a list of individual patients with a specific illness, since hospitals serve as natural clusters of patients with that condition (Indrayan & Holt, 2016, p. 108).

3.3.3.3.2 Demerits

1. **Higher Sampling Error:** Cluster sampling generally produces higher sampling error compared to SRS. However, smaller clusters can make this method approach the accuracy of simple random sampling with lower sampling error. When there is intraclass correlation among the variables of interest (e.g., in the study of infectious diseases such as COVID-19), a larger sample size is required compared to other sampling methods to achieve the same level of precision.
2. **Misinterpretation of Results:** A common error researchers make when analysing cluster samples is treating them as if they were simple random samples. This misconception often results in reported standard errors that are smaller than they should be, thereby creating the false impression that the survey results are more precise than they actually are (Lohr, 2021, p. 166).

Conclusion: For novice researchers, three practical aspects of cluster sampling should be emphasised:

1. When units within all clusters exhibit the same variability with respect to the measure of interest as the overall target population, reliable estimates can be obtained from a small number of clusters. However, if there is moderate variability within clusters but considerable variability between clusters, smaller clusters may be necessary to ensure stability (Lavrakas, 2008, p. 98).
2. For a given sample size, smaller units generally yield more precise results than larger ones. For instance, a simple random sample of 600 houses may cover a town more evenly than 20 city blocks, each containing approximately 30 houses. However, the field costs associated with locating 600 individual houses and travelling between them are higher than those required to identify 20 blocks and visit all residences within them. Therefore, when both cost and precision are considered, larger units may sometimes prove superior (Cochran, 1977, p. 233).
3. To achieve equal confidence and precision, the overall sample size in cluster sampling often needs to be increased. Nonetheless, the time and resources required for data collection must be carefully evaluated to ensure that the sampling design remains efficient.

Figure 3.5 illustrates the process of selecting a cluster sample from a hypothetical population.

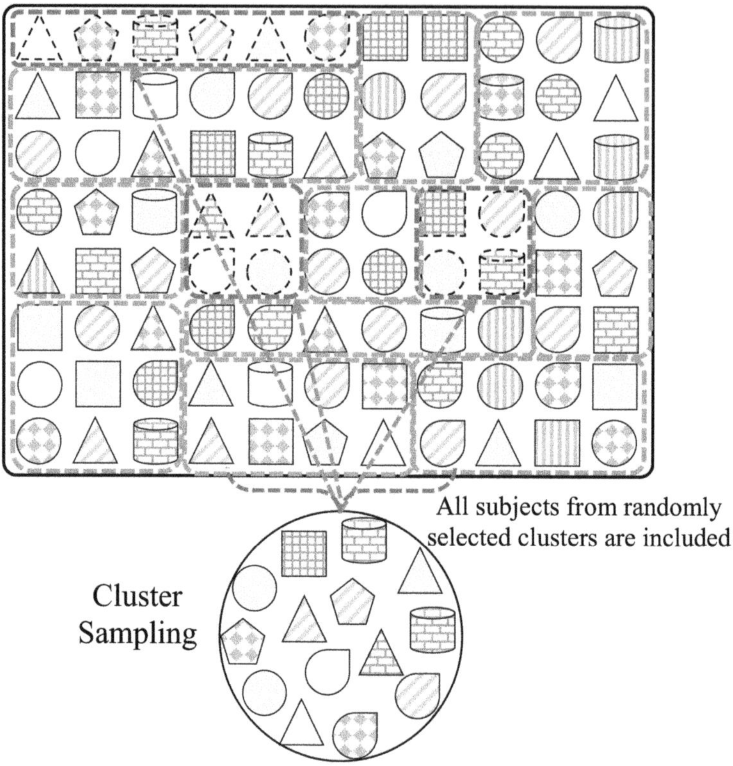

FIGURE 3.5
Schematic presentation of cluster sampling.

3.3.3.4 Cluster Sampling Selection Method

1. **Determine Clustering:** Identify an appropriate method for clustering the population. The elements within each cluster should exhibit similarities in terms of location and physical proximity.
2. **List Population Clusters:** Compile a comprehensive list of all population clusters to serve as the sampling frame for the study.
3. **Estimate Sample Size:** Calculate the required sample size (n) for the research project based on the study's objectives and statistical considerations.
4. **Select Random Cluster:** Randomly select one cluster and include all subjects or elements within that selected cluster in the sample.
5. **Gather Additional Clusters:** Continue randomly selecting additional clusters and collecting all subjects within them until the required sample size (n) is reached.

These steps are illustrated in Figure 3.6.

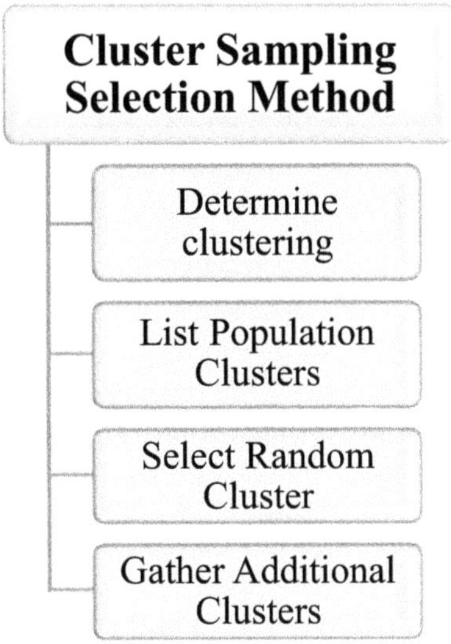

FIGURE 3.6
Cluster sampling selection procedure.

3.3.3.5 Two-Stage Cluster Sampling

Two-stage cluster sampling is used when developing a sampling frame for all units within a selected cluster or when interviewing and administering questionnaires to every unit in a cluster is not feasible. In this approach, a simple random sample of larger clusters is first selected. These clusters are then subdivided into smaller units, from which a second simple random sample is drawn. All members of the clusters chosen in this second stage are subsequently contacted or have their questionnaires completed. This process results in the creation of a sampling frame or membership list specific to the sampled clusters in the second stage. A researcher aims to estimate the prevalence of uncontrolled diabetes among adults in a large metropolitan region. In the first stage of two-stage cluster sampling, a simple random sample of districts within the metropolitan area is selected from the full list of administrative districts. Each chosen district is then divided into smaller clusters, such as registered family medicine practices or outpatient diabetes clinics. In the second stage, a simple random sample of clinics from each selected district is drawn. All eligible diabetic patients attending the sampled clinics during the study period are invited to participate in the survey and undergo clinical assessments. This approach reduces the cost and logistical burden of recruiting participants while enabling the collection of data from diverse clinical settings across the region.

3.3.3.6 Usefulness of Cluster Sampling

Cluster sampling is particularly useful when the units in the overall population are not more homogeneous than the enumeration units within the clusters with respect to the variables being measured in the sample survey. This implies that each cluster should exhibit significant variance, while the overall variance should be minimal. In other words, although each cluster may consist of distinct or heterogeneous individual units, the clusters themselves should be similar and homogeneous.

In certain circumstances, cluster sampling can significantly reduce travel expenses and the costs associated with frame construction without increasing sample errors. Armitage notes that enumeration units within clusters are typically much more homogeneous than the population as a whole, making such situations uncommon. Consequently, cluster sampling, which involves sampling every enumeration unit within a sampled cluster, can lead to considerable redundancy (Levy, 2005, p. 1031).

To mitigate this redundancy, researchers often prefer multistage sampling. By taking subsamples of enumeration units within each sample cluster, multistage designs reduce the sampling redundancy associated with including every enumeration unit. As a result, cluster sampling is becoming less common than multistage sampling in practice.

3.3.4 Stratified Random Sampling

Stratified random sampling (StRS), commonly referred to as *stratified sampling*, is a probability sampling technique frequently employed in survey research. This method involves classifying elements of a population (or, in practice, members of the sampling frame) into several mutually exclusive and exhaustive strata or groups based on shared characteristics relevant to the survey. Sampling is then conducted independently within each stratum. Each partition of the frame is termed a *stratum* (singular of *strata*), and the process of dividing the population is known as *stratification*.

By employing independent sampling procedures for each stratum, researchers can obtain unbiased estimates of the means or totals within each stratum. The overall population total can be estimated by summing the estimated totals for all strata. To calculate the overall population, mean, a stratum-weighted average of the estimated means is used (Palmer, 1999, p. 5697). When a simple random sample is drawn from each stratum, the process is referred to as *stratified random sampling* (Cochran, 1977, p. 89; Levy & Lemeshow, 2013, p. 121).

TIP

Stratified random sampling improves precision and cost-effectiveness by dividing a population into distinct strata based on shared characteristics. This approach ensures that each subgroup is properly represented, leading to more accurate and unbiased estimates compared to simple random sampling.

3.3.4.1 Example of Stratified Populations

A straightforward example of stratified populations can be found in a country's hospital-discharged patient population, which may be divided by region and by hospital size, based on the number of available beds. For instance, one typical stratum might consist of hospitals located in the southern region with 500 or more beds.

3.3.4.2 Advantages over Simple Random Sampling

One of the primary drawbacks of simple random sampling (SRS) is its potential inability to adequately represent one or more relevant subgroups within the population (Indrayan & Holt, 2016, p. 608). Consequently, stratified random sampling is often regarded as a more precise sampling technique than SRS (Salkind, 2006, p. 967). Stratification enhances both the cost-effectiveness and precision of a sampling design (Parsons, 2005, p. 5697).

The characteristic selected for stratification should either produce groups of particular interest that require separate analysis or be suspected of influencing the variable under study. Although the resulting sample may not perfectly represent other important variables, it will accurately reflect the characteristic used for stratification.

For example, research on diabetes mellitus mortality rates may yield a non-representative sample if participants are not grouped according to relevant factors such as maximum plasma glucose levels, age, gender, coexisting conditions, and patient compliance. Any of these variables could substantially influence the outcome or prognosis, underscoring the importance of careful stratification – even after the results have been extrapolated (Indrayan & Holt, 2016, p. 608).

3.3.4.3 Basic Foundations for Stratification

Typically, researchers begin with a set of analytical survey objectives that define study domains and specify the precision requirements for target estimators. Costs and administrative constraints also play crucial roles in the survey design process. Cochran identifies four primary justifications for employing a stratified design (Cochran, 1977, p. 89):

1. **Separate Parameter Estimates:** Researchers may wish to obtain distinct population parameter estimates for each subdomain within a larger population, effectively treating each subpopulation as a separate "population".
2. **Administrative Purposes:** Stratification may also be used for administrative reasons. For example, a survey organisation may have regional field offices responsible for conducting surveys within specific demographic or geographic segments.
3. **Ensuring Representativeness:** It is essential to ensure that the sample accurately represents the target population. Population subgroups can vary considerably and present distinct sampling challenges. For instance, individuals residing in different regions of a country often possess different characteristics, necessitating diverse sampling techniques. In such cases, stratified sampling may be the only feasible approach to achieving adequate representation.
4. **Increased Precision:** Stratification can improve the precision of sample estimators across the population. By dividing a heterogeneous population into internally homogeneous strata, researchers can achieve substantially lower sampling variability within each stratum. Consequently, population estimates obtained by combining estimates from all strata are generally more precise than those derived from a simple random sample of the same overall size.

The precision gains achieved through stratification, as described in Reason 4, can theoretically justify many widely used sampling techniques (Parsons, 2005, p. 5697).

In the example population described, there are strata containing 4, 5, 6, 8, 9, and 10 members. A total of 22 samples are allocated proportionally based on the size of each stratum, resulting in allocations of 1 sample, 1.25 samples, 1.5 samples, 2 samples, 2.25 samples, and 2.5 samples, respectively. Following standard rounding procedures, these values are adjusted accordingly. For the stratum corresponding to 1.5 samples, rounding is performed alternately up and down, and the same alternating approach applies to strata with 2.5 samples.

Figure 3.7 illustrates the process of selecting a systematic sample from a hypothetical population.

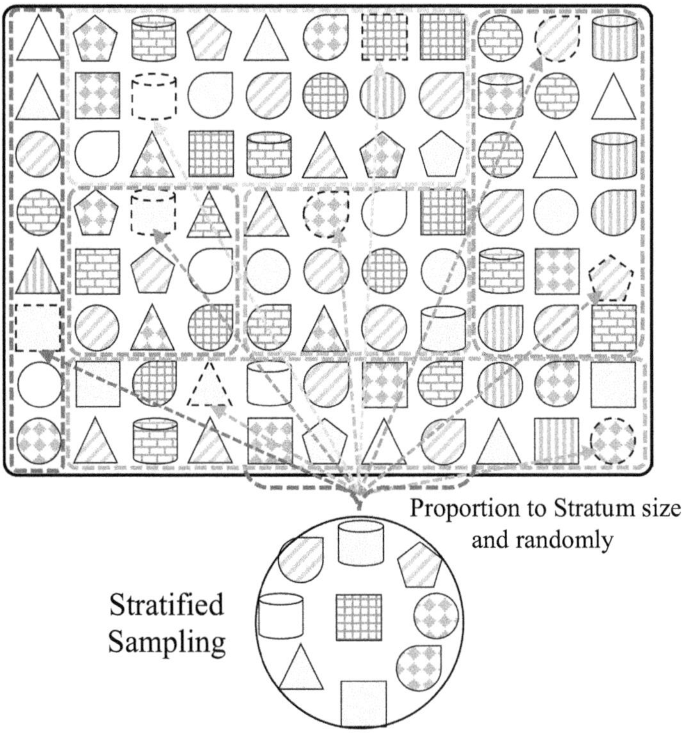

FIGURE 3.7
Schematic presentation of stratified random sampling.

3.3.4.4 Defining and Constructing Strata

A key question in stratified sampling is: *"How are strata constructed?"* Researchers also frequently ask which characteristics are most suitable for defining strata and how to establish appropriate boundaries between them.

The formation of strata is fundamental to the process of stratified random sampling. Strata should be constructed based on shared characteristics of the elements within each group, with the goal of achieving *homogeneity within strata* and *heterogeneity between strata*. This deliberate organisation is often guided by prior experience and the researcher's professional judgement (Kothari, 2004, p. 59)

3.3.4.5 Phases of Stratum Construction

The strategy for constructing strata typically involves two main phases:

1. **Identifying the Population Parameter:** The first step is to determine the population parameter that needs to be estimated.

2. **Dividing the Population:** Next, divide the population into groups based on a variable that appears to be related to the variable of interest. This ensures that the resulting strata are homogeneous with respect to the characteristic being studied (Levy & Lemeshow, 2013, p. 126). If the criterion chosen for stratification is strongly associated with the target variable, it enhances the precision of population estimates (Frey, 2021). Researchers may use a single criterion or a combination of criteria to define the boundaries of each stratum.

The frequency distribution of the variable under investigation provides the most effective basis for stratification. When such information is unavailable, the frequency distribution of another parameter closely correlated with the variable of interest serves as the next best alternative (Cochran, 1977).

For example, if the goal is to determine the average daily cost of a hospital bed, hospitals can be stratified by geographic location. Hospitals in economically thriving regions may charge higher fees than those in economically disadvantaged areas.

Stratifying populations based on qualitative characteristics such as gender, race, or geographic location is straightforward. Researchers can also use quantitative or ordinal characteristics, like age groups or income levels. The cumulative square root of frequencies (CSRF), introduced by Dalenius and Hodges, has proven effective in these cases (Dalenius & Hodges Jr, 1959). Using this method, it is recommended to divide the population into three to nine strata.

3.3.4.6 Steps for Stratifying Quantitative Data

To stratify classified quantitative data in a table, follow these steps:

1. **Calculate Square Roots:** Compute the square root of the frequency for each item in the second column of the table.
2. **Compute Cumulative Square Root Frequency (CSRF):** For each row, sum the square root values of all preceding rows to determine the CSRF. For example, to calculate the CSRF for the third row, sum the square root values of the first, second, and third rows, and continue this process for all subsequent rows.
3. **Determine Interval Class:** Divide the CSRF value of the last class by the desired number of sample strata (typically between three and nine) to establish the interval class. This calculation yields the cumulative square root value for each stratum (Sinha et al., 2018).
4. **Define Stratum Boundaries:** The cumulative square root frequency (CSRF) value closest to each interval determines the boundaries of each stratum.

TABLE 3.2

Distribution of 1,600 Residents in a Specific Region Categorised by Age Groups

Strata	Cumulative	Square Root	Frequency	Age Class
Children	14.49	14.49	210	00–04
	28.77	14.28	204	05–09
Teenager	49.04	20.27	411	10–19
Young	72.28	23.24	540	20–29
	92.28	20.00	400	30–39
Middle aged	108.71	16.43	270	40–49
	122.35	13.64	186	50–59
Elderly	132.25	9.90	98	60–69
	139.67	7.42	55	70–79
	145.15	5.48	30	80+
	–	–	2400	Sum

Example 3.1: Consider the frequency distribution of 1,600 residents in a specific region, categorised by age groups, as shown in the first and second columns of Table 3.2. Using the CSRF method, we will define five strata for stratified sampling.

Dividing the final CSRF value of 145.15 by 5 yields 29.03, 58.06, 87.09, 116.12, and 145.15. The boundaries of each stratum are then determined by selecting the cumulative values closest to these calculated figures.

3.3.4.7 Allocation

A common question in stratified sampling is: *"How will sample sizes be distributed across each stratum?"* Allocation refers to the size of the sample selected from each stratum. Once the strata are defined, it is essential to determine the sample size allocated to each one. Sample allocation can typically be done in three ways: equal allocation, proportional allocation, and optimal allocation, as described below.

3.3.4.7.1 Equal Allocation

Equal allocation involves selecting the same number of samples from each stratum, regardless of the stratum's size. This means the sample is uniformly distributed across all strata. The number of samples (n_i) for each stratum can be calculated using the formula:

$$n_1 = n_2 = \cdots = n_K = \frac{n}{K}$$

For example, if a population is divided into four strata with sizes $N_1 = 700$, $N_2 = 400$, $N_3 = 300$, and $N_4 = 600$, and we decide to use equal allocation with a total sample size of $n = 88$, each stratum will contribute:

$$n_1 = n_2 = n_3 = n_4 = \frac{88}{4} = 22$$

Equal allocation is particularly useful when estimates for individual strata or differences between strata are required. However, it may not be the best choice for estimating the overall population mean or total unless the sampling costs, stratum variances, and stratum sizes are approximately equal across strata. In such cases, equal, proportional, and optimal allocations yield similar results (Malec, 2005, p. 5694).

3.3.4.7.2 Proportional Allocation

As the name suggests, proportional allocation distributes the total sample size in proportion to the sizes of the strata. This technique ensures that the sample reflects the population's structure by maintaining a consistent ratio of the sample size to the population size within each stratum. If $P_i = n_i / N_i$ represents the proportion of the population included in stratum i, and n is the total sample size, the number of elements selected from stratum i is given by:

$$n_i = \frac{N_i}{N} \times n$$

Example 3.2: Consider a university with 10,000 students divided among various schools: 3,500 in Health Sciences, 2,000 in Rehabilitation, 1,500 in Psychology, and 3,000 in Nursing. If the administrator desires a sample size of 200 students (2%), the allocation would be:

- **Health Sciences:** 70 students (2% of 3,500)
- **Rehabilitation:** 40 students (2% of 2,000)
- **Psychology:** 30 students (2% of 1,500)
- **Nursing:** 60 students (2% of 3,000)

3.3.4.7.3 Optimal Allocation

Optimal allocation is designed to minimise variance when estimating a population mean or total for a given sample size and fixed cost (Lavrakas, 2008, p. 553). This allocation method is also known as Neyman allocation, named after J. Neyman, who demonstrated its effectiveness in 1934.

For K strata, total sample size n, and variance σ_j^2 within stratum j, the optimal allocation within stratum j is calculated as:

$$n_j = n\left(\frac{N_j \times \sigma_j}{\Sigma N_i \times \sigma_i}\right) = \frac{n \times N_j \times \sigma_j}{N_1 \times \sigma_1 + N_2 \times \sigma_2 + \cdots + N_K \times \sigma_K}$$

Example 3.3: To illustrate how to divide a sample of size $n = 88$ among four strata using optimal allocation, the sample sizes are calculated as follows:

- For stratum 1:

$$n_1 = \frac{88 \times 700 \times 15}{(700 \times 15) + (400 \times 18) + (300 \times 9) + (600 \times 5)} = \frac{924,000}{23,400} \approx 40$$

- For stratum 2:

$$n_2 = \frac{88 \times 400 \times 18}{(700 \times 15) + (400 \times 18) + (300 \times 9) + (600 \times 5)} = \frac{633,600}{23,400} \approx 27$$

- For stratum 3:

$$n_3 = \frac{88 \times 300 \times 9}{(700 \times 15) + (400 \times 18) + (300 \times 9) + (600 \times 5)} = \frac{237,600}{23,400} \approx 10$$

- For stratum 4:

$$n_4 = \frac{88 \times 600 \times 5}{(700 \times 15) + (400 \times 18) + (300 \times 9) + (600 \times 5)} = \frac{264,000}{23,400} \approx 11$$

The costs associated with sampling can vary significantly among strata, depending on the sampling techniques employed. For instance, accessing one stratum may be easier and less costly than another. If c_j represents the cost per element in stratum j, the total cost can be expressed as:

$$C = c_1 n_1 + c_2 n_2 + \cdots + c_K n_K = \sum n_j c_j$$

The *optimal allocation considering cost* for stratum j can then be calculated as:

$$n_j = n\left(\frac{\frac{N_j.\sigma_j}{\sqrt{c_j}}}{\sum \frac{N_j.\sigma_j}{\sqrt{c_j}}}\right) = n\left(\frac{\frac{N_1.\sigma_1}{\sqrt{c_1}}}{\frac{N_1.\sigma_1}{\sqrt{c_1}} + \frac{N_2.\sigma_2}{\sqrt{c_2}} + \cdots + \frac{N_k.\sigma_k}{\sqrt{c_k}}}\right)$$

If the standard deviations of the strata are similar, optimal and proportional allocations will yield comparable sample sizes for each stratum. However, as differences in standard deviations increase, optimal allocation becomes more efficient.

3.3.4.7.4 Comparing Allocations

The choice of allocation method in stratified sampling depends on the research objectives, stratum variances, and sampling costs, with each method—equal, proportional, and optimal allocation—offering distinct advantages under different conditions.

Proportional allocation is often regarded as the optimal approach for estimating the population mean or total. It is particularly effective when the variabilities within strata and the associated sampling costs are consistent. This method is frequently employed when there is limited information about strata variances or collection costs, as effective stratification can yield homogeneous strata with similar variances.

When the objective is to estimate the population value of a characteristic, proportional allocation is considered the most effective and ideal design, especially when within-stratum variances are similar and the cost of selecting an item is uniform across strata.

In contrast, equal allocation is preferred when estimates for individual strata or differences between strata are required. If the aim is to compare differences among strata, selecting an equal number of samples from each stratum may be more appropriate, even if the strata differ in size.

In situations where strata differ in both size and variability, a "disproportionate sampling design" can be advantageous. This approach allows for larger samples to be drawn from more variable strata and smaller samples from less variable strata, effectively accounting for both stratum size and variability differences.

Selecting items from each stratum is a critical aspect of stratified sampling that requires careful handling. Simple random sampling is the most common method for choosing sample items within each stratum. However, if circumstances warrant, systematic sampling may also be applied (Kothari, 2004, p. 553).

3.3.4.8 Advantages and Disadvantages of Stratified Sampling

Stratification offers three primary benefits over simple random sampling (Levy & Lemeshow, 2013, p. 126):

- **Increased Precision:** In many cases, stratified sampling can yield higher precision than simple random sampling, resulting in lower standard errors for estimates.
- **Separate Estimates:** It allows for separate estimation of parameters within each stratum as well as for the overall population, achieving a specified degree of precision.
- **Simplified Data Collection:** For administrative, logistical, or political reasons, collecting data through stratified sampling may be

less complicated than gathering data via simple random sampling. Consequently, stratified sampling generally provides standard errors that are smaller than those obtained from simple random samples.

The main drawback of stratified sampling is that each enumeration unit must be classified into strata before sampling can commence. This requirement can be impractical if the necessary information is not readily accessible (Levy & Lemeshow, 2013, p. 126).

3.3.4.9 Quota and Stratified Sampling

One non-random strategy often used in opinion and market research surveys to maintain proportionality is "quota sampling". This method involves calculating the required sample size for each stratum in advance. Enumerators are then instructed to continue sampling until the necessary "quota" for each stratum is achieved. Common stratification variables include geographic location, age, gender, race, and income indicators.

If enumerators randomly select individuals within geographic areas and classify them into the appropriate strata, the process closely resembles "stratified random sampling". Quota sampling can thus be defined as stratified sampling in which units within strata are selected in a somewhat non-random manner. As a result, standard sampling-error calculations cannot be confidently applied to quota sample results.

Although quota samples often correlate well with probability samples on opinion and attitude questions, they tend to produce biased estimates for variables such as income, education, and occupation (Cochran, 1977, p. 135).

3.3.5 Multistage Random Sampling (MRS)

Probability sampling methods can be categorised as either "single-stage" or "multistage". Single-stage samples include simple random sampling, systematic random sampling, cluster sampling, and stratified random sampling. In single-stage sampling, elements in the target population are gathered into a sampling frame, from which a sample is directly selected.

In contrast, "multistage sampling" (or multistage random sampling, MRS) involves selecting samples in stages, considering the "hierarchical structure" of the population. This method proceeds from larger to smaller units, sampling in two or more hierarchical levels (Lavrakas, 2008, p. 492).

The target population is first divided into "primary sampling units" (PSUs), which are sampled initially. The selected PSUs are then subdivided into "secondary sampling units" (SSUs), from which samples are taken next. This process continues until the "ultimate sampling units" are identified (Lavrakas, 2008, p. 492). When the selection at each stage is random, the method is referred to as multistage random sampling (Indrayan & Holt, 2016).

Multistage sampling extends cluster sampling by organising sampling units in a hierarchical structure with primary, secondary, tertiary, and so on, based on the number of stages in the design. For clarity, consider a population divided into primary sampling units (PSUs), initially without stratification. Suppose a frame contains M PSUs, from which a random sample of m PSUs is selected at the first stage. Within each selected PSU i, the population consists of N_i secondary units, and a random sample of n_i units is drawn, where $n_i < N_i$. Sampling within each PSU is independent of the others, and additional stages may be added as needed. Any probability sampling method – such as cluster sampling or stratified sampling – can be applied at any stage and may vary across PSUs. The units chosen at the final stage serve as the enumeration or listing units for surveys (Shimizu, 2005, p. 3742).

Multistage sampling is also known as "nested sampling" or "k-stage sampling", where k denotes the number of stages in the design. A key feature is that the sample selected at one stage forms the population for the next stage, which is commonly referred to as subsampling. It is important to distinguish multistage sampling from "multiphase sampling": nested sampling units appear in multistage designs, whereas multiphase sampling uses the *same* set of units at each phase. Both methods can be incorporated into complex survey designs.

For example, to estimate smoking prevalence among females aged 25 and under in a county with thousands of families, one might:

1. Randomly select five cities,
2. Select 12 census blocks within each city, and
3. Select 50 households within each block.

Although the sampling units include cities, census blocks, and households, the study population would consist of all females aged 25 or younger in the selected households. This design could yield up to $5 \times 12 \times 50 = 3000$ families. While this may be small relative to the county's total number of families, it can still produce precise estimates of smoking prevalence for the target group.

Finally, it is important to note that standard error formulas from simple random sampling do not apply to such designs. Instead, variance estimation methods appropriate for complex sample designs must be used (Lavrakas, 2008, p. 492).

3.3.5.1 Advantages of Multistage Random Sampling (MRS)

The primary advantages of multistage random sampling include cost reduction and time savings during data collection, largely because it typically requires less travel. For example, in a multistage sample where city blocks serve as PSUs, listing activities may be restricted to only those sampled blocks. In contrast, a single-stage household sample across an entire city would require listing every household.

Another advantage is that smaller sampling units do not need to rely on the complete sampling frame. This is particularly useful when a comprehensive list of all members of the target population is either unavailable or too costly to construct. For instance, while a list of hospitals may be accessible, a corresponding list of hospital patients may not exist. In multistage sampling, the sampling frame is constructed in partial units at each stage, making the design more manageable than most single-stage approaches.

However, the operational benefits of multistage sampling come at the cost of reduced sampling efficiency. For equivalent estimations, the sampling error of a multistage sample is generally larger than that of a simple random sample of the same size. Although multistage sampling can reduce variances for a given cost unit (Palmer, 1999, p. 3742), it may also produce larger sampling errors compared with simpler sampling designs.

In addition, sequential clustering enables a larger number of units to be sampled at a lower cost within a multistage framework, a benefit that is often not achievable in simple designs (Kothari, 2004, p. 65).

3.3.6 Area Sampling

Area sampling, also known as geographic sampling, is a sampling method that employs well-defined geographical regions as the primary sampling units. The sampling frame, or *area frame*, can be conceptualised as a map divided into N non-overlapping subareas that collectively cover the entire region of interest. These subareas serve as the fundamental sampling units. Although often represented as a map, the sampling frame can also be expressed as a list of locations. These sampling units are commonly referred to as *segments* or *area segments*, with the area frame effectively comprising a list of all segments.

Area sampling is a form of multistage sampling (Valliant et al., 2013, p. 257). Any partition of the area frame into segments will yield unbiased estimates of population parameters; however, the efficiency of these estimates depends on the specific partitioning. An efficient area sample design requires that the subareas be as equal in size as possible. Although the underlying concept is straightforward, its effective implementation demands substantial expertise. Enumerators (field workers) must accurately identify the boundaries of each area segment, using natural features such as roads, rivers, and fences whenever feasible. Materials used in area sampling may include aerial photographs, county highway maps, and street maps, with aerial photography being particularly valuable for studies conducted in sparsely populated areas (Kotz et al., 2005, p. 228).

3.3.6.1 Application of Area Sampling

Area sampling has diverse applications across many fields. It is commonly employed in agricultural and forestry research to study land characteristics within the sampling area, such as acres planted in specific crops or the extent of forest coverage. In behavioural research, area sampling is used when a complete or up-to-date sampling frame for observational units (households, individuals, firms, etc.) is unavailable. In such cases, data are collected from all units located within the sampled areas. This method has been successfully applied in countries lacking maintained resident lists; moreover, even when population registries are available, area sampling can serve as the initial stage in a two-stage sampling process (Everitt & Howell, 2021, p. 137).

3.3.6.2 Challenges and Considerations of Area Sampling

A major challenge in area sampling lies in accurately defining the primary sampling units (the areas) and establishing clear rules for associating population elements with them. Administrative boundaries (e.g., villages, counties) are frequently used to delineate primary sampling units, provided their size is appropriate for the study's objectives. Individuals and households are typically linked to area segments based on their primary residences, though complications may arise when individuals or households maintain multiple residences (Everitt & Howell, 2021, p. 137).

Caution must be exercised when generalising results from area sampling to the reference population, and internal correlations among sampling units should be carefully considered. Because neighbouring individuals may influence each other, sample estimates must account for the strength of these correlations, which may not fully represent the characteristics of the reference population. This issue is particularly relevant in studies of communicable diseases and social behaviours.

3.3.6.3 Relationship to Other Sampling Methods

Area sampling can be considered a variation of cluster sampling (Indrayan & Holt, 2016, p. 20). Although both methods involve dividing a population into groups – areas or clusters – the key distinction lies in the sampling procedure within these groups. In area sampling, a random sample of units is selected from within each randomly chosen area. In contrast, cluster sampling involves randomly selecting clusters and then including *all* units within those clusters, effectively conducting a complete census of each selected cluster.

Both approaches involve grouping the population into smaller, more manageable units that are then sampled randomly. However, the essential difference is the method of selecting units within the groups: area sampling extracts a subsample from each selected area, whereas cluster sampling includes every unit within each selected cluster. Both techniques aim to reduce the cost and effort associated with sampling large populations.

Area sampling assumes relative homogeneity within each area, while cluster sampling assumes that clusters are internally heterogeneous but collectively representative of the population. The choice between the two methods depends on factors such as the geographic distribution of the population, the availability of a sampling frame, and the research objectives.

From another perspective, area sampling is a specific instance of multistage sampling. Although area sampling can be categorised as a type of multistage sampling, there are distinctions that differentiate it from other forms. Area sampling is a particular case of multistage sampling in which the initial stages involve geographic divisions (Valliant et al., 2013, p. 257). However, multistage sampling represents a broader concept and can be applied to various types of units, potentially involving more than two stages, especially when subareas exist within the selected areas. For example, a study may involve selecting schools, then classrooms within those schools, and finally students within those classrooms.

Figure 3.8 illustrates the process of selecting a systematic sample from a hypothetical population.

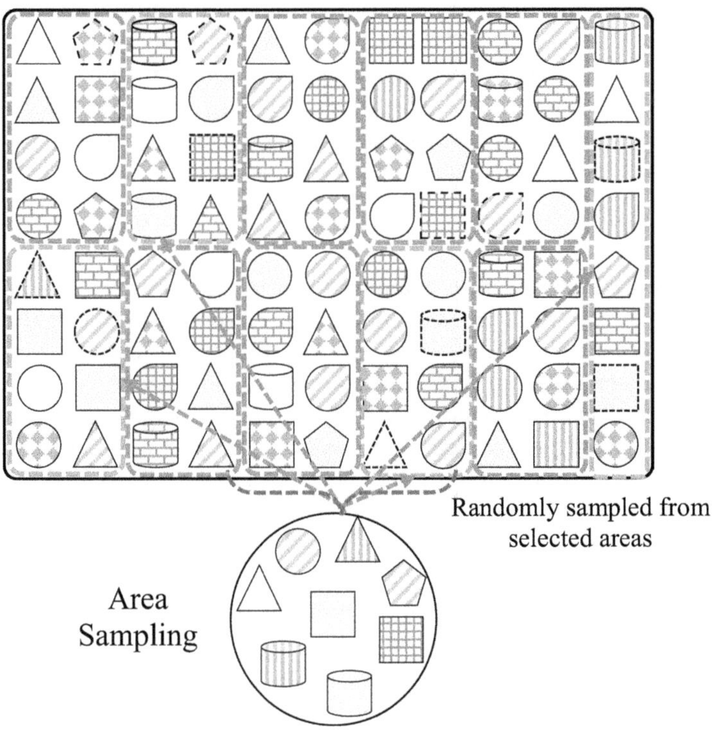

FIGURE 3.8
Schematic presentation of area sampling.

3.3.7 Probability Proportional to Size (PPS) Sampling

Probability proportional to size (PPS) sampling is a method that enhances simple random sampling (SRS) by incorporating the size of clusters or blocks into the selection process. In this context, clusters may include cities, schools, colleges, or hospitals, while units may consist of individuals, students, or patients. In simple random sampling, each block in the population has an equal chance of selection; however, blocks may differ substantially in size, and equal-probability selection may not adequately represent the entire population.

When selecting clusters, it is therefore important to account for their size, introducing a distinct probability of selection known as PPS. This method ensures that larger blocks have a higher likelihood of being chosen, particularly when block sizes vary greatly.

TIP

Probability proportional to size (PPS) sampling improves upon conventional random sampling by assigning selection probabilities to clusters based on their relative size. This technique is especially effective when cluster sizes vary widely, as it ensures that larger clusters are more likely to be included in the sample. By aligning selection likelihood with cluster magnitude, PPS sampling enhances representativeness and leads to more accurate population estimates.

To illustrate PPS, consider an example from Indrayan et al. (2024, p. 467), which resembles a method recommended by the World Health Organization (WHO) for estimating immunisation coverage in developing countries. This example also incorporates a systematic sampling component.

Suppose *cluster random sampling* (*CRS*) is used to investigate the prevalence of poor vision among elderly individuals (aged 50 and older) in a census-block region with a total population of 500,000. The goal is to select 20 clusters, each consisting of 30 individuals (one cluster per block). The following procedure is applied:

1. **Listing the Population:** The population of each census block is listed, and cumulative totals are calculated.
2. **Determining the Sampling Fraction:** The sampling fraction is set at one cluster per 25,000 residents, derived from the goal of selecting 20 clusters from a population of 500,000. A random number between 1 and 25,000 is generated. A sample of 20 numbers is then created by

adding 25,000 sequentially and systematically to this initial number. The 20 census blocks corresponding to these selected numbers are included in the sample.

3. **Conducting Home Visits:** Starting from a geographically random point in each selected block, home visits are conducted. The first 30 residents aged 50 or older in neighbouring households are identified, and their visual acuity is assessed. This yields one cluster of 30 individuals from each selected block.

To illustrate the PPS selection process, Table 3.3 presents data for only 10 blocks.

TABLE 3.3

Illustration of PPS Sampling

Block Number	Block Size (Population)	Cumulative Block Size	Selected Blocks by PPS (Random Number)
1	4387	4387	
2	12,275	16,662	
3	8931	25,593	3(18,789)
4	5365	30,958	
5	7987	38,945	
6	2361	41,306	
7	4580	45,886	7(43,789)
8	15,439	61,325	
9	9438	70,763	
10	6753	77,516	10(68,789)

Example 3.4: To conduct a survey on the prevalence of poor vision among individuals aged 50 years and older in a district with a population of 500,000, we will select 20 clusters. Each cluster will consist of 30 individuals, following the procedure outlined below.

Solution: We illustrate this approach using the first three blocks out of 25, with their sizes shown in Table 3.3. The first randomly drawn number is 18,789. This number corresponds to block number 3, as all numbers from 16,663 to 25,593 fall within this block. Next, we add 25,000 to 18,789, resulting in 43,789. This number falls within block number 7, making it the second block selected. Adding 25,000 again yields 68,789, which belongs to block number 10, making it the third block selected. This systematic selection process continues until all 20 clusters have been chosen.

3.3.7.1 Features of Probability Proportional to Size (PPS) Sampling

Probability proportional to size (PPS) sampling possesses several important characteristics that distinguish it from simple random or standard cluster sampling:

- **Population Size Consideration:** The population size of each block is used to determine the probability of its selection, as described in step (2).
- **Increased Probability for Larger Blocks:** Blocks with larger populations have a higher likelihood of being included in the sample. This principle, known as probability proportional to size (PPS), ensures that larger clusters are adequately represented. In this example, the size refers to the population within the census blocks, while the sampling units are individuals aged 50 years and older.
- **Self-Weighting Sampling:** By employing PPS, the sample becomes self-weighting, which simplifies the estimation process. Unlike stratified random sampling, weighted computations are not required with this type of PPS design.
- **Flexible Cluster Sizing:** The sampling approach allows for practical flexibility in cluster size. For example, if a team can efficiently manage 30 individuals in a single day, clusters of this size are selected. If 40 individuals can also be handled within the same timeframe, clusters of that size may be chosen instead. This operational flexibility facilitates efficient survey implementation without compromising the PPS design.

3.3.7.2 Limitations of Probability Proportional to Size (PPS) Sampling

There are several limitations to consider when using probability proportional to size (PPS) sampling:

- **Applicability:** PPS is relevant only in situations where the primary sampling unit consists of a block containing multiple inquiry units. It is not suitable for populations where such hierarchical structures do not exist.
- **Data Availability:** Accurate information on the size of every block in the population must be accessible. In many cases, this may pose a challenge, requiring the use of a surrogate measure. For example, in our scenario, block size was determined based on the total population; however, the ideal criterion should focus on individuals aged 50 years and older. In cases where the exact number of patients is not readily available, an alternative measure such as the bed capacity of a hospital can serve as a proxy for the total number of patients.

TABLE 3.4

Calculation of Selecting Beds in Ten Wards Using the PPS Method

Cumulative Probability	Cumulative Range	No. of Beds	Wards
0.140	1–21	21	A
0.167	22–46	25	B
0.067	47–56	10	C
0.087	57–69	13	D
0.067	70–79	10	E
0.30	80–109	30	F
0.060	110–118	9	G
0.073	119–129	11	H
0.060	130–138	9	I
0.080	139–150	12	J
1.00	–	150	Sum

Example 3.5: Consider a hospital with 10 wards, where the goal is to estimate the number of unoccupied beds by randomly selecting four wards. This example initially utilises a simple random sampling approach.

Solution: The total number of beds in the wards is as follows: 21, 25, 10, 13, 10, 30, 9, 11, 9, and 12, as indicated in the second column of Table 3.4. The hospital contains a mix of larger wards with more beds and smaller wards with fewer beds. Consequently, using simple random sampling may not produce an accurate estimate of the total number of unoccupied beds. To improve precision, it is preferable to assign larger wards a higher probability of selection, while smaller wards are given proportionally fewer opportunities. This method is known as probability proportional to size (PPS) sampling and ensures that larger units are adequately represented in the sample, resulting in more reliable estimates.

We define N as the total number of hospital beds and N_i as the number of beds in the i_{th} ward. Thus, we have

$$N = N_1 + N_2 + ... + N_{11} + N_{12}$$

The probability of selecting the i_{th} ward in the sample is given by

$$P_i = \frac{N_i}{N}.$$

3.4 Some Concerns About Sampling Approaches

There is a common misconception that probability sampling methods are always superior in capturing the main characteristics of a population, but this is not necessarily the case. When using probability sampling techniques, the sampling frame must include all participants, and the population size should be known or closely estimated. Probability sampling methods perform best in large populations, where deviations from true population parameters can be more readily identified. Sampling errors are deviations from these true parameters, and their detection is most effective when sufficiently large samples are selected. We will now revisit the earlier discussion on choosing the most appropriate sampling design for specific circumstances (Berndt, 2020, p. 370; Scheaffer et al., 2011).

- **Simple Random Sampling (SRS):** In this method, each individual has an equal chance of being selected, making the process straightforward and generally perceived as fair. However, a significant limitation is the frequent lack of an up-to-date list of all population members. SRS serves as the fundamental building block and point of reference for all other sampling designs discussed in this chapter. Nevertheless, few large-scale surveys rely solely on SRS, as alternative methods typically offer greater precision, efficiency, or both.
- **Systematic Sampling:** This method is easier to implement and provides a more even distribution of selections across the population compared to SRS. However, using a systematic algorithm may overlook important population characteristics, particularly if the data have inherent periodic patterns that align poorly with the systematic interval.
- **Stratified Random Sampling (StRS):** Stratified sampling involves selecting samples based on shared or unique characteristics, making them generally more representative of the population. StRS produces estimators with lower variance than SRS for a given sample size, especially when measurements are homogeneous within strata but differ across strata. This method can enhance the study's external validity and generalisability. For StRS to be effective, measurements should be similar within each stratum, with variances becoming more apparent across strata.

While systematic sampling is valued for its practical simplicity, it may outperform SRS in terms of estimated error limits when there is a negative correlation between paired items within the same systematic sample. For instance, this occurs with periodic data containing alternating high and low values. Conversely, if a systematic sample consists only of extreme values (e.g., all highs), the results may be misleading. Stratified sampling is particularly advantageous for populations with linear trends or poorly understood periodic structures. For example, economic time series can be stratified by month or quarter, with random samples drawn from each stratum. While both stratified and systematic sampling require coverage across the entire population, the stratified design allows for a more randomised selection process and often results in smaller estimation errors. However, stratified sampling is ineffective if the population cannot be divided into meaningful strata or if proportional allocation across strata is not feasible.

- **Cluster Sampling:** Cluster sampling is widely used due to its cost-effectiveness and practicality when a complete sampling frame of individual elements is unavailable. Cluster random sampling (CRS) is particularly efficient for large populations. If measurements within clusters are heterogeneous and cluster means are approximately equal, cluster sampling may be preferable to SRS or StRS. The ideal scenario for cluster sampling occurs when each cluster contains a wide range of measurements while maintaining roughly equal cluster means. Unlike stratified sampling, which requires homogeneous strata with differing means, cluster sampling can accommodate heterogeneous clusters.

To compare the final three designs, consider a population organised into k systematic samples of size n. Systematic sampling selects one of the k clusters of size n, representing $n \cdot k$ items. Effective systematic sampling requires heterogeneous clusters. Alternatively, the $n \cdot k$ elements can be viewed as n strata, each containing k elements, from which one element is chosen systematically. In this case, the means of the strata should differ significantly, while elements within strata should be as homogeneous as possible. This design provides an optimal environment for systematic sampling and aligns with the conceptual framework of cluster sampling. Despite their differences, these three designs share fundamental sampling concepts.

- **Quota Sampling:** Quota sampling is faster and simpler than stratified sampling because it does not require random selection. It facilitates comparisons within subgroups. However, because randomisation is absent, sampling errors cannot be calculated, and there is a higher risk of bias, making population generalisations difficult.
- **Purposive Sampling:** Purposive sampling allows researchers to select units based on theoretical, logical, or analytical reasoning. This method is particularly useful in qualitative research with multiple phases or objectives. However, it may introduce bias if selection criteria are not clearly defined or documented, making it difficult to ensure that the population remains representative.
- **Self-Selection Sampling:** This approach saves time and often results in more honest responses, with participants demonstrating greater engagement. However, it is prone to selection bias, which can produce inaccurate or exaggerated results and a non-representative sample

- **Snowball Sampling:** Snowball sampling is especially useful for populations that are difficult to locate or recruit. Nevertheless, because random selection is not employed, this method may introduce biases that affect the validity of the results.

References

Berndt, A. E. (2020). Sampling methods. *Journal of Health Law, 36*(2), 224–226.

Boslaugh, S. (2007). *Encyclopedia of epidemiology.* Sage Publications.

Cochran, W. G. (1977). *Sampling techniques.* John Wiley & Sons, Inc.

Dalenius, T., & Hodges Jr, J. L. (1959). Minimum variance stratification. *Journal of the American Statistical Association, 54*(285), 88–101.

Everitt, B., & Howell, D. C. (2021). *Encyclopedia of statistics in behavioral science.* Sage Publications.

Frey, B. B. (2021). *The Sage encyclopedia of research design.* Sage Publications.

Indrayan, A., & Holt, M. P. (2016). *Concise encyclopedia of biostatistics for medical professionals.* Chapman and Hall and CRC Press.

Indrayan, A., Mishra, A., & Bhaskarapillai, B. J. (2024). Simplified sample size formulas for detecting a medically important effect. *Indian Journal of Community Medicine, 49*(3), 464–471.

Kothari, C. (2004). *Research methodology: Methods and techniques.* New Age International.

Kotz, S., Balakrishnan, N., Read, C. B., Vidakovic, B., & Johnson, N. L. (2005). *Encyclopedia of statistical sciences* (Vol. 1). John Wiley & Sons.

Lavrakas, P. J. (2008). *Encyclopedia of survey research methods.* Sage Publications.

Levy, P. S. (2005). *Encyclopedia of biostatistics* (ArmitageP. & T. Colton, Eds., 2nd ed.). Wiley.

Levy, P. S., & Lemeshow, S. (2013). *Sampling of populations: Methods and applications.* John Wiley & Sons.

Lohr, S. L. (2021). *Sampling: Design and analysis.* Chapman and Hall and CRC Press.

Machin, D., Campbell, M. J., Tan, S. B., & Tan, S. H. (2018). *Sample sizes for clinical, laboratory and epidemiology studies.* John Wiley & Sons.

Malec, D. (2005). *Encyclopedia of biostatistics* (M. H. Gail, P. Armitage, & T. Colton, Eds., Vol. 2, 2nd ed.). Wiley.

Palmer, C. (1999). Encyclopedia of biostatistics. *BMJ, 318*(7182), 542.

Parsons, V. (2005). *Encyclopedia of biostatistics* (M. H. Gail, P. Armitage, & T. Colton, Eds., Vol. 2, 2nd ed.). Wiley.

Peregrine, P. N. (2018). Sampling theory. *The Encyclopedia of Applied Statistics, 1*, 1–3.

Salkind, N. J. (2006). *Encyclopedia of measurement and statistics.* Sage Publications.

Saneii, S. H., & Doosti, H. (2024). *Practical biostatistics for medical and health sciences.* Springer.

Scheaffer, R. L., Mendenhall III, W., Ott, R. L., & Gerow, K. G. (2011). *Elementary survey sampling.* Cengage Learning.

Shimizu, I. (2005). *Encyclopedia of biostatistics* (M. H. Gail, P. Armitage, & T. Colton, Eds., Vol. 2, 2nd ed.). Wiley.

Sinha, S., Sankhala, G., & Lal, S. P. (2018). Profile characteristics and analysis of the constraints faced by the dairy farmers of urban and peri-urban areas of Indian National Capital Region vis-a-vis using mobile android application "Eco-Dairy". *International Journal of Current Microbiology and Applied Sciences, 7*(3), 2335–2342.

Valliant, R., Dever, J. A., & Kreuter, F. (2013). *Practical tools for designing and weighting survey samples* (Vol. 1). Springer.

4

Key Factors in Determining Sample Size

4.1 Introduction

Every observation collected from a population provides valuable information about the variable or variables under study. However, researchers must also consider the costs they are willing to incur for this information, as both sample collection and data processing can be resource-demanding. Collecting insufficient data may lead to inaccurate or unreliable estimates of population parameters, whereas collecting excessive data can result in unnecessary expenditure of time and resources during the research process.

Selecting an appropriate sample size is therefore crucial for ensuring the precision and certainty of research results, in accordance with the specific purpose and subject matter of the study. The sample size directly influences whether the findings of a research project are accepted or rejected, regardless of the clinical effectiveness of the intervention (Gupta et al., 2016). By calculating the appropriate sample size, medical researchers can better evaluate the cost, time requirements, feasibility, scientific validity, and justification of their studies (Andrade, 2020). Consequently, determining the correct sample size can be challenging for researchers, as it depends on multiple factors and requires specific details to provide statisticians with accurate and sufficient information.

TIP

Sample size is an important consideration for both scientific and economic reasons. An undersized study may waste resources because it lacks sufficient power to produce meaningful results, whereas an oversized study consumes more resources than necessary (Lenth, 2001).

DOI: 10.1201/9781003749783-4

4.2 Factors Affecting Sample Size Calculation

In general, determining the appropriate sample size for a trial or research project involves consideration of at least four fundamental components:

- **Variability or dispersion** of the studied variable,
- **Effect size** (estimation error),
- **Significance level**, and
- **Power of the test.**

However, additional factors must also be considered when determining the optimal sample size. These include the method used to select participants, the size of the reference population, the type of significance test (one-tailed or two-tailed), and anticipated participant dropout rates. Each of these factors plays a critical role in sample size determination.

The required sample size is also influenced by the type of hypothesis test employed in the research. In this book, the Z test (Z criterion) will be applied unless otherwise specified. Three key parameters influence sample size in hypothesis testing: the *p*-value (dependent on alpha), power (related to beta), and **effect size** (a clinically relevant assumption). It is important to note that sample size is inversely related to effect size (Das et al., 2016).

TIP

Formulas for sample size, hypothesis testing, and confidence intervals are interrelated and can be derived from or converted into one another. In general, sample size is obtained by combining the measure of variability with the confidence level and dividing by the estimation error. It increases when variability (σ^2), the confidence level ($1 - \alpha$), or the power of the test ($1 - \beta$) increases and also when the estimation error (d) decreases.

4.3 Standard Deviation or Event Rate

The nature and homogeneity of the variable distribution in the population from which a sample is drawn also affect the required sample size. A more uniform population, in which members are similar, results in decreased variance (or dispersion). In sample size formulas, variance is typically included in the numerator, indicating that sample size and variance are directly proportional. Consequently, sample size increases in dispersed, heterogeneous populations with higher variance.

TIP

To determine sample size, use the largest plausible variance and select proportions closest to 0.5, since $p(1 - p)$ is maximised at that value. For example, use $p = 0.29$ for values between 0.25 and 0.29, $p = 0.50$ for values between 0.45 and 0.53, and $p = 0.62$ for values between 0.62 and 0.70.

If the variance of x is not available from prior studies or expert opinion, the final way to overcome this challenge is to conduct a pilot study to obtain it.

The dispersion of quantitative data, whether discrete or continuous, is measured by the standard deviation (σ), which represents the mean of deviations from the population mean (μ). Some studies – particularly those comparing survival rates or determining the presence or absence of a condition – utilise qualitative scales instead of quantitative measurements. In such studies, where the outcome variable follows a binomial distribution, the variance of the proportion of subjects with the condition of interest is calculated as $p(1 - p)$, where p is the proportion and $(1 - p)$ is its complement.

Estimating population variance (σ^2) and proportion (p) can be challenging. Researchers may employ the following four methods to estimate population variance for sample size determination:

- Relying on previous sampling of the same population (Cochran, 1977, p. 78), provided that the nature, conditions, and structure of the population have not changed significantly.
- Using results from studies conducted in similar populations (Cochran, 1977, p. 78),
- Consulting expert opinion or informed estimates about the population structure from knowledgeable and experienced individuals, and
- Conducting a pilot study and utilising its results (Cochran, 1977, p. 78).

TIP

Any variation in the values of factors that may affect the study's objectives will impact the calculated sample size. Accordingly, researchers must exercise careful judgment when selecting appropriate values for these components.

When multiple values for variance are available, researchers should select the largest value when calculating the sample size to ensure that the resulting estimate is sufficiently conservative. Similarly, if different proportion values emerge during sample size estimation, the value closest to 0.5 should be chosen, as this maximises $p(1 - p)$ and helps ensure that the calculated sample size is adequate, since $p(1 - p)$ increases as p approaches 0.5. For example:

- Select $p = 0.29$ if p is between 0.25 and 0.29.
- Choose $p = 0.50$ if p is between 0.45 and 0.53.
- Select $p = 0.62$ if p falls within the range of 0.62 to 0.70.

The point at which $p(1 - p)$ reaches its maximum is critical for determining a conservative sample size.

4.4 Effect Size

The primary objective of most research studies is to compare a parameter between two or more populations or to estimate the value of a parameter. The closer an estimate of a parameter is to its true value in the population, the more accurate it is considered to be. The difference between this estimate and the actual population value is referred to as the *estimation error.* These terms are sometimes used interchangeably. For instance, in a sampling study estimating disease prevalence in a population, the estimated value may differ from the actual prevalence, with a smaller difference indicating greater estimation precision and lower estimation error.

This difference typically decreases as the sample size or number of participants increases; conversely, it increases as the sample size decreases, leading to a larger estimation error. This relationship implies that estimation error and required sample size are inversely related – when one increases, the other decreases. This relationship is reflected in the sample size formula's denominator, represented by the symbol *"d"*.

If a study aims to compare the mean or proportion between two populations, the effect size is defined as the absolute difference between the two means $|\mu_1 - \mu_2|$ or the absolute difference between the two proportions $|p_1 - p_2|$.

Before calculating the sample size in clinical research, investigators must predict the clinically important effect size, which represents the minimum difference that a treatment must produce to justify a change in practice (Gogtay, 2010). The sample size is based on the expected effect size for the primary outcome. When multiple equally important outcomes are present, the sample size is calculated for each endpoint of interest, and the largest feasible sample size is selected for the study (Machin et al., 2018).

The value of d can be expressed as either an absolute (fixed and specific) or a relative error when determining sample size. For example, if the actual prevalence rate in the population is less than 6% (a fixed value), there may be circumstances where parameters must be expressed proportionate to their actual values (relative precision) rather than as fixed absolute values. Relative precision is calculated by dividing the difference between the estimated and true values by the true value.

For instance, if the researcher aims to estimate the prevalence rate within 25% of the actual rate, and the true population prevalence is 20%, the estimated rate would range from 15% to 25%. This range is obtained by applying the formula:

$$20\% \pm (25\% \times 20\%) = 20\% \pm 5\% = 15\% \textit{ to } 25\%.$$

Similarly, if the actual prevalence is 10%, the estimated rate would range from 7.5% to 12.5%, calculated as:

$$10\% \pm (25\% \times 10\%) = 10\% \pm 2.5\% = 7.5\% \textit{ to } 12.5\%.$$

4.5 Clinically Important Difference and Effect Size

The clinically important difference and effect size reflect the magnitude of a specific effect. When determining sample size, these metrics indicate the size of the effect that can be detected by a test with a specified power. They also measure how distinct the alternative hypothesis is from the null hypothesis. Generally, their values represent the smallest effect considered clinically significant or the hypothesised population effect size (StataCorp, 2023, p. 8).

The definition of what constitutes "clinically important" is determined by the researcher and can vary between studies. For example, in clinical trials lacking prior information about the effectiveness of a specific clinical procedure, a standardised effect size (adjusted for the standard deviation) between 0.25 and 0.5 may be deemed clinically significant.

Effect size definitions can differ based on study design, analysis endpoint, and the statistical model and tests employed. For instance, when comparing two independent proportions, effect size can be represented by the difference between the two proportions, their ratio, or the odds ratio. The magnitude of effect sizes can vary significantly across studies. A treatment effect of 1% that leads to increased mortality may be considered clinically significant, whereas a 10% treatment effect resulting in decreased ankle circumference due to oedema might be perceived as less important. Effect size is typically defined such that power increases as its value (or absolute value) increases.

When determining sample size, effect size quantifies the difference between the alternative and null sampling distributions, which represent the distributions under the alternative and null hypotheses, respectively, of a test statistic. A smaller effect size indicates greater overlap between these two distributions, making it more challenging to reject the null hypothesis and resulting in lower power to detect an effect.

For example, consider conducting a z-test to compare a mean μ with 0 from a population with a known standard deviation σ. The null hypothesis is $H_0 : \mu = 0$, while the alternative hypothesis is $H_A :\ \mu \neq\ 0$. The test statistic is the sample mean, which follows a normal distribution with a mean of 0 and standard deviation σ under the null hypothesis. In contrast, it follows a normal distribution with a mean μ (different from 0) and standard deviation σ under the alternative hypothesis. The extent of overlap between these distributions is determined by the mean difference $\mu - 0 = \mu$ and the standard deviation σ.

The larger the absolute value of μ, the greater the difference between the two populations, which results in less overlap between their distributions and higher statistical power to detect differences in μ. Conversely, a larger standard deviation σ increases the overlap between the distributions, thereby reducing the power to detect differences. Statistical power can be expressed as a function of μ and σ or as a function of their combination, represented by the standardised difference $\delta = \frac{(\mu - 0)}{\sigma}$. The larger the absolute value of $|\delta|$, the greater the power; conversely, the smaller $|\delta|$, the lower the power. Thus, effect size is defined as the standardised difference δ.

4.6 Significance Level

The significance level in statistical hypothesis testing is a predetermined maximum threshold for the probability of a Type I error, which is the probability of incorrectly rejecting the null hypothesis H_0, often referred to as a false-positive conclusion. When conducting a hypothesis test, the values observed in the sample serve as evidence for deciding whether to reject H_0 (Indrayan & Malhotra, 2017; Malone et al., 2016).

In hypothesis testing, the area under the sampling distribution curve that distinguishes significant from non-significant results is defined by the significance level, or α (alpha). If a statistical test yields a *p*-value less than α, the result is considered statistically significant. Results are typically regarded as significant if $p < 0.05$, corresponding to a significance level of 5% ($\alpha = 0.05$). This α value is also used in sample size software and calculation formulas.

The Type I error, also known as the *alpha error*, represents the risk of incorrectly concluding that a treatment is effective when it is not. Formally, it refers to rejecting the null hypothesis H_0 when it is in fact true.

For most statistical purposes, a conventional α level of 0.05, or equivalently a 95% confidence level, is adequate (Noordzij et al., 2010), unless the project proposal specifies an alternative level such as $\alpha = 0.01$ or $\alpha = 0.10$. A p-value less than 0.05 indicates that a Type I error is expected to occur five times out of 100 trials. Similarly, $p < 0.01$ suggests that a Type I error would be expected to occur once for every 100 repetitions of the experiment. Although $\alpha = 0.05$ is usually the default threshold, $\alpha = 0.01$ can be selected to reduce the risk of a Type I error. Adjusting the significance threshold affects the estimated sample size; for example, increasing the significance level from 5% to 10% will decrease the required sample size.

The sample size is directly influenced by this component, whose value is derived from the standard normal distribution $Z_{1-\frac{\alpha}{2}}$. The corresponding Z-values for 90%, 95%, and 99% significance levels are 1.645, 1.96, and 2.58, respectively. Therefore, achieving a larger sample size and a higher confidence level results in a lower significance level.

4.7 One-Sided Test versus Two-Sided Test

Another factor influencing sample size is whether the test is directional (upper or lower one-sided) or non-directional (two-sided). Two-sided tests require more subjects than their one-sided counterparts. Although choosing a one-sided test may be appealing because it requires a smaller sample size, one-sided tests are generally less common than two-sided tests. In many applications, the direction of the effect – whether it is greater or smaller than a hypothesised value – is unknown, necessitating the use of a two-sided test.

Using a one-sided test even when the direction of the effect may be known remains controversial. Selecting a one-sided test eliminates the possibility of detecting an effect in the opposite direction, which may be undesirable in certain studies. It is therefore crucial to exercise caution when deciding to use a one-sided test, as doing so restricts the ability to rule out the opposite effect (StataCorp, 2023, p. 9).

4.8 Power of the Test

The Type II error (β), also known as a *false negative,* occurs when a study fails to reject a false null hypothesis H_0. This situation arises when the study cannot detect a significant difference because the available data provide insufficient evidence. Statistical power, defined as (1 − β), is the complementary probability of a Type II error. Thus, the power of a statistical test represents the probability of correctly rejecting a false null hypothesis H_0. It reflects how often similar samples would yield *p*-values less than α when the alternative hypothesis (H_1) is true. More formally, it involves rejecting H_0 when (H_1) is actually true.

The power of a test indicates its ability to detect a specific difference or effect size. A test is considered to have high power if it can confidently reject the null hypothesis H_0 and identify small differences. In essence, power refers to the likelihood that a statistical test will produce a significant result when a true difference exists. It is also described as the probability of correctly identifying a true positive effect.

TIP

Practically, Test power (1–β) represents the probability of correctly rejecting a false null hypothesis and reflects a test's ability to detect clinically important differences and true positive effects. Type II error (β) indicates the risk of missing such effects. Power can be calculated retrospectively to assess how likely a completed study was to detect a true effect or used prospectively to determine an appropriate sample size (Altman, 1980).

Power is influenced by the researcher's desired level of certainty in detecting a real difference or effect, commonly referred to as a *true positive.* Typically, power levels of 0.80 (80%), 0.90 (90%), and 0.95 (95%) are used, with corresponding one-tailed values of 0.84, 1.28, and 1.645 derived from the standard normal distribution $Z_{1-\beta}$. These values are commonly applied when calculating sample size for most statistical purposes.

To illustrate the concepts of Type I error, Type II error, significance level, and the power of the test, we refer to Table 4.1.

The most commonly used values for test power and significance level, along with their squared sums for use in the numerator of the sample size formula, are presented in Table 4.2.

TABLE 4.1

Illustration of Type I and Type II Errors in Hypothesis Testing

Hypothesis Testing Outcomes		Reality (Population) H$_0$ is True	Reality (Population) H$_1$ is True
Research Data (Sample)	H$_0$ is True	Accurate $(1-\alpha)$ **True positive**	Type II error (β) **False negative**
	H$_1$ is True	Type I error (α) **False positive**	Accurate Power $(1-\beta)$ **True negative**

Tables 4.1 and 4.2 illustrate the relationships between Type I and Type II errors, as well as the coefficients used in sample size calculations based on various significance levels and power values. Understanding these concepts is crucial for designing effective studies and ensuring that the results obtained are both reliable and valid.

Note: The sample size is typically calculated for two primary purposes: estimating parameters within a population or comparing means or proportions between two populations, as discussed below.

When the sample size is calculated to estimate parameters in a population, the research outcomes involve both point estimation and interval estimation, often referred to as confidence intervals. This process entails adding and subtracting the margin of error (estimation error).

Importantly, when calculating confidence intervals, the power of the test is not a factor; instead, it is sufficient to consider the significance level, variance, and margin of error within the sample size formula. Therefore, adjusting the corresponding coefficients based on the power of the test lacks a logical and scientific basis.

TABLE 4.2

The Coefficients of $\left(z_{1-\frac{\alpha}{2}} + z_{1-\beta}\right)^2$ for Sample Size Calculations

Significance level of α						
000.1	0.01	0.05	0.10	Level		
(3.29)	(2.58)	(1.96)	(1.645)	Value	Level	The value for power of test $(1-\beta)$ is one tailed
10.82	6.66	3.84	2.69	(0.000)	0.50	
12.56	8.03	4.90	3.58	(0.253)	0.60	
14.56	9.64	6.17	4.68	(0.524)	0.70	
17.08	11.71	7.85	6.16	(0.842)	0.80	
18.71	13.08	8.99	7.19	(1.036)	0.85	
20.91	14.92	10.51	8.54	(1.282)	0.90	
24.31	17.81	12.96	10.76	(1.645)	0.95	
34.46	26.63	20.61	17.81	(2.58)	0.99	

TIP

Balancing the significance level and power of the test is essential for determining an appropriate sample size. Researchers should avoid relying solely on default values such as 0.80 or 0.05 and instead consider the specific research question and the potential consequences of Type I and II errors. Conducting a power analysis assists in selecting optimal values, enabling informed decisions about the trade-offs between significance level and power.

Conversely, when determining the sample size to compare a parameter between groups or to assess a parameter in a population against a fixed value, statistical hypothesis tests are employed. It is essential to recognise that both Type I (α) and Type II (β) errors are inherent in hypothesis testing and serve as critical components of this methodology. Strictly speaking, power is a characteristic of statistical tests and does not influence estimation or confidence intervals. Consequently, when calculating the sample size for comparisons using hypothesis tests, it is imperative to include the power of the test ($1 - \beta$) in the sample size formula, alongside the three aforementioned factors: significance level, variance, and estimation error.

Readers are often interested in understanding how to effectively balance the significance level and the power of a test when determining the sample size for a study. In essence, they seek guidance on selecting appropriate values for test power and significance level, rather than merely relying on conventional defaults such as 0.80 or 0.05.

To choose optimal values for both the significance level and power of a test, it is essential to maintain a balance between these two factors. This requires careful consideration of the specific research question, the potential consequences of Type I and Type II errors, and the resources available for the study.

TIP

Strictly speaking, power is a property of statistical tests and does not influence estimation or the construction of confidence intervals.

One effective method for selecting the significance level and power of a test is to conduct a power analysis. A power analysis involves determining

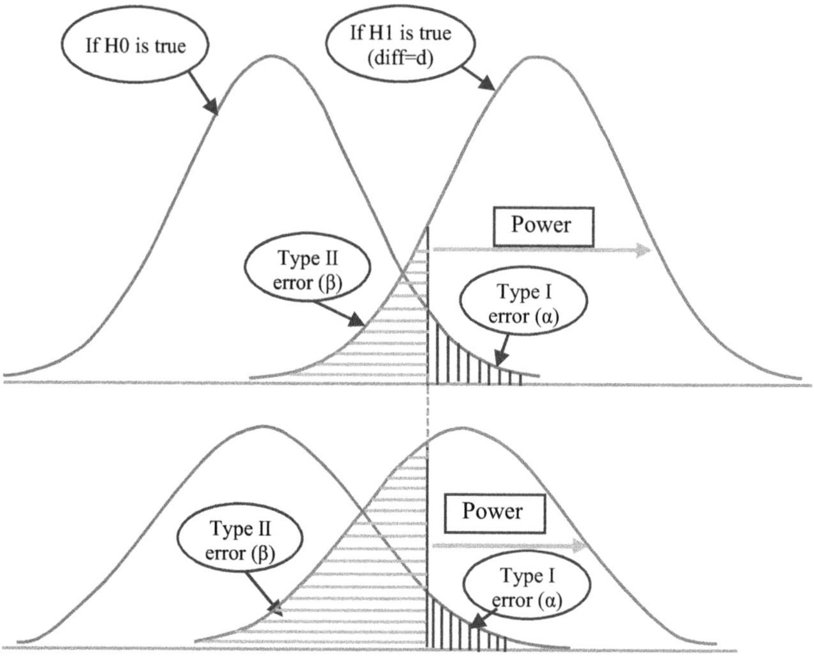

FIGURE 4.1
The relationship between the significance level and power of the test.

the sample size required to achieve a desired level of power for a given effect size and significance level. This approach allows researchers to make informed decisions regarding the trade-offs between significance level and power, thereby selecting optimal values tailored to the specific research context.

As illustrated in Figure 4.1, the height of the upper curve exceeds that of the lower normal curve. Additionally, the increased kurtosis of the upper curve indicates that its variance and dispersion are smaller compared to those of the lower curve. Increasing the sample size reduces the variance of the distribution, which leads to greater data accumulation and density at the centre of the distribution. Consequently, the likelihood of Type II errors decreases, thereby enhancing the power of the test.

TIP

As the overlap between the two distributions increases, the effect size decreases, which makes it more challenging to reject the null hypothesis and lowers the statistical power to detect a true effect.

4.9 Sampling Method or Design Effect (Deff)

The process of collecting sample units for a research study, known as the sampling strategy, has a significant impact on the calculation of sample size. The formulas presented in this book assume that sampling is conducted using the simple random sampling (SRS) technique.

However, in practice, sample units are often collected through alternative methods, which can necessitate a larger sample size. For example, if a cluster sampling approach is employed, the sample size may need to be multiplied by the intraclass correlation coefficient of the clusters (e.g., 0.33). This indicates that 33% more participants are required in cluster sampling to achieve the same level of accuracy as in simple random sampling.

The effect of the sampling method on sample size is referred to as the design effect (Deff). It is defined as the ratio of the variance of the estimate obtained from the sampling method to the variance of the estimate obtained from a simple random sample (SRS) of the same size (Cochran, 1977). Mathematically, this can be expressed as:

$$Deff = \frac{Var(\bar{x})}{Var(\bar{x}_{SRS})} \tag{4.1}$$

To determine the final sample size, the sample size calculated using the formulas must be multiplied by the design effect (*Deff*).

4.10 Finite Population Correction

Consider a scenario in which you want to estimate the value of a single parameter in two populations: one with 100,000 individuals and another with 1,000 individuals. Assuming that other characteristics of both populations are similar, both would yield the same initial sample size calculation (e.g., 150 participants). The sample proportion of the larger population is 0.00150, whereas for the smaller population it is 0.150. With the smaller population, the data provide more precise information. This illustrates that sample size is influenced by the size of the reference population. Consequently, when determining the sample size, it is essential to consider the population size and adjust the sample size accordingly.

This adjustment is known as the "Finite Population Correction (FPC)", which modifies the sample size calculation by a factor of $1-\frac{n_0}{N}$. Therefore, if the initial sample size estimate is $\boldsymbol{n_0}$, the corrected sample size using FPC should be calculated as follows (Lohr, 2021):

$$n = \frac{n_0}{1 + \frac{n_0}{N}} = \frac{N \times n_0}{N + n_0} \tag{4.2}$$

When n is small relative to the population size N, the finite population correction (FPC) approaches unity. Practically, the FPC can be disregarded when the sampling fraction is less than 5%, and in some cases, up to 10% (Cochran, 1977). Specifically, if $n \leq 0.05 \times N$ or $1 - \frac{n}{N} \geq 0.95$, it can be safely ignored (Scheaffer et al., 1990, p. 83), resulting in $n = n_0$.

For larger populations, the FPC is 0.9985, which is greater than 0.95, allowing it to be disregarded. Thus, the corrected sample size remains:

$$n = \frac{100000 \times 150}{100000 + 150} = 150$$

In the case of the smaller population mentioned earlier, the FPC is 0.85, which is less than 0.95. Therefore, the corrected sample size should be:

$$n = \frac{1000 \times 150}{1000 + 150} = 131$$

4.11 Dropout Rate

In addition to the factors discussed previously, researchers should consider the dropout rate when determining the sample size for a research study, as it can have a significant impact. The dropout rate refers to the expected proportion of participants who will not complete the study – due to non-response or other reasons – relative to the anticipated response rate (1 – d).

Typically, sample size calculations determine the number of study subjects required to achieve statistical significance for a given hypothesis. However, in clinical practice, it is often necessary to enrol additional participants to account for potential dropouts. The dropout rate can be estimated using previous research, pilot studies, or the researcher's own experience (Charan et al., 2021). If d represents the dropout rate and n is the sample size calculated from the formula, then the adjusted sample size N_1 can be calculated as follows:

$$N_1 = \frac{n}{1 - d} \tag{4.3}$$

Some researchers suggest that in such circumstances, neighbours, friends, or coworkers could serve as replacements. However, this strategy reduces the randomness of the sampling method to some extent and may introduce bias.

TIP

To adjust the calculated sample size for the design effect of the sampling method, multiply the sample size by the design effect (Deff).

To account for the anticipated non-response or dropout rate, divide the adjusted sample size by the expected response rate $(1 - d)$.

4.12 Additional Factors for Determining Sample Size

To accurately determine the sample size, researchers must identify the factors that influence it. Understanding their expectations for the sample is crucial for estimating an appropriate sample size. Nonetheless, the established sample size should be sufficient and feasible given the available resources and facilities for the research. Various constraints can hinder the collection of an adequate sample, including study costs, time limitations, manpower, facilities, equipment, and the limited number of cases. In such instances, researchers may need to adjust their expectations for the study – such as the significance level, test power, or estimation error – by modifying some of the previously mentioned components, ensuring that the necessary sample size aligns with the available research resources.

Most statistical sources, including this book, employ formulas for calculating sample size that are generally applicable and consider four main factors: estimation error, test power, variability, and significance level. However, these formulas often overlook additional considerations such as population size, dropout rate, and design effect. In the second step, after calculating the primary sample size n_0 using standard formulas, the researcher can apply coefficients or multipliers to adjust the sample size. For example, when accounting for the effects of design, reference population, and the combined impact of both factors, the sample size can be adjusted as follows:

$$n = Deff \times n_0 \tag{4.4}$$

$$n = FPC \times n_0 \tag{4.5}$$

$$n = Deff \times FPC \times n_0 \tag{4.6}$$

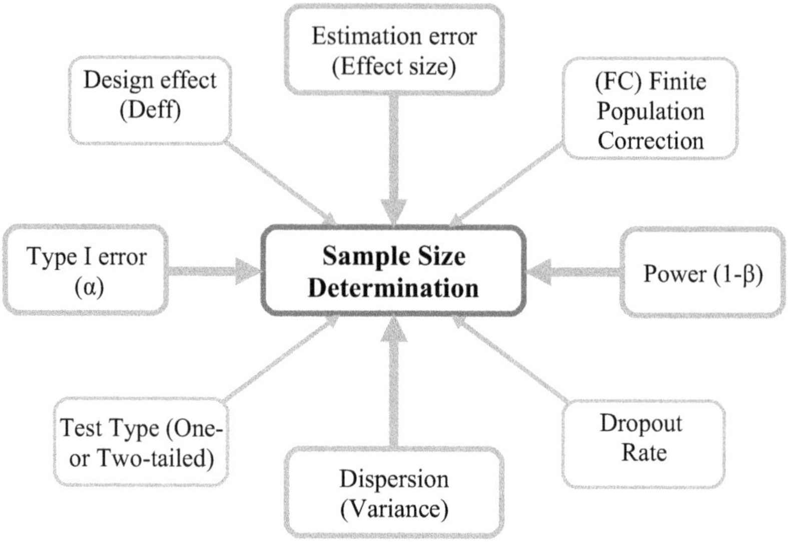

FIGURE 4.2
Factors affecting sample size determination.

Overall, the effect size, significance level, test power, and variability are typically regarded as the most important factors influencing sample size determination. These factors are schematically represented in Figure 4.1 as the four main directions: North, South, East, and West. Additionally, four other factors – namely, the type of statistical test (one-tailed or two-tailed), sampling method or design (Deff), finite population correction (FPC), and dropout rate – have a lesser impact on sample size and are represented as four sub-directions (North-west, North-east, South-east, and South-west) in the schematic representation (Figure 4.2).

Researchers should carefully consider these factors when planning a study and determining an appropriate sample size to achieve valid and reliable results. While this classification provides a general framework, it is important to note that the relative importance of these factors can vary depending on the specific context of the study.

4.13 Calculating Sample Size Using a Cost Model

The implementation of any research project is influenced by various factors, including funding, human resources, facilities, and equipment. In essence, research projects are not independent of these elements. Many researchers aspire to conduct specific studies but find themselves unable to do so due to limitations in facilities, funding, or other constraints that prevent them from collecting the minimum number of samples required by statistical formulas. Since each observation incurs costs, important questions arise: Should the project be postponed due to insufficient funding? Should it proceed with fewer facilities and resources? How does sample size relate to the budget? To achieve optimal precision and minimise estimation errors, researchers must strive to conduct their studies using all available resources.

Assuming a linear model for research facilities and cost factors, the following equations can be used to determine the sample size:

$$C_T = C_0 + nC_0$$

$$n = \frac{C_T - C_0}{C_U} \tag{4.7}$$

In these equations, C_T represents the total research budget, C_0 denotes the initial fixed costs of the research, and C_U is the per capita cost of each sampling unit.

The sample size does not influence the initial fixed costs of the study, as these costs are largely independent of the number of participants. Initial and ongoing research costs include designing and planning the study, creating questionnaires and guidelines, statistical training, conducting pilot studies, creating and measuring variables, programming and coding for data analysis and interpretation, reporting, and publishing.

Conversely, the cost per unit (C_U) reflects the per capita cost of each sampling unit and is directly proportional to the sample size. Costs associated with the sample size may include transportation, reaching each sampling unit, administering and completing the questionnaire, editing and coding responses, data entry into the database, data extraction, and data analysis. Any reduction or increase in the sample size (n) will impact these costs; therefore, C_U should be multiplied by n.

Budget, time, and resource constraints are major obstacles in most research projects, making it challenging to achieve the minimum sample size needed to generalise results from the sample to the reference population.

Example 4.1: The total budget allocated for a health research project is $55,000, while the fixed and initial costs amount to $52,000. If the per capita cost for each sampling unit is $110, how many participants should be included in the sample size?

Solution: The information provided for this project is as follows:

$$C_T = 55000,\ C_0 = 30000, C_U = 110$$

The required sample size is calculated as:

$$n = \frac{55000 - 52000}{110} = \frac{3000}{110} = 27.27 \cong 28$$

Thus, the sample size needed is **28 participants.**

TIP

When multiple outcomes of equal importance are present, the sample size should be calculated for each endpoint of interest, and the largest feasible sample size should be used for the study (Machin et al., 2018).

4.14 Sample Calculation for Multiple Outcomes of Interest

Up to this point, our sample size calculations have been based on the assumption of a single identifiable outcome (endpoint). However, in most surveys, information is collected on multiple items. For instance, many studies include several endpoints of interest, such as blood pressure, body mass index, blood sugar, and cholesterol levels. In these situations, three approaches to determining sample size are commonly proposed:

- **Specify Margins of Error:** First, estimate the sample size required separately for each of the most critical items considered in the survey (Cochran, 1977, p. 81).
- **Identify a Primary Outcome:** Determine which endpoint is more important than the others and designate it as the primary outcome. The sample size can then be calculated based on this primary endpoint (Indrayan & Holt, 2016, p. 548; Machin et al., 2018). The remaining outcomes may or may not be measured with sufficient precision.
- **Equal Importance of Outcomes:** If each outcome measure is considered equally important, a common strategy is to calculate the sample size for each outcome separately and select the largest value. This ensures that the sample size is adequate to address all study questions. While this approach meets all requirements, some parameters may be overestimated relative to others (Indrayan & Holt, 2016, p. 548; Machin et al., 2018).

4.15 Ethical Considerations in Sample Size Determination

Ethical considerations in sample size calculation are critical in research study design, particularly in clinical trials where patient safety is paramount. It is essential to weigh the risks of conducting underpowered trials, which may not adequately address the research question, against the ethical concerns of overpowered trials that could expose participants to unnecessary risks. The decision between continuing to use inadequately evaluated treatments outside of controlled trials and conducting trials to gather useful data may seem straightforward; however, there are arguments both for and against conducting trials with low statistical power. Small trials can contribute to meta-analyses and provide valuable insights.

Striking a balance between the study's scientific value and the burden on participants is important, as increasing the sample size does not necessarily enhance the study's value. Additionally, having a well-defined sample size calculation prior to initiating the study can help prevent data dredging and ensure meaningful results. Prior power calculations assist researchers in identifying the primary outcome variable, guiding the interpretation of study results, and preventing selective reporting.

Reporting practical constraints and achievable power in the study protocol and final report is essential, particularly when resources are limited.

Researchers must justify their sample size calculations and be transparent about any limitations that may affect the ability to achieve high statistical power. Ultimately, ethical research should include sample size calculations and clearly communicate any constraints that may impact the study's power.

Overall, ethical considerations in sample size determination are vital for ensuring the validity and reliability of research studies. In summary, while sample size calculations are crucial for ethical research, their application should balance scientific rigour with available resources to uphold ethical standards (Bacchetti et al., 2005; Machin et al., 2018, p. 38).

4.16 Summary

Creating a precise schematic diagram to illustrate the influence of various factors on sample size can be challenging due to their complex interactions. However, a simplified representation can be provided that ranks these factors according to their general importance in determining sample size. It should be noted that the actual impact of each factor may vary depending on the specific context and study design.

1. **Effect Size:** The magnitude of the difference or relationship you aim to detect. Larger effects typically require smaller sample sizes to be detected with sufficient power.
2. **Significance Level (Alpha):** The probability of incorrectly rejecting the null hypothesis when it is true. A lower significance level

(e.g., 0.01 instead of 0.05) generally requires a larger sample size to achieve the same power.

3. **Power of the Test:** The probability of correctly rejecting the null hypothesis when it is false. A higher desired power (e.g., 0.80 or 0.90) usually necessitates a larger sample size.
4. **Dispersion (Variance):** The variability within the sample. Higher variance typically requires a larger sample size to achieve the same level of precision in estimation or hypothesis testing.
5. **Type of Statistical Test:** Statistical tests can be conducted as either one-tailed or two-tailed. Two-tailed tests typically require a higher corresponding value for alpha compared to one-tailed tests. For instance, a two-tailed significance level of 0.05 corresponds to 1.96, whereas a one-tailed significance level of 0.05 corresponds to 1.645.
6. **Sampling Methods or Design (Deff):** The method used to select participants or units from the population. Complex or less efficient sampling methods may require larger sample sizes to achieve representative results.
7. **Finite Population Correction (FPC):** Necessary when sampling from a finite population rather than an effectively infinite one. If the population is small relative to the sample size, adjustments are made to the sample size calculation.
8. **Dropout Rate:** Relevant in longitudinal or intervention studies where participants may drop out before study completion. A higher expected dropout rate may require a larger sample size to ensure adequate power.

References

Altman, D. G. (1980). Statistics and ethics in medical research: III How large a sample? *British Medical Journal, 281*(6251), 1336.

Andrade, C. J. (2020). Sample size and its importance in research. *Indian Journal of Psychological Medicine, 42*(1), 102–103.

Bacchetti, P., Wolf, L. E., Segal, M. R., & McCulloch, C. E. (2005). Ethics and sample size. *American Journal of Epidemiology, 161*(2), 105–110.

Charan, J., Kaur, R., Bhardwaj, P., Singh, K., Ambwani, S. R., & Misra, S. (2021). Sample size calculation in medical research: A primer. *Annals of the National Academy of Medical Sciences, 57*(02), 074–080.

Cochran, W. G. (1977). *Sampling techniques.* John Wiley & Sons, Inc.

Das, S., Mitra, K., & Mandal, M. (2016). Sample size calculation: Basic principles. *Indian Journal of Anaesthesia, 60*(9), 652–656.

Gogtay, N. J. (2010). Principles of sample size calculation. *Indian Journal of Ophthalmology, 58*(6), 517–518.

Gupta, K. K., Attri, J., Singh, A., Kaur, H., & Kaur, G. (2016). Basic concepts for sample size calculation: critical step for any clinical trials! *Saudi Journal of Anaesthesia, 10*(3), 328–331.

Indrayan, A., & Holt, M. P. (2016). *Concise encyclopedia of biostatistics for medical professionals.* Chapman and Hall and CRC Press.

Indrayan, A., & Malhotra, R. K. (2017). *Medical biostatistics.* Chapman and Hall and CRC Press.

Lenth, R. V. (2001). Some practical guidelines for effective sample size determination. *The American Statistician, 55*(3), 187–193.

Lohr, S. L. (2021). *Sampling: Design and analysis.* Chapman and Hall and CRC Press.

Machin, D., Campbell, M. J., Tan, S. B., & Tan, S. H. (2018). *Sample sizes for clinical, laboratory and epidemiology studies.* John Wiley & Sons.

Malone, H. E., Nicholl, H., & Coyne, I. (2016). Fundamentals of estimating sample size. *Nurse Researcher, 23*(5), 21–25.

Scheaffer, R. L., Mendenhall, W., Ott, L., & Gerow, K. (1990). *Elementary survey sampling* (Vol. 501). Duxbury Press California.

StataCorp LLC. (2023). *Stata power, precision, and sample-size reference manual.* StataCorp LLC.

5

Population Size Estimation Techniques

5.1 Introduction

Understanding population size – the total number of individuals within a population – is a fundamental concept across numerous fields of study. In many cases, population size can be assumed to be known or sufficiently large such that it has a negligible impact on parameter estimates, allowing researchers to omit it from analyses. However, accurately determining population size is often essential to a study's objectives, particularly when the size is unknown.

Indeed, estimating population size is both a primary goal and a critical component of research projects across disciplines such as health, psychology, ecology, sociology, and wildlife management. Accurate population estimates are vital for funding allocation, study design and implementation, assessment evaluations, and intervention strategies. For example, estimating population size is a core objective in many epidemiological and ecological studies and animal monitoring programmes.

Mobile and motile organisms pose unique challenges for population estimation. Their capacity to move, disperse, and evade detection makes them more difficult to count, even though they may represent abundant members of their species. Fortunately, a variety of well-established methods exist for estimating the size of mobile populations. Each approach has its own advantages and limitations, making it more suitable for certain contexts than others (Mielke Jr et al., 1999).

TIP

Accurately estimating population size is essential across fields like health, psychology, ecology, sociology, and wildlife management. Reliable estimates support effective funding decisions, study design, programme evaluation, and intervention planning – especially in epidemiology, ecological research, and wildlife monitoring.

DOI: 10.1201/9781003749783-5

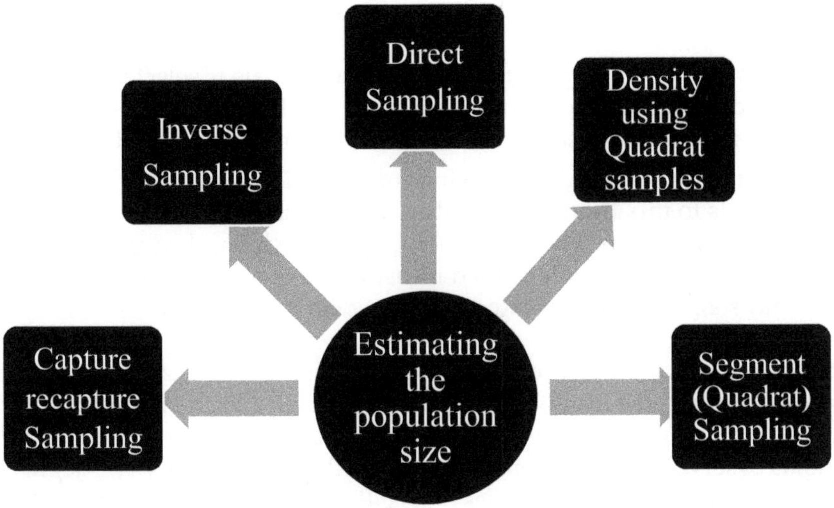

FIGURE 5.1
Different ways of estimating the size of population.

Moreover, these estimation techniques can be applied to analogous scenarios, such as estimating the number of defects in a bolt of material or counting attendees at a concert or sporting event (Scheaffer et al., 2011, p. 313). This chapter will present and discuss five methods of population size estimation: Capture–Recapture, Inverse, Direct, Density using Quadrat, and Segment or Quadrat Sampling, as illustrated in Figure 5.1.

5.2 Capture–Recapture Sampling

5.2.1 General Concepts

Capture–recapture is a straightforward method for estimating total population size through a form of resampling. Originally developed to count animals within a confined area (Indrayan & Holt, 2016, p. 70), the method was first applied by Laplace in 1786 to estimate the population of France using birth records from selected parishes. Capture–recapture sampling is also known as *capture–mark–recapture* or *mark–release–recapture* (Lavrakas, 2008, p. 80).

In many situations, manually counting every individual in a population is impractical due to constraints such as time, labour, and cost. Compared with a full census, capture–recapture sampling can produce statistically valid estimates of population size more quickly and efficiently (Lavrakas, 2008, p. 80).

The basic procedure of capture–recapture sampling consists of two stages:

1. **Capture Stage:** A random sample of individuals is selected (or captured) from the target population – such as fish in a pond – marked or tagged, and subsequently released back into the population.
2. **Recapture Stage:** After allowing sufficient time for the marked individuals to mix thoroughly within the population, a second random sample is drawn. The proportion of previously marked individuals in this second sample is then measured. It is essential that the second-stage sample is obtained independently of the first.

The total population size can be estimated using information from both stages, including the number of individuals marked in the first sample, the total number captured in the second sample, and the number of marked individuals observed in that second sample (Mielke Jr et al., 1999). The degree of overlap between the two samples – specifically, the number of individuals identified in both – plays a critical role in determining the accuracy of the population size estimate (Chao et al., 2001).

To obtain a valid estimate of population size using capture–recapture sampling, the following four assumptions must be met (Lavrakas, 2008, p. 80; Mielke Jr et al., 1999):

1. All members of the population have an equal chance of being captured in both samples, meaning that both samples are obtained through simple random sampling without replacement.
2. The selection of subjects for the second sample is unaffected by whether they were identified in the first sample.
3. During the sampling interval, the ratio of marked to unmarked individuals remains constant, indicating that the population is closed and its size and composition do not change over time.
4. Marked individuals can be accurately matched between the first and second stage samples.

Capture–recapture methods have been widely applied to estimate the abundance of various animal populations, including birds, mammals, fish, reptiles, and insects. These methods have also been used to assess the detectability of animals for other survey techniques and to estimate survival rates and additional population parameters. Furthermore, capture–recapture techniques have been applied to estimate the size of elusive human populations, such as the homeless, to adjust for census undercounts of minority groups, and to estimate the frequency of vital events such as accidents (Thompson, 2012, p. 263).

The capture–recapture method operates under the assumption that the ratio of the total number of unidentified population elements (N) to the number of sample elements in the first stage (marked elements, n_1) is equal to the ratio of the number of sample elements in the second stage (n_2) to the number of marked elements in that sample (i.e., recaptures, s). In other words, if the second sample is representative, the proportion of marked subjects in that sample should approximately match the proportion of marked subjects in the population (Thompson, 2012, p. 265).

An estimate of the total population can then be obtained by solving for N using simple arithmetic:

$$\hat{N} = \frac{n_1 \times n_2}{s} \tag{5.1}$$

The two primary types of capture–recapture methods arise from an unidentified parameter in the second sampling stage. The technique is termed "direct sampling" when the number of marked subjects in the second sample is unknown, but the sample size is fixed. Conversely, it is referred to as the "inverse method" when the sample size in the second stage is unknown, but the number of previously identified subjects is fixed.

TIP

Capture–recapture is an efficient alternative to a full census when a population is too large or difficult to count. By marking individuals in an initial sample and measuring how many are recaptured in a second sample, researchers can estimate total population size – provided key assumptions are met, including equal capture probability, independent samples, a closed population, and correct identification of marked subjects.

In direct sampling, a random sample is taken from the target population, with each subject identified and returned to the population (Mielke Jr et al., 1999). A fixed-size random sample is then taken from the population, and the previously identified subjects that are "recaptured" from the first sample are counted again. In inverse sampling, the process is reversed: the number of previously identified subjects – rather than the sample size – serves as the fixed factor in the second sample. Thus, the second sampling continues until a predetermined number of subjects from the first sample have been selected.

The following notation should be used for both direct and inverse sampling:

- N: estimated size of the population,
- t: total number of subjects found in the first sample,

- n: total number of subjects found in the second sample,
- s: number of recaptured subjects in the second sample.

5.2.2 Direct Sampling

Assume that a researcher selects and identifies n_1 subjects at random from a total population of size N during an initial sampling. The researcher then selects a second random sample of size n_2, from which s subjects were previously identified in the first sampling. In direct sampling, also referred to as *"single capture"* (Thompson, 2012, p. 265), and conducted without replacement, the random variable of interest is s. The probability $P(s)$ of observing s previously identified subjects in the second sample follows the hypergeometric distribution (Mielke Jr et al., 1999), expressed as:

$$p(s) = \frac{\binom{n_2}{s}\binom{N-n_1}{n_2-s}}{\binom{N}{n_2}} \tag{5.2}$$

To obtain a statistically unbiased estimate over the long run, one can add 1 to each of the parameters and then subtract 1 from the final estimate (Indrayan & Holt, 2016; Mielke Jr et al., 1999). Thus, the total population size N can be estimated using:

$$\hat{N} = \frac{(n_1+1)\times(n_2+1)}{(s+1)} - 1 \tag{5.3}$$

For this estimation, the unbiased estimated standard deviation is given by (Mielke Jr et al., 1999):

$$\hat{\sigma}(\hat{N}) = \sqrt{\frac{(n_1+1)(n_2+1)(n_1-s)(n_2-s)}{(s+2)(s+1)^2}}$$

Note: When s is small relative to n_1 and n_2, the total population size $\hat{N}$ can be approximated using the simpler formula:

$$\hat{N} = \frac{n_1 \times n_2}{s}$$

and the approximate standard error is given by

$$\hat{d}(\hat{N}) = 2\sqrt{\frac{n_1^2.n_2(n_2-s)}{s^3}}$$

This approximate standard error is sufficient for practical purposes but is slightly less accurate than the Chapman formula, especially when the number of recaptures (s) is small relative to the sample sizes.

A 95% confidence interval for the estimated total population size can then be calculated using

$$\hat{N} \pm 1.96 \times \hat{\sigma}\left(\hat{N}\right) \tag{5.4}$$

TIP

Direct sampling is a capture–recapture method where a researcher takes a first sample, marks the individuals, and then draws a second fixed-size sample to count how many marked individuals are recaptured. This count is used to estimate the total population size.

Example 5.1: Consider a sample of 48 deer ($n_1 = 48$) that have been marked, captured, and released back into their natural habitat. After mixing with the rest of the population, a second sample of 35 deer ($n_2 = 35$) is collected from the same area, and 16 of these ($s = 16$) are found to have been previously marked. Estimate the total number of deer.

Solution: The data are as follows:

$$n_1 = 35, \quad n_2 = 48, \quad s = 16$$

$$N = \frac{n_1 \times n_2}{s} = \frac{35 \times 48}{16} = 105$$

Using the adjusted (Chapman) estimator:

$$N = \frac{(n_1 + 1) \times (n_2 + 1)}{(s + 1)} - 1 = \frac{(35 + 1) \times (48 + 1)}{(16 + 1)} - 1 = 102.76 \approx 103$$

Rounding up, the estimated population size is 103, which may be more realistic than the earlier estimate of 105 (Indrayan & Holt, 2016, p. 70).

McCarty et al. evaluated the prevalence of childhood diabetes in Madrid, Spain, using the same capture–recapture methodology. A population-based registry identified 432 cases from hospital inpatient records. Data from the Spanish Diabetes Association contributed 138 additional cases, with 119 cases shared between the two sources. The total number of paediatric diabetes cases is estimated as follows:

$$N = \frac{(n_1+1)\times(n_2+1)}{(s+1)} - 1 = \frac{(432+1)\times(138+1)}{(119+1)} - 1 = 500.558 \approx 501$$

Rounding up, the estimated total number of paediatric diabetes cases is 501.

Example 5.2: Suppose an organisation aims to estimate the number of smokers in a specific area who are part of the general population. To achieve this, 3,500 smokers are randomly selected and identified. After two months, another random sample of 2,400 smokers is chosen, with 634 individuals recaptured from the first sample. Determine the total size of the population.

Solution: The data are as follows:

$$n_1 = 3500, \quad n_2 = 2400, \quad s = 634$$

The approximate total smoking population is estimated using the basic capture–recapture formula:

$$N = \frac{n_1 \times n_2}{s} = \frac{2400 \times 3500}{634} = 13249.21 \approx 13250$$

The approximate standard error of the estimate is calculated as:

$$\hat{d}(\hat{N}) = 2\sqrt{\frac{n_1^2.n_2(n_2-s)}{s^3}} = 2\sqrt{\frac{3500^2 \times 2400(2400-634)}{634^3}} = 902.75$$

The 95% confidence interval for the total number of smokers in the population is then:

$$\hat{N} \pm 1.96 \times \hat{d}(\hat{N}) = 13250 \pm 1.96 \times 902.75 = [11481,\ 15020]$$

Thus, the estimated total number of smokers in the area is approximately 13,250, with a 95% confidence interval ranging from 11,481 to 15,020.

Example 5.3: The Department of Labor and Social Affairs conducted a study to estimate the total number of unemployed persons in the country. For the initial sample, 480 unemployed individuals were randomly selected and identified using their national identity numbers. Three months later, another sample of 950 individuals was chosen, from which 120 unemployed persons were recaptured. Estimate the total size of the population.

Solution: The relevant data for this study are:

$$n_1 = 480, \quad n_2 = 950 \quad and \quad s = 120$$

The approximate total number of unemployed individuals is calculated as follows:

$$\hat{N} = \frac{n_1 \times n_2}{s} = \frac{950 \times 480}{120} = 3800$$

The approximate standard error of the estimate is given by:

$$\hat{d}\left(\hat{N}\right) = 2\sqrt{\frac{n_1^2.n_2\left(n_2 - s\right)}{s^3}} = 2\sqrt{\frac{480^2 \times 950\left(950 - 120\right)}{120^3}} = 648.49$$

The 95% confidence interval for the total number of unemployed individuals in the population is calculated as:

$$\hat{N} \pm 1.96 \times \hat{\alpha}\left(\hat{N}\right) = 3800 \pm 1.96 \times 648.49 = 3800 \pm 1271.03 == \left[2528.97 \textit{ to } 5071.03\right]$$

5.2.3 Inverse Sampling

Inverse sampling, an adaptive sampling method developed by J. B. S. Haldane in 1945, is particularly useful for estimating the frequency of a feature in populations that are significantly larger than the sample size. This approach is often employed when the population size is considered infinite (Lavrakas, 2008, p. 393).

In inverse sampling (sometimes referred to as standard inverse sampling), cases are selected until a predetermined event occurs a specified number of times. This method is advantageous when the total number of samples to be taken is unknown (Mielke Jr et al., 1999). Unlike direct sampling, in inverse sampling, the size of the second sample is not fixed in advance; sampling continues until a predetermined number of subjects from the first sample are drawn.

TIP

Inverse sampling is an adaptive capture–recapture method in which sampling continues until a predetermined number of "successes" (such as previously marked individuals) are observed. Instead of fixing the sample size in advance, the total number of observations becomes a random variable. This approach is especially useful for very large or effectively infinite populations where the event of interest is rare.

To clarify, inverse sampling relies on the negative binomial distribution and involves conducting a series of Bernoulli trials until a set number of successful cases are collected. Typically, the desired number of cases (r) is chosen from the population in which the probability of having the desired trait is lowest. Consequently, the total sample size becomes a random variable in this design, leading to biased conventional estimates of the occurrence of a characteristic derived from the binomial distribution (Lavrakas, 2008, p. 393).

In inverse sampling without replacement, the random variable is n_2, and the probability P of observing n_2 is given by

$$p(s) = \frac{\binom{n_2 - 1}{s - 1}\binom{N - n_1}{n_2 - s}}{\binom{N}{n_2}} \tag{5.5}$$

After solving this equation, a statistically unbiased estimate can be obtained by adding 1 to each of the parameters and then subtracting 1 from the final result (Indrayan & Holt, 2016; Mielke Jr et al., 1999). Thus, the total population size N can be estimated using:

$$\hat{N} = \frac{n_2(n_1 + 1)}{(s+1)} - 1 \tag{5.6}$$

The unbiased estimated standard deviation is given by (Mielke Jr et al., 1999):

$$\hat{\sigma}(\hat{N}) = \sqrt{\frac{(n_1 + 1)(n_1 - s + 1)n_2(n_2 - s)}{s^2(s+1)}}$$

Alternatively, as Scheaffer stated:

$$\hat{N} = \frac{n_2.n_1}{s} - 1 \quad \text{and} \quad \hat{\sigma}(\hat{N}) = \sqrt{\frac{(n_1^2)n_2(n_2 - s)}{s^2(s+1)}} \tag{5.7}$$

We can then estimate a 95% confidence interval for the total population size using:

$$\hat{N} \pm 1.96 \times \hat{\sigma}(\hat{N})$$

Example 5.4: This example is adapted from Scheaffer et al. 2011, p. 317). Authorities at a large wildlife preserve are concerned about the population of a specific bird species. A random sample of 150 birds is tagged and released. A second sample is drawn in the same month until 35 tagged birds are recaptured (s = 35). In total, 100 birds are recaptured. Find the total size of the birds.

Solution: Given information:

$$n_1 = 150, \quad n_2 = 100, \quad s = 35$$

The total number of birds is estimated as:

$$N = \frac{n_1 \times n_2}{s} = \frac{150 \times 100}{35} = 428.57 \approx 429$$

The approximate error of the estimate is calculated using

$$\hat{d}\left(\hat{N}\right) = 2\sqrt{\frac{\left(n_1^2\right) n_2 \left(n_2 - s\right)}{s^2 \left(s+1\right)}} = 2\sqrt{\frac{150^2 \times 100\left(100-35\right)}{35^2 \times 36}} = 115.17$$

The 95% confidence interval for the total bird population is therefore:

$$429 - 115.17 = 314 \ \ and \ \ 429 + 115.17 = 544$$

Thus, we can be quite confident that the true population size lies between 314 and 544 birds.

Example 5.5: In another scenario, 20 individuals were identified as illegal immigrants in the local population. A month later, 825 additional locals were selected through inverse sampling for a second sample. No replacements were allowed until all ten illegal immigrants from the initial sample were identified. Estimate the total number of illegal immigrants.

Solution: The provided information is as follows:

$$n_1 = 20, \ n_2 = 825, \ s = 10$$

The total number of immigrants is estimated as:

$$N = \frac{n_1 \times n_2}{s} = \frac{20 \times 825}{10} = 1650$$

The estimation error is calculated using

$$\hat{d}\left(\hat{N}\right) = 2\sqrt{\frac{\left(n_1^2\right) n_2 \left(n_2 - s\right)}{s^2 \left(s+1\right)}} = 2\sqrt{\frac{20^2 \times 825\left(825-10\right)}{10^2 \times 11}} = 989$$

The 95% confidence interval for the total immigrant population is

$$1650 - 989 = 661 \quad and \quad 1650 + 989 = 2639$$

We can be quite confident that the true population size lies between 661 and 2639 individuals.

5.2.3.1 Advantages and Disadvantages of Inverse Sampling

Inverse sampling generally yields more precise estimates than direct sampling, particularly when the sample size required to obtain the desired number of individuals is small relative to the total population size N (Scheaffer et al., 2011). However, the uncertain and potentially variable sample size can introduce additional complexities in the analysis.

Inverse sampling is particularly recommended for rare outcomes, as a fixed sample size may not yield enough cases of interest to support reliable conclusions. For example, when studying adult epilepsy – a rare condition – even a sample of several thousand individuals from the general population may not provide a sufficient number of cases to draw valid inferences. In such situations, the sampling scheme may involve including every epilepsy case observed in a clinic and continuing data collection until, for instance, 30 cases have been obtained. In this design, the number of outcomes of interest is fixed, whereas the sample size becomes a random variable determined by chance (Indrayan & Holt, 2016, p. 308).

This sampling method is appropriate for counting attributes or events but is unsuitable for quantitative measurements. For example, we cannot ensure that sampling can continue until the mean direct bilirubin level falls within a particular range (0.15–0.17 mg/dL). However, we can specify that sampling will continue until 50 cases with elevated direct bilirubin levels (above 0.20 mg/dL) have been identified. This effectively converts a quantitative measure into a qualitative one (Indrayan & Holt, 2016, p. 388).

5.2.4 Additional Uses for Capture–Recapture

The applications of capture–recapture estimation extend well beyond ecology, where it is commonly used to estimate wildlife populations. This method can be applied across a wide range of fields. Chao et al. identified three major types of capture–recapture models: ecological models, log-linear models, and the sample coverage technique (Chao et al., 2001). In the following, we highlight several key applications:

- **Estimating Census Under-coverage:** One important application of capture–recapture techniques is estimating under-coverage in census data. In this setting, the census acts as sample 1, while an independent probability sample drawn from the population serves as sample 2.
- **Estimating Eye Disease Cases:** Capture–recapture models have proven effective for estimating the total number of eye disease cases using limited register data, as demonstrated by Ramos et al.

(2020). These models incorporate various list structures, including three independent lists, three dependent lists, and two dependent lists. Chao et al. (2001) also endorsed the 17 recommendations proposed by Hook and Regal for applying capture–recapture methods in epidemiology. However, several key assumptions must be satisfied before determining whether the method is appropriate.

- **Estimating Foreign Immigrants:** The total number of foreign immigrants entering a country can be estimated by comparing two lists: one from the Interior Ministry (IM) of the host country and another from the United Nations (UN). In this context, generating one list is considered the "capture", while creating the second list is the "recapture", as both lists represent samples drawn from the same population. Assuming the method's underlying assumptions hold, each immigrant either appears on the UN list or does not, and likewise for the IM list. Although additional lists may exist, we focus on these two for simplicity (Lohr, 2021; Ramos et al., 2020).

Let n_1 represent the number of individuals on the UN list, n_2 the number on the IM list, and s the number of immigrants appearing in both lists. The total immigrant population can then be estimated using the following formula (Figure 5.2):

$$N = \frac{n_1 n_2}{s} \tag{5.8}$$

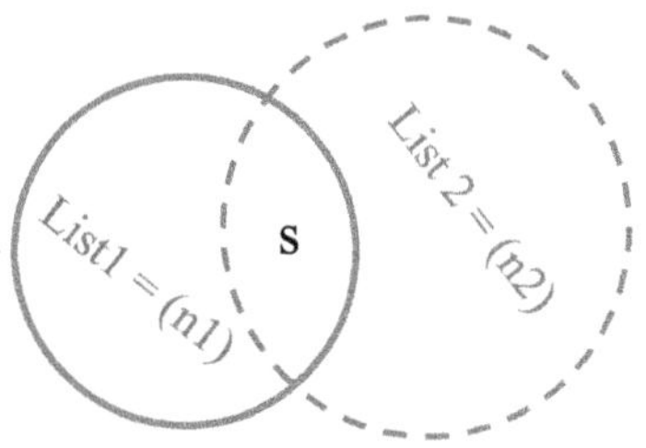

FIGURE 5.2
Venn diagram illustrating how two lists overlap to produce matched cases.

This estimate is based on the same assumptions used in the wildlife estimation example, with one minor difference noted below. Interested readers may refer to Lohr (Lohr, 2021, p. 499) for further details:

- The population is closed.
- Each list provides a simple random sample (SRS) from the immigrant population.

- The two lists are independent.
- The lists allow individuals to be matched. Although this may appear straightforward, it is often quite challenging in practice.

Example 5.6: A study conducted by the Department of Labor and Social Affairs aimed to estimate the total number of unemployed individuals in the country. Initially, a sample of 480 unemployed people was identified using their national identification numbers. Three months later, a new sample was drawn, revealing that 120 of the previously identified unemployed individuals were still without employment. The size of the second random sample was then expanded to 950 individuals, with 120 of them having appeared in the initial sample. How many unemployed people are in the country?

Solution: In this study, $n_1 = 480$, $n_2 = 950$, and $s = 120$. Thus, the approximate total number of unemployed individuals is

$$N = \frac{n_2(n_1+1)}{s+1} - 1 = \frac{950(480+1)}{120+1} - 1 = 3776.$$

For this estimator, the unbiased estimated standard deviation given by Mielke is

$$\hat{\sigma}(\hat{N}) = \sqrt{\frac{(n_1+1)(n_1-s+1)n_2(n_2-s)}{s^2(s+1)}}$$

$$= \sqrt{\frac{(480+1)(480-120+1)950(950-120)}{120^2(120+1)}} = \sqrt{\frac{136{,}915{,}928{,}500}{1{,}742{,}400}}$$

$$= 280.32$$

Alternatively, a brief calculation using Scheaffer's approximation gives:

$$\hat{N} = \frac{n_2(n_1)}{s} - 1 = \frac{950 \times 480}{120} - 1 = 3799$$

and

$$\hat{\sigma}(\hat{N}) = \sqrt{\frac{(n_1^2)n_2(n_2-s)}{s^2(s+1)}} = \sqrt{\frac{480^2 \times 950(950-120)}{120^2(120+1)}} = 322.90$$

We can then estimate a 95% confidence interval for the total size of the population using the first estimator:

$$\hat{N} \pm 1.96 \times \hat{\sigma}(\hat{N}) = 3776 \pm 1.96 \times 280.32 = (3227,\ 4326).$$

Example 5.7: A statistician is attempting to estimate how many people attended a protest meeting. To support the estimation, he distributed 500 free orange sunhats to attendees who chose to wear them. He then went to a nearby tower building and selected a random sample of 300 attendees, of whom 28 were wearing the orange sunhats. Estimate the total number of people who attended the protest meeting.

Solution: The available data are

$$n_1 = 500, n_2 = 300, s = 28.$$

The estimated total number of attendees using the capture–recapture estimator is

$$\hat{N} = \frac{n_1 n_2}{s} = \frac{500 \times 300}{28} = 5357.14.$$

The unbiased estimated standard deviation is given by

$$\hat{d}\left(\hat{N}\right) = 2\sqrt{\frac{n_1^2\, n_2\left(n_2 - s\right)}{s^3}} = 2\sqrt{\frac{500^2 \times 300\left(300 - 28\right)}{28^3}} = 1928.00.$$

A 95% confidence interval for the total population may then be calculated as

$$\hat{N} \pm \hat{d}\left(\hat{N}\right) = 5357.14 \pm 1928.00,$$

which gives

$$(3429,\ 7285)$$

Example 5.8 (Estimating Active Cars During Peak Hours): A traffic research centre seeks to estimate the number of cars in use in a city during peak hours. The study focuses on 850 registered taxis within the taxi organisation. Typically, 10% of these taxis do not operate during peak hours because of breakdowns or driver illness. Estimate the total number of active taxis during peak hours.

Solution: This scenario uses the capture–recapture method, where the registered taxis act as the initial sample.

- Total registered taxis: $n_0 = 850$.
- Percentage operating during peak hours: $90\% = 100\% - 10\%$.
- Number of active taxis during peak hours: $n_1 = n_0 \times 0.90 = 850 \times 0.90 = 765$.
- Total number of observed cars: $n_2 = 627$.
- Number of taxis identified in the second sample: $s = 56$.

The estimate of the total number of active cars during peak hours is

$$\hat{N} = \frac{n_1 n_2}{s} = \frac{765 \times 627}{56} = 8565.27.$$

Thus, the estimated number of active cars in the city during peak hours is approximately 8565.

5.3 Choosing Sample Sizes for Direct and Inverse Sampling

When selecting between direct and inverse sampling techniques, it is important to consider their strengths and weaknesses. Scheaffer notes that although both methods are viable, direct sampling is generally less reliable than inverse sampling, particularly when the second sample size n_2 required to recapture s tagged individuals is small relative to the total population size N; that is, when $\frac{n_2}{N}$ is small.

For example, if inverse sampling is used without prior knowledge of N, a poor choice of n_1 may lead to an inflated estimate of N. To obtain exactly $s = 10$ recaptured animals, a substantially larger second sample size n_2 is required when $N = 10{,}000$, but only $n_1 = 50$ individuals are initially captured (Scheaffer et al., 2011, p. 317).

The sampling fractions for the first and second capture sessions (p_1 *and* p_2) are defined as:

$$p_1 = \frac{n_1}{N}, p_2 = \frac{n_2}{N}.$$

This leads to the following expression for the relative variance:

$$\frac{V(\hat{N})}{N} = \frac{1 - p_1}{p_1 p_2}.$$

To simplify sample size determination, the proportion $V(\hat{N})/N$ can be expressed for various values of p_1 and p_2. The resulting values are displayed in Table 5.1.

Table 5.1 shows that increasing either p_1 or p_2 results in a decrease in the ratio $\frac{V(\hat{N})}{N}$. This trend reflects the principle that, for fixed N, the variance $V(\hat{N})$ decreases as sample sizes increase, leading to more precise estimates.

Once an approximate value of N is available and a target variance $V(\hat{N})$ is specified, identifying the necessary sampling fractions becomes straightforward when one of the two fractions is known. However, the challenge – and

TABLE 5.1

Proportion $\frac{V(N)}{N}$ in Terms for Different p_1 *and* p_2 Values

	p_1									
p_2	**0.005**	**0.01**	**0.05**	**0.10**	**0.15**	**0.25**	**0.333**	**0.40**	**0.50**	**0.75**
0.005	39800	19800	3800	1800	1134	600	400	300	200	67
0.01	19900	9900	1900	900	567	300	200	150	100	34
0.05	3980	1980	380	180	114	60	40	30	20	6.6
0.10	1990	990	190	90	57	30	20	15	10	3.3
0.15	1327	660	127	60	38	20	14	10	7	2.2
0.25	796	396	76	36	23	12	8	6	4	1.3
0.333	597	297	57	27	17	9	6	5	3	1
0.40	498	248	48	23	15	8	5	4	3	0.8
0.50	398	198	38	18	12	6	4	3	2	0.7
0.75	266	132	25	12	8	4	2.7	2	1.3	0.4

the central interest – lies in determining the optimal combination of p_1 and p_2 that achieves the desired precision with the smallest total sample size.

Figure 5.3 illustrates the sampling fractions p_1 *and* p_2 that produce a standard deviation of approximately 100 for the scenario described in Example 5.9a. The cross indicates the combination that yields the smallest total sample size.

> **Example 5.9a:** A research team wants to estimate the current deer population, which they believe is approximately the same as last year's estimate of 800 to 1,000 deer. The objective is to determine the sampling fractions p_1 and p_2 that yield a margin of error of 200 while minimising the total sample size.

Solution: The most straightforward approach is to use the graphical output from the tool (see Figure 5.3). If the researcher tags 315 animals, this corresponds to a sampling fraction of $p_1 = 31.5\%$. Subsequently, capturing 215 more animals results in a second sampling fraction of $p_2 = 21.5\%$.

This setup produces a standard deviation of approximately 100. The calculations proceed as follows:

$$\frac{V(\hat{N})}{N} = \frac{1-p_1}{p_1 p_2}$$

Substituting the values:

$$V(\hat{N}) = N \cdot \frac{1-p_1}{p_1 p_2} = 1000 \times \frac{1-0.315}{0.315 \times 0.215} = 10114.5.$$

The standard error is then:

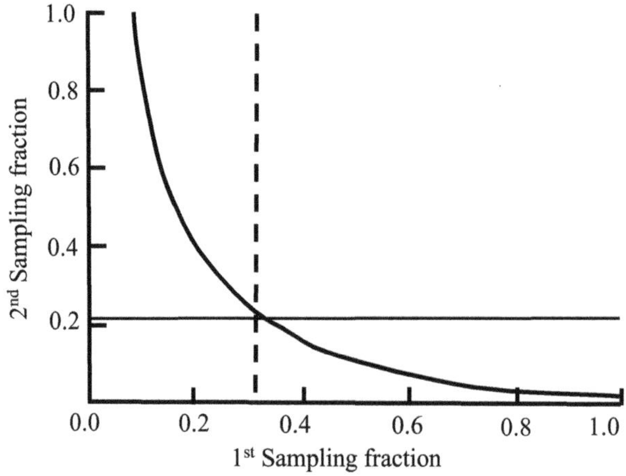

FIGURE 5.3
Optimal sampling fractions.

$$SE(\hat{N}) = \sqrt{10114.5} = 100.57$$

It is worth noting that sample size calculations for inverse sampling are nearly identical to those for direct sampling. Consequently, the tool developed for this purpose functions similarly for both approaches.

> **Example 5.9b:** In this scenario, the research team again estimates that the deer population this year mirrors last year's estimate of 800 to 1,000 deer. The goal is to determine the sampling fraction p_1 and the number of recaptures s that would yield a margin of error of 200 while minimising the total sample size.

Solution: Following the approach used in Example 5-9a, an initial sampling fraction of 31.5% is selected, with a target number of recaptures of 68.5 (rounded up to 69 in practice). This corresponds to a second sampling fraction of 21.5%.

The similarity between the two solutions arises because, with sufficiently large sample sizes, the random variability of s in direct sampling becomes small. Under these conditions, the two methods are virtually indistinguishable in terms of efficiency.

Furthermore, the tag–recapture techniques described here can be extended beyond two stages. In the second stage, the $(n-s)$ untagged animals may be tagged, and all n animals can be returned to the population. A third sample can then be taken, repeating the counting and tagging operations. This multistage approach results in a more accurate estimator of N and is particularly useful in ongoing studies where samples may be collected weekly. These methods can also be adapted to account for births and deaths within the population, as well as varying capture probabilities at each stage.

5.4 Estimating Population Density Using Quadrat Samples

A key concept in this approach is *element population density*, which refers to the average number of elements or organisms per unit (volume, area, or quadrat). The predicted population density should then be multiplied by the total area of the research region. A group of components or living organisms can be conceptualised as a unit. A biological community consists of multiple organism populations that interact with one another. Biologists often attempt to estimate population densities in their study areas. Variations in population density are common, but substantial fluctuations may indicate underlying issues that could threaten the entire community. For example, researchers may aim to estimate the number of microorganisms in a specific liquid, the number of fish in a lake, or the number of trees in a forest.

This method is applicable not only in ecology and biology but also in social, industrial, and medical research. Examples include estimating waste production in the textile industry or the volume of calls received at a call centre.

Let a region of total size "A" be divided into sub-regions $a_1, a_2, \ldots, a_k$, where n_i is the number of elements in the i-th sub-region, and the k sub-regions together have a total area exactly equal to A.

$$a_1 + a_2 + \cdots + a_k = \sum_{i=1}^{k} a_i = A \tag{5.9}$$

For simplicity, we refer to any sub-region as a *quadrat*, even if it is not square. For a sample of n randomly selected quadrats, let m_i represent the number of elements in the i-th quadrat, $\bar{m}$ the average number of elements per quadrat, and $\hat{\lambda}$ the element density, defined as the predicted mean number of elements per unit area (Scheaffer et al., 2011, p. 320).

$$m_1 + m_2 + \cdots + m_k = \sum_{i=1}^{k} m_i = M \tag{5.10}$$

$$\bar{m} = \frac{\sum_{i=1}^{k} m_i}{n} \tag{5.11}$$

$$\hat{\lambda} = \frac{M}{A} = \frac{\bar{m}}{\bar{a}} \tag{5.12}$$

where $\bar{a}$ is the average quadrat area.

The variance of $\bar{m}$ is estimated by:

$$S_m^2 = \frac{\sum_{1}^{n} (m_i - \bar{m})^2}{n-1} = \frac{1}{n-1}\left[\sum_{i=1}^{n} m_i^2 - \frac{(\bar{m})^2}{n}\right] \tag{5.13}$$

The variance of $\hat{\lambda}$ is then:

$$Var\left(\hat{\lambda}\right) = \frac{1}{a.n} \times \frac{S_m^2}{a} = \frac{S_m^2}{a^2.n} \tag{5.14}$$

where a is the area of a quadrat.

This variance corresponds to the sample variance of the number of elements in the selected n quadrats. A rough estimate of the total population is

$$\hat{M} = \hat{\lambda}.A$$

where A is the entire study region. The variance of $\hat{M}$ is computed as follows:

$$Var\left(\hat{M}\right) = Var\left(A.\hat{\lambda}\right) = A^2 \times Var\left(\hat{\lambda}\right) = A^2 \times \frac{S_m^2}{a^2.n} \quad (5.15)$$

As usual, the bound on the estimation error at the 95% confidence level is

$$\hat{d}\left(\hat{\lambda}\right) = \mathbf{1.96}\sqrt{Var\left(\hat{\lambda}\right)} \cong \mathbf{2}\sqrt{Var\left(\hat{\lambda}\right)}$$

$$\hat{d}\left(\hat{M}\right) = A.\hat{d}\left(\hat{\lambda}\right) = \mathbf{1.96} \times \hat{A}\sqrt{Var\left(\hat{\lambda}\right)} \cong \mathbf{2}\hat{A}\sqrt{Var\left(\hat{\lambda}\right)}$$

Example 5.10 (Estimating Fire Ant Hills): A state is currently facing a serious issue with fire ants. Accurately estimating the number of ant hills per unit area at specific locations is crucial for monitoring population growth. The data in the table below were collected from 50 sample quadrats, each measuring approximately 16 m². This example is adapted from Scheaffer et al. (p. 321).

Number of Hills	Frequency
0	13
1	8
2	12
3	10
4	5
5	2
Sum	50

Based on the data above, estimate the number of ant hills per unit area.

Solution: The estimated density of ant hills per unit area is

$$\Sigma f_i.m_i = (13\times 0)+(8\times 1)+(12\times 2)+(10\times 3)+(5\times 4)+(2\times 5) = 92$$

The average number of hills per quadrat is

$$\bar{m} = \frac{\Sigma f_i.m_i}{n} = \frac{92}{50} = 1.84$$

To estimate the variance of $\bar{m}$, we first need to compute the sum of squares:

$$\Sigma f_i.m_i^2 = \left(13\times 0^2\right)+\left(8\times 1^2\right)+\left(12\times 2^2\right)+\left(10\times 3^2\right)+\left(5\times 4^2\right)+\left(2\times 5^2\right) = 276$$

Now compute the sample variance:

$$S_m^2 = \frac{1}{50-1}\left[276 - \frac{92^2}{50}\right] = 2.178$$

Each quadrat has area $a = 16\ \text{m}^2$. The estimated number of ants per meter (density) is

$$\hat{\lambda} = \frac{\overline{m}}{a} = \frac{1.84}{16} = 0.115$$

This is the estimated number of hills per m².

Variance of the density estimator is

$$Var\left(\hat{\lambda}\right) = \frac{S_m^2}{a^2.n} = \frac{2.178}{(16)^2 \times 50} = 0.00017$$

The bound on the estimation error is

$$\hat{d}\left(\hat{\lambda}\right) = 2\sqrt{0.00017} = 0.0261$$

Thus, the 95% confidence interval for the density is

$$0.115 \pm 0.0261 = (0.0889,\ 0.1411)$$

Alternative variance estimator: Assuming that the ant hills are randomly dispersed throughout the study area, the variance of $\hat{\lambda}$ can be estimated as:

$$\text{Var}\left(\hat{\lambda}\right) = \frac{\hat{\lambda}}{an} = \frac{0.115}{16 \times 50} = \frac{0.115}{800} = 0.00014375 \approx 0.000144$$

$$\hat{d}\left(\hat{\lambda}\right) = 2\sqrt{0.000144} = 0.024$$

The similarity between the two variance estimates suggests that the assumption of random dispersion may be reasonable for these data.

It is important to note that under the randomness assumption, both $\hat{\lambda}$ and $\hat{d}\left(\hat{\lambda}\right)$ depend on the data solely through $\overline{m}$.

Example 5.11 (Call Centre Analysis): An organisation that answers calls would like to determine the average number of calls it receives per hour. The table below displays the number of calls recorded over a randomly selected 12-quarter-hour period. Calculate the estimated number of calls per hour and the estimation error.

period (f_i)	Number of calls (m_i)
2	0
3	1
6	2
1	3
12	Sum

Number of Calls Received in a Call Centre

Solution: First, compute the total number of calls:

$$\Sigma f_i.m_i = (2\times 0)+(3\times 1)+(6\times 2)+(1\times 3) = 18$$

The average number of calls per quarter-hour period is

$$\bar{m} = \frac{\Sigma f_i.m_i}{n} = \frac{18}{12} = 1.5$$

Since each unit corresponds to a quarter-hour ($\boldsymbol{a} = \frac{\mathbf{1}}{\mathbf{4}}$ hour), the estimated number of calls per hour is

$$\hat{\lambda} = \frac{\bar{m}}{a} = \frac{1.5}{\frac{1}{4}} = 6$$

To estimate the variance of $\hat{\lambda}$, we first need to compute the sum of squares:

$$\Sigma f_i.m_i^2 == (2\times 0^2)+(3\times 1^2)+(6\times 2^2)+(1\times 3^2) = 36$$

The sample variance of calls per quarter-hour can be estimated by

$$S_m^2 = \frac{1}{n-1}\left(\Sigma f_i m_i^2 - \frac{(\Sigma f_i m_i)^2}{n}\right) == \frac{1}{n-1}\left[36 - \frac{18^2}{12}\right] \approx 0.818$$

The variance of $\hat{\lambda}$ (calls per hour) is

$$Var\left(\hat{\lambda}\right) = \frac{S_m^2}{a^2.n} = \frac{0.818}{(\frac{1}{4})^2 \times 12} = 1.091$$

The estimation error is

$$\hat{d}(\hat{\lambda}) = 2\sqrt{\mathrm{Var}(\hat{\lambda})} = 2\sqrt{1.091} = 2.089$$

Assuming 24 hours of operation, the estimated total number of calls per day is

$$\hat{M} = \hat{\lambda} \times 24 = 6 \times 24 = 144$$

The corresponding estimation error is

$$\hat{d}(\hat{M}) = 24 \times \hat{d}(\hat{\lambda}) = 24 \times 2.089 \approx 50.14$$

The call centre receives an estimated 6 calls per hour, with an estimation error of approximately 2.09 calls per hour. Over a full 24-hour period, the estimated total number of calls is 144, with an error of about 50 calls.

Example 5.12 (Estimating Street Vendors): The municipality is trying to determine how many street vendors operate in a metropolis covering 652 km². One-way street junctions are generally not cost-effective for vendors; thus, experts recommend that they set up business only at intersections of two major roads or highways. There are 848 large junctions in the city suitable for peddlers. A statistician randomly selects 27 crossings, and the following table displays the frequency of the number of vendors observed at these intersections.

Number of Intersection (f_i)	Number of Vendors (m_i)
3	4
2	5
4	6
5	7
6	10
4	11
2	13
1	14
27	Sum

Frequency of Vendors in the Samples

Solution: In this instance, all intersections are assumed to be of equal area ($a = 1$).

First, compute the total number of vendors in the sampled intersections:

$$\sum_{i=1}^{k} f_i.m_i = (3\times4)+(2\times5)+(4\times6)+(5\times7)+(6\times10)+(4\times11)+(2\times13)+(1\times14)=225$$

The average number of vendors per sampled intersection is

$$\bar{m} = \frac{\Sigma f_i.m_i}{n} = \frac{225}{27} = 8.33$$

Thus, the estimated density of vendors per intersection is

$$\hat{\lambda} = \frac{\bar{m}}{a} = \frac{8.33}{1} = 8.33$$

To estimate the variance of $\hat{\lambda}$, we first need to compute the sum of squares:

$$\Sigma f_i.m_i^2 = (3\times4^2)+(2\times5^2)+(4\times6^2)+(5\times7^2)+(6\times10^2)$$
$$+(4\times11^2)+(2\times13^2)+(1\times14^2)=2105$$

The sample variance of vendors per intersection is

$$S_m^2 = \frac{1}{n-1}\left(\Sigma f_i m_i^2 - \frac{(\Sigma f_i m_i)^2}{n}\right) = \frac{1}{27-1}\left[2105 - \frac{225^2}{27}\right] = 8.85$$

The variance of the density estimate ($\hat{\lambda}$) is

$$Var\left(\hat{\lambda}\right) = \frac{S_m^2}{a^2.n} = \frac{8.85}{(1)^2\times27} = 0.328$$

The estimation error is

$$\hat{d}\left(\hat{\lambda}\right) = 2\sqrt{\text{Var}\left(\hat{\lambda}\right)} = 2\sqrt{0.328} = 1.14$$

The estimated total number of vendors in the city is

$$\hat{M} = 848\times\hat{\lambda} = 848\times8.85 = 7063.8 \approx 7064$$

The corresponding estimation error is

$$\hat{d}\left(\hat{M}\right) = 848\times\hat{d}\left(\hat{\lambda}\right) = 848\times1.14 = 966.7$$

The estimated total number of vendors in the city is approximately **7,064**, with a 95% confidence interval of

$$\hat{M} \pm \hat{d}\left(\hat{M}\right) = 7063.8 \pm 966.7 \approx \left(6097.1, 8029.5\right)$$

5.5 Segment (Quadrat) Sampling

Segment sampling refers to the use of sample units in area probability sampling, a specific type of cluster sampling (Lavrakas, 2008, p. 802). This method, which is a form of area frame sampling, closely resembles the third approach (estimating population density) but focuses solely on counting the number of segments that contain the desired feature, rather than the exact number of features within each segment. Detecting the presence or absence of a species is generally easier than counting individuals; therefore, simply determining whether a species exists within a sample segment (quadrat) can provide a reliable estimate of population density and size.

Segment sampling involves partitioning a region into sections or segments, which can be either regular or irregular in shape (Gallego, 1995). This technique divides a population into "n" segments. While segment areas may not always be equal, their sizes must be known. The total size of the population is then estimated based on the fraction of segments exhibiting specific characteristics. Let A_i represent the size of the i-th segment, and let $A = a_1 + a_2 + \cdots + a_n$ denote the total area of interest. A segment (quadrat) that contains the species of interest is termed a *"stocked quadrat"*.

Let k denote the number of non-stocked (i.e., lacking the desired features) sampled quadrats from the population within region A. The proportion of unstocked quadrats in the population can be approximated as $e^{-\lambda a}$, assuming the elements are randomly distributed. As previously established, a good estimator of the population proportion is the sample proportion of unstocked quadrats. Consequently, $\frac{k}{n}$ serves as an estimator for $e^{-\lambda a}$. This leads to the following estimates for λ and M:

$$\hat{\lambda} = -\frac{1}{a} ln(\frac{k}{n})$$

$$\widehat{Var}\left(\hat{\lambda}\right) = \frac{1}{na^2}\left(e^{\hat{\lambda}a} - 1\right)$$

Here, **a** represents the area of each segment (not the total number of segments), **n** denotes the number of sampled segments, **k** is the number of segments lacking the characteristic of interest, and **ln** refers to the natural (Napierian) logarithm.

$$\hat{M} = \hat{\lambda}.A$$

$$\widehat{Var}\left(\hat{M}\right) = A^2.\widehat{Var}\left(\hat{\lambda}\right) = \frac{A^2}{n.a^2}\left(e^{\hat{\lambda}a} - 1\right)$$

$$\hat{d}\left(\hat{M}\right) = A.\hat{d}\left(\hat{\lambda}\right)$$

Example 5.13 (Estimating Vehicles During Peak Hours): A traffic research centre aims to estimate the number of cars in use in a city during peak hours. With 850 cabs registered with the taxi organisation, it is observed that typically only 10% of taxis are not operational during the busiest hours due to breakdowns or driver illness. Estimate the total number of vehicles on the road during peak hours.

Solution: To estimate the number of cars in the city, we treat the registered cabs as an initial "marked" sample in a capture–recapture model. During peak hours, 90% of the registered taxis are operational.

$$n_0 = 850. \quad n_1 = n_0 \times (100 - \%10) = 850 \times (\%90) = 765.$$

A random sample of vehicles is observed continuously until the 56th taxi is encountered. The 56th taxi appears as the 627th vehicle in the sample.

$$n_2 = 627, s = 56$$

Using the standard capture–recapture estimator:

$$\hat{N} = \frac{n_1 \times n_2}{s} = \frac{765 \times 627}{56} = 8565.3 \approx 8566$$

The estimation error is calculated as follows:

$$\hat{d}_{(\hat{N})} = 2\sqrt{\frac{n_1^2 n_2 (n_2 - s)}{s^2 (s+1)}} = 2\sqrt{\frac{765^2 \times 627(627 - 56)}{56^2 \times (56+1)}} = 2165.3$$

Thus, during the busiest period of the day, the estimated number of cars on the road in the city is between:

$$\hat{N} \pm \hat{d}(N) = 8566 \pm 2165.3 \Rightarrow [6400.7, 10731.3] \approx [6401, 10732]$$

Example 5.14 (Estimating Polluting Vehicles): The Environmental Protection Agency (EPA) seeks to estimate the total number of polluting vehicles in an 80 km² city. To accomplish this, the city is segmented into areas of 0.25 km², and agents are instructed to note the presence of polluting cars during the same hours. Reports indicate that a sample of $n = 20$ segments was examined, with $k = 4$ of these segments showing no polluting vehicles. Estimate the total number of vehicles causing pollution.

Solution: The total number of segments in the city is

$$a = 0.25,\ \ k = 4,\ \ n = 20,\ \ and\ \ A_{\text{total segments}} = \frac{80}{0.25} = 320,$$

where

- $a = 0.25\text{km}^2$ is the area of a single segment,
- $A = 80\text{km}^2$ is the total city area,
- $n = 20$ is the number of sampled segments, and
- $k = 4$ is the number of segments with no polluting vehicles.

Using the segment-sampling formula, the estimated number of polluting vehicles in each segment is

$$\hat{\lambda} = -\frac{1}{0.25} ln(\frac{4}{20}) == -\frac{1}{0.25} ln\left(\frac{4}{20}\right) = 6.43$$

The estimation error is

$$\hat{d}\left(\hat{\lambda}\right) = 2\sqrt{\frac{1}{na^2}\left(e^{\hat{\lambda}a} - 1\right)} = 2\sqrt{\frac{1}{20 \times 0.25^2}\left(e^{6.43 \times 0.25} - 1\right)} \approx 3.57$$

The estimated total number of polluting vehicles in the city is

$$\hat{M} = \hat{\lambda} \cdot A_{\text{total segments}} = 6.43 \times 320 \approx 2057.6$$

The corresponding estimation error is

$$\hat{d}\left(\hat{M}\right) = A_{\text{total segments}} \cdot \hat{d}\left(\hat{\lambda}\right) = 320 \times 3.57 \approx 1142.4$$

Thus, the 95% confidence interval for the total number of polluting vehicles in the city is

$$(2057.6 \pm 1142.4) \approx 916 \text{ to } 3200$$

Conclusion: Based on this segment sampling, the city likely has between 916 and 3,200 polluting vehicles, with an estimated mean of approximately 2,058 vehicles.

> **Example 5.15 (Estimating Bodies Under Rubble):** In a city affected by an earthquake, remnants may still be present under the debris. The Red Crescent Society divided the 54 km² city into segments of 0.25 km² each. Trained dogs were then used to investigate $n = 18$ of these segments, with only $k = 2$ segments showing *no trace of bodies* beneath the rubble. Estimate the total number of bodies under the rubble at a 95% confidence level.

Solution: The total number of segments in the city is

$$k = 2\ ,\ n = 18\ and\ A_{\text{total}} = \frac{54}{0.25} = 216$$

$$\frac{A_{\text{total}}}{a} = \frac{54}{0.25} = 216$$

where $a = 0.25$ km² is the area of a single segment, $A = 54$ km² is the total city area, $n = 18$ is the number of sampled segments, and $k = 2$ is the number of segments with no detected bodies.

Using the segment-sampling formula, the estimated number of bodies visible under the debris, along with its standard deviation in each segment, is

$$\hat{\lambda} = -\frac{1}{a}\ln\left(\frac{k}{n}\right) = -\frac{1}{0.25} \times \ln\left(\frac{2}{18}\right) = 8.79 \approx 9$$

The estimation error is

$$\hat{d}\left(\hat{\lambda}\right) = 2\sqrt{\frac{1}{n.a^2}\left(e^{\hat{\lambda}a} - 1\right)} = 2\sqrt{\frac{1}{18 \times 0.25^2}\left(e^{8.79 \times 0.25} - 1\right)} \approx 5.33$$

5.5.1 Estimating the Total Number of Bodies in the City

The estimated total number of bodies under the rubble is

$$\hat{M} = \hat{\lambda} \cdot A_{\text{total segments}} = 8.79 \times 216 \approx 1896.6$$

The corresponding estimation error is

$$\hat{d}\left(\hat{M}\right) = A_{\text{total segments}} \cdot \hat{d}\left(\hat{\lambda}\right) = 216 \times 5.33 \approx 1151.3$$

The total number of remnants visible under the debris, along with their estimation error for the city, is calculated as follows:

$$\hat{M} = 8.79 \times 216 = 1896.6 \approx 1897$$

$$\hat{d}\left(\hat{M}\right) = A \times \hat{d}\left(\hat{\lambda}\right) = 216 \times 5.33 = 1151.3$$

The 95% confidence interval for the total number of remnants visible under the debris in the city is

$$\hat{M} \pm \hat{d}\left(\hat{M}\right) = \left(1896.6 \pm 1151.28\right) = 745 \text{ to } 3047.88$$

Based on this segment sampling, the estimated number of bodies under the rubble in the city is approximately 1,897, with a 95% confidence interval ranging from 745 to 3,048.

References

Chao, A., Tsay, P., Lin, S. H., Shau, W. Y., & Chao, D. Y. (2001). The applications of capture-recapture models to epidemiological data. *Statistics in Medicine, 20*(20), 3123–3157.

Gallego, F. J. (1995). *Sampling frames of square segments.* European Commission Luxembourg.

Indrayan, A., & Holt, M. P. (2016). *Concise encyclopedia of biostatistics for medical professionals.* Chapman and Hall and CRC Press.

Lavrakas, P. J. (2008). *Encyclopedia of survey research methods.* Sage Publications.

Lohr, S. L. (2021). *Sampling: design and analysis.* Chapman and Hall and CRC Press.

Mielke Jr, P. W., Berry, K. J. J. P., & Skills, M. (1999). Capture-recapture methodology: Direct and inverse sampling. *Perceptual and Motor Skills, 89*(3), 748–752.

Ramos, P. L., Sousa, I., Santana, R., Morgan, W. H., Gordon, K., Crewe, J., Rocha-Sousa, A., & Macedo, A. F. (2020). A review of capture-recapture methods and its possibilities in ophthalmology and vision sciences. *Ophthalmic Epidemiology, 27*(4), 310–324.

Scheaffer, R. L., Mendenhall III, W., Ott, R. L., & Gerow, K. G. (2011). *Elementary survey sampling.* Cengage Learning.

Thompson, S. K. (2012). *Sampling* (Vol. 755). John Wiley & Sons.

6

Sample Size for Estimating and Comparing Means and Totals

6.1 Introduction

When we refer to the mean, we are discussing the average value of a quantitative variable within a population or comparing the means of a quantitative variable across two populations in which that variable can be measured. The concept of *total value* pertains to the sum of the values of a quantitative variable within a population. In this chapter, we outline the methodology for calculating the required sample size for each of these scenarios, accompanied by illustrative examples.

6.2 Estimating the Mean of a Single Population

To estimate the mean of a quantitative variable in a single population, the minimum required number of participants must be determined using the significance level (α), a measure of dispersion, and a specified estimation error (d). Notably, the power of the test is *not* included in this calculation. The formula for estimating the minimum sample size under a simple random sampling (SRS) design is

$$n = \frac{z^2_{1-\frac{\alpha}{2}} \times \sigma^2}{d^2} \tag{6.1}$$

where

- σ represents the standard deviation, as described in Chapter 5. It may be derived from prior studies, expert opinion, or pilot data.
- d denotes the desired precision of the estimate, reflecting how close the sample mean should be to the true population mean.

DOI: 10.1201/9781003749783-6

- $Z_{1-\frac{\alpha}{2}}$ is the standard normal deviate corresponding to a two-tailed test at the chosen significance level.

Precision (or estimation error) is typically defined as the maximum acceptable difference between the estimated mean and the true population mean. This tolerance is determined by the researcher based on available resources, logistical constraints, and the study's scientific objectives.

In most research contexts – including social, industrial, management, medical, health, and epidemiological studies – a significance level of 5% is commonly considered sufficient. However, specific conditions may warrant using a significance level of 1% or 10%. When such adjustments are made, and when hypotheses about mean differences are being tested, the power of the test should also be incorporated into the sample size calculation.

TIP

If the calculated sample size (n) is not a whole number and results in a decimal, it should always be rounded up to the next whole number, rather than following standard mathematical rounding rules. This practice ensures that the sample size is sufficient to achieve the desired levels of statistical power and significance. For example, both 84.02 and 84.65 should be rounded up to 85.

Example 6.1: A study was conducted to estimate the level of serum cholesterol in men from a specific population. The research question was: How many samples are needed to estimate this level within 5 mg/100 ml of its actual value with 95% confidence? This requirement means that the maximum acceptable difference between the estimated serum cholesterol level and the true population value is 5 mg.

Solution: In this example, $d = 5$, and the significance level is 5%. The corresponding value from the standard normal distribution for a two-tailed test at the 5% significance level is 1.96.

To determine the sample size, we also need an estimate of the population standard deviation. Based on studies in similar populations, as cited in the literature review, the standard deviation of serum cholesterol is approximately 40 mg/100 ml.

By substituting these values into the formula, the minimum sample size required to estimate serum cholesterol is calculated as follows:

$$n = \frac{1.96^2 \times 40^2}{5^2} = 245.9 \approx 246$$

In any case where the calculated sample size is a decimal, it should always be rounded up. Therefore, both 245.9 and 245.2 would be rounded to 246.

> **Example 6.2:** An insurance company aims to estimate the average blood pressure of women aged 18 years and older in a small city with a population of 5,000 women. Their goal is to achieve this estimation with 99% confidence and a maximum estimation error of 2 mmHg. Previous studies conducted in similar populations have indicated that the standard deviation for this population does not exceed 18 mmHg.

Solution: In this example, the relevant parameters include $d = 2$, a 1% significance level (corresponding to 99% confidence) with a z-value of 2.58, and an estimated standard deviation of $\sigma = 17$ mmHg.

Thus, the initial sample size is calculated as follows:

$$n_o = \frac{2.58^2 \times 17^2}{(2)^2} = 480.92 \approx 481$$

Since the sampling fraction is

$$\frac{n_o}{N} = \frac{481}{5000} = 0.096$$

and this value is *greater than 0.05*, the finite population correction (FPC) must be applied:

$$n = \frac{481}{1 + \dfrac{481}{5000}} = 438.79 \approx 439$$

Thus, the final required sample size, after applying the finite population correction, is 439.

> **Example 6.3:** An authorised ambulance service agency seeks to estimate the average amount of money received from each ambulance that enters their garage for services. Although the variance in the amount received is unknown, it is understood that most amounts fall within a range of **$600** (the difference between the maximum and minimum amounts). Given that the total number of records in this agency is N = 1,600 ambulances, the question arises: How many records should be reviewed (sample size) to estimate the average amount received within a maximum difference of $30?

Solution: To calculate the sample size, it is essential to know the standard deviation, which may not always be readily available to the researcher. However, based on empirical rules, we can estimate that $R = 4\sigma$. This indicates that the range (maximum amount minus minimum amount) is approximately equal to four times the standard deviation ($R \cong 4SD$) (Scheaffer et al., 2011, p. 89). Therefore, the standard deviation can be estimated as follows:

$$\sigma = \frac{R}{4} = \frac{600}{4} = 150$$

Now, the initial sample size can be calculated using the formula:

$$n_o = \frac{z^2 \times \sigma^2}{d^2} = \frac{(1.96)^2 \times (150)^2}{(30)^2} = 96.04 \approx 97$$

Since the sampling fraction is

$$\frac{n_o}{N} = \frac{97}{1600} = 0.0606$$

and this value exceeds **0.05**, the finite population correction (FPC) must be applied:

$$n = \frac{97}{1 + \frac{97}{1600}} = 92$$

Thus, the final sample size required for this study is 92 ambulances.

6.3 Sample Size for Confidence Intervals of One Mean

This section outlines the procedure for calculating the sample size necessary to achieve a specified distance (margin of error, E) from the mean to the confidence limits at a designated confidence level for a single mean, assuming that the underlying data distribution is normal.

The margin of error (E) for a confidence interval concerning a population mean is defined as:

$$E = \frac{z \times \sigma}{\sqrt{n}}$$

In this equation:

- z represents the z-score corresponding to the area under the standard normal distribution between $-z$ and z, reflecting the desired confidence level.
- σ denotes the population standard deviation.
- n is the sample size.

We can rearrange this equation to solve for the required sample size (n) as follows:

$$n = \left(\frac{z \times \sigma}{E} \right)^2 \tag{6.2}$$

To effectively apply this formula and calculate the sample size required for a specified margin of error, we must know the values of z, E, and σ.

> **Example 6.4:** A nutritionist plans to estimate the mean weight of mice after they have been fed a special diet. The objective is to determine how many mice must be weighed so that a 95% confidence interval will have a margin of error of 1 g. Previous studies have indicated that the weight of the mice is normally distributed with a standard deviation of 4 g.

Solution: To calculate the sample size, we will use the information provided. For a significance level of 5%, the corresponding z-value is $z_{1-\frac{\alpha}{2}} = 1.96$.

Given that $E = 1$ g and $\sigma = 4$ g, the sample size is computed as follows:

$$n = z^2_{1-\frac{\alpha}{2}} \times \left(\frac{\sigma}{E} \right)^2 = 1.96^2 \times \left(\frac{4}{1} \right)^2 = 61.47 \cong 62$$

We round up to *62 mice* to ensure that a 95% confidence interval is achieved with a margin of error of 1 g.

If the goal is to decrease the margin of error of a confidence interval without altering the confidence level, this can be achieved by increasing the sample size. Increasing the sample size enhances the precision of the estimate, thereby reducing the margin of error.

6.4 Estimating the Total Value of a Population

To estimate the total value of a variable within a population, a formula similar to that used for estimating the mean may be applied, with a minor adjustment regarding the estimation error. Because the estimation error contributes to the total estimate, it should be divided by the number of individuals in the population (Thompson, 2012, p. 54). This leads to the following sample size formula for estimating a population total:

$$\hat{\tau} = N \times \bar{y}$$

$$n_0 = \frac{z^2_{1-\frac{\alpha}{2}} \times \sigma^2}{\left(\frac{d}{N}\right)^2} = \frac{N^2 \times z^2_{1-\frac{\alpha}{2}} \times \sigma^2}{d^2} \tag{6.3}$$

The details of this calculation are illustrated in the example below.

> **Example 6.5:** A poultry farmer aims to estimate the total weight gain over four weeks resulting from a new diet for 3,000 chicks. The farmer is concerned about the time, costs, and potential casualties among the chickens. To accurately estimate the total weight gain, a sample of chicks should be weighed at a 5% significance level. The farmer considers a difference of up to 20,000 grams (20 kg) between the estimated and actual total weight gain to be acceptable. Previous studies indicate that the weight gain of chicks varies between 60 g and 180 g.

Solution: In this study, an estimation error or precision of 20,000 grams for the total of 3,000 chicks is considered. The range of weight gain per chick is

$$R = 180 - 60 = 120 \text{ grams}$$

Since the standard deviation is unknown, we estimate it as a quarter of the range:

$$\sigma = \frac{R}{4} = \frac{120}{4} = 30 \text{ g per chick}$$

The standard deviation for the total population should be scaled by the total number of chicks (3,000), and then the sample size for estimating the total weight gain can be calculated using the formula for the total:

$$n_o = \frac{z^2 . \sigma^2}{d^2} = \frac{(1.96)^2 \times (30 \times 3000)^2}{20000^2} = 77.79 \approx 78$$

Since the sampling fraction is

$$\frac{n_o}{N} = \frac{78}{3000} = 0.0259 < 0.05$$

Since the finite population correction (FPC) can be ignored, the final sample size is n = 78 chicks. Thus, the farmer needs to weigh 78 chicks to accurately estimate the total weight gain from this diet.

Example 6.6: A researcher aims to estimate the average weight of 90 rats on a specific diet. The most suitable sampling method for this study is stratified sampling, dividing the rats into male and female groups. Since the variance within each group is unknown, the researcher selects and weighs the heaviest and lightest rat in each group. The range of weight differences for male and female rats is 10 g and 18 g, respectively. The question arises: How many rats should be sampled to estimate the average weight with 95% confidence interval?

Solution: For a normal distribution, the range is approximately four times the standard deviation. Assuming the weights of the rats are normally distributed, we estimate the standard deviation for each category:

$$\sigma_1 = \frac{10}{4} = 2.5(\text{male rats}) \ \textit{and} \ \sigma_2 = \frac{18}{4} = 4.5(\text{female rats})$$

The pooled variance is calculated as:

$$S_p^2 = \frac{(N-1)\sigma_1{}^2 + (N_2-1)\sigma_2{}^2}{N_1 + N_2 - 2} = \frac{(50-1)\times 2.5^2 + (40-1)\times 4.5^2}{40+50-2} = 12.45$$

Next, the initial sample size is determined using:

$$n_o = \frac{z^2 S_p^2}{d^2} = \frac{1.96^2 \times 12.45}{1} = 47.8 \approx 48$$

Since the sampling fraction is

$$\frac{n_o}{N} = \frac{48}{90} = 0.53 > 0.05$$

We must apply the finite population correction (FPC). Thus, the final sample size is

$$n = \frac{48}{1 + \frac{48}{90}} = 31.3 \approx 32$$

This sample size can be divided into male and female groups using the optimum allocation method:

$$n_i = n\left(\frac{N_i\sigma_i}{\sum_{i=1}^{2} N_i\sigma_i}\right)$$

Calculating for each group:

$$n_1 = 32\times\left(\frac{50\times 2.5}{(50\times 2.5)+(40\times 4.5)}\right) = 13$$

$$n_2 = 32\times\left(\frac{40\times 4.5}{(50\times 2.5)+(40\times 4.5)}\right) = 19$$

Thus, the sample should consist of 13 male rats and 19 female rats, with weights for each stratum proportional to their variability: $w_1 = 0.41$ *and* $w_2 = 0.59$.

6.5 Comparing the Means of Two Independent Populations

The comparison of means between two independent groups implies that the samples have been randomly drawn from two independent populations, or that participants have been randomly assigned to two groups: control and intervention. For example, in a study comparing the average blood pressure levels of individuals who exercise regularly versus those who do not, the mean blood pressure levels in the two groups are independent and can be calculated and compared.

The sample size required for each group to detect a difference in means can be determined using the following formula (Malone et al., 2016, p. 3):

$$n = \frac{(z_{1-\frac{\alpha}{2}} + z_{1-\beta})^2\left(\sigma_1^2 + \sigma_2^2\right)}{(\mu_1 - \mu_2)^2} \tag{6.4}$$

where μ_1 *and* μ_2 are the population means, and σ_1^2 *and* σ_2^2 are the population variances for groups 1 and 2, respectively.

If we assume that the variances of the two groups are equal ($\sigma_1^2 = \sigma_2^2 = \sigma^2$), this formula can be simplified to:

$$n = \frac{2\sigma^2(z_{1-\frac{\alpha}{2}} + z_{1-\beta})^2}{(\mu_1 - \mu_2)^2} \qquad (6.5)$$

Example 6.7: It is believed that infants born to mothers who smoke weigh less than those born to non-smoking mothers. To investigate the effect of maternal smoking during pregnancy on infant weight, a study has been designed. If there is an expected average weight difference of 300 grams between the two groups of infants, how many samples are needed in each group to detect this weight difference with 99% confidence interval and 95% power?

Solution: In this example, the following parameters are specified:

- The weight difference between the two groups that is considered clinically important (cannot be ignored) is 300 grams ($\mu_1 - \mu_2 = 300$ g).
- The standard deviation of infant weight in the two groups is based on data from previous studies: $\sigma_1 = 0.49$ kg for infants born to smoking mothers and $\sigma_0 = 0.37$ kg for infants born to non-smoking mothers.
- The corresponding z-values from the standard normal distribution are $z_{1-\beta} = 1.64$ for 95% power and $z_{1-\frac{\alpha}{2}} = 2.58$ for a significance level of 0.01.

The required sample size for each group is calculated using the formula for comparing two independent means:

$$n = \frac{(z_{1-\frac{\alpha}{2}} + z_{1-\beta})^2\left(\sigma_1^2 + \sigma_2^2\right)}{(\mu_1 - \mu_2)^2} = \frac{(1.64 + 2.58)^2 \times \left(0.49^2 + 0.37^2\right)}{0.3^2} = 74.60$$

Thus, at least 75 random samples are needed in each group to detect a weight difference of 300 grams with 99% confidence and 95% power.

To facilitate sample size calculations, the term $(z_{1-\frac{\alpha}{2}} + z_{1-\beta})^2$ is calculated for different values of α and β and presented in Table 6.1. For example, the squared coefficient for 80% power and a significance level of 0.05 is 7.84, which is the most commonly used value in this table.

TABLE 6.1

The Square of the Sum of the Corresponding Standard Normal for α and β from the $(z_{1-\frac{\alpha}{2}} + z_{1-\beta})^2$

0.001	0.002	0.01	0.02	0.05	0.10	0.20	α	
3.29	**3.09**	**2.58**	**2.33**	**1.96**	**1.64**	**1.28**	Z	$1-\beta$
10.82	9.55	6.66	5.43	3.84	2.71	1.64	**0.00**	**0.50**
12.55	11.18	8.03	6.67	4.90	3.58	2.35	**0.253**	**0.60**
14.55	13.07	9.64	8.15	6.18	4.69	3.26	**0.525**	**0.70**
15.72	14.18	10.60	9.03	6.94	5.36	3.84	**0.675**	**0.75**
17.06	15.44	11.67	10.02	7.84	6.17	4.50	**0.84**	**0.80**
18.75	17.06	13.10	11.36	9.00	7.18	5.38	**1.04**	**0.85**
20.91	19.11	14.88	13.02	10.51	8.57	6.57	**1.28**	**0.90**
24.36	22.42	17.82	15.77	12.99	10.82	8.57	**1.64**	**0.95**
28.52	26.42	21.44	19.18	16.08	13.62	11.09	**2.05**	**0.98**
31.55	29.33	24.03	21.64	18.37	15.77	13.02	**2.33**	**0.99**
40.72	38.19	32.10	29.33	25.50	22.42	19.11	**3.09**	**0.999**

6.6 Comparing the Means of Two Dependent Groups (Paired Data)

A paired design may employ naturally matched pairs (often referred to as "matched siblings"), artificially created pairs (in which subjects are matched based on important characteristics), or self-pairing (the same subject measured before and after an intervention). The calculated sample size determines the number of pairs required for the study. Because the appropriate statistical test is the paired *t*-test, the relevant standard deviation is the *standard deviation of the differences,* denoted as σ_d. This quantity represents the standard deviation of the difference scores calculated as $d = x_1 - x_2$, where the two measurements correspond to pre- and post-treatment values.

To calculate the sample size required to detect a mean difference $\Delta = \mu_1 - \mu_2$ at a two-sided significance level α with power $(1-\beta)$, where the clinically relevant effect size is defined as the difference between post-treatment and pre-treatment measurements, the required sample size (number of pairs) is given by (Julious & Campbell, 1998):

$$n = \frac{(z_{1-\frac{\alpha}{2}} + z_{1-\beta})^2 \times \sigma_d^2}{(\mu_1 - \mu_2)^2} \tag{6.6}$$

However, obtaining an accurate estimate of σ_d from published data can be challenging. It is therefore recommended to derive a preliminary estimate at the outset of the study or by conducting a pilot study.

> **Example 6.8 (Sample Size Calculation for a Heart Rate Study):** A study was conducted to identify a 10-beats-per-minute (bpm) increase in heart rate when standing compared to sitting. The researchers needed to determine the sample size required to detect this difference using a two-sided 5% significance level and 90% power. Because no published estimate of the standard deviation of the difference was available, experts provided an opinion that the standard deviation of the sitting–standing difference would be no more than 25 bpm. How many samples are required to detect the difference of 10-beats-per-minute (bpm) increase in heart rate?

Solution: In this example, an effect size (difference to be detected) of 10 bpm is specified. A significance level of 5% and a power of 90% correspond to z-values of 1.96 and 1.28 from the standard normal distribution, respectively. The expert-based estimate of the standard deviation of the differences is taken as $\sigma = 25$. The required sample size is calculated using the paired-samples formula:

$$n = \frac{\left(z_{1-\frac{\alpha}{2}} + z_{1-\beta}\right)^2 \times \sigma_d^2}{(\mu_1 - \mu_2)^2} = \frac{(1.96 + 1.28)^2 \times 25^2}{10^2} = 65.61 \approx 66$$

Thus, approximately 66 paired observations are required to detect a 10-bpm increase in heart rate when transitioning from sitting to standing.

6.7 Unequal or Imbalanced Sample Sizes

In parallel, crossover, or case–control studies comparing two or more treatments, the sample sizes in each treatment group may not be equal. For example, in a clinical trial involving severely ill patients or individuals with life-threatening diseases, it may be considered unethical to assign too many participants to the placebo group. In such cases, researchers may prefer to allocate fewer patients to the placebo arm to more effectively evaluate the drug's safety and efficacy. A commonly used allocation ratio is 1:2, meaning that each patient has a one-third probability of being assigned to the placebo group and a two-thirds probability of receiving the active treatment.

For different allocation ratios, the sample size formulas can still be applied with appropriate adjustments to the degrees of freedom (Chow et al., 2017, p. 32). This type of allocation is referred to as *imbalanced* or *unequal sample size.*

The required sample sizes for the two groups, under a general allocation ratio $k = \frac{n_2}{n_1}$, are:

$$n_1 = \frac{\left(\sigma_1^2 + \frac{\sigma_2^2}{K}\right)(z_{1-\frac{\alpha}{2}} + z_{1-\beta})^2}{(\mu_2 - \mu_1)^2} \tag{6.6}$$

and

$$n_2 = \frac{\left(K.\sigma_1^2 + \sigma_2^2\right)(z_{1-\frac{\alpha}{2}} + z_{1-\beta})^2}{(\mu_2 - \mu_1)^2} \tag{6.7}$$

It is evident that

$$n_2 = k.\, n_1$$

$$n_2 = k.\, n_1 = \frac{\left(K.\, \sigma_1^2 + \sigma_2^2\right)(z_{1-\frac{\alpha}{2}} + z_{1-\beta})^2}{(\mu_2 - \mu_1)^2}$$

If the variances of the two groups are equal, such that ($\sigma_1^2 = \sigma_2^2 = \sigma^2$), then the formulas simplify as follows:

$$n_1 = \frac{K+1}{k} \times \frac{\sigma^2(z_{1-\frac{\alpha}{2}} + z_{1-\beta})^2}{(\mu_2 - \mu_1)^2} \tag{6.8}$$

and

$$n_2 = (K+1) \times \frac{\sigma^2 \times (z_{1-\frac{\alpha}{2}} + z_{1-\beta})^2}{(\mu_2 - \mu_1)^2} \tag{6.9}$$

It is important to note that unequal treatment allocation can introduce bias into the randomisation process in clinical trials, particularly in multicentre designs (Chow et al., 2017, p. 32; Rosner, 2006, p. 308). Therefore, consulting a statistician is advisable before implementing unequal sample sizes.

Example 6.9: Continuing from Example 6.7, suppose that the number of non-smoking mothers is assumed to be three times the number of smoking mothers. We need to determine how many samples should be taken in each group.

Solution: In this case, $k = 3, \sigma_1 = 0.49 \; and \; \sigma_0 = 0.37$. The sample sizes for smokers (n_1) and non-smokers (n_2) are calculated as follows:

$$n_1 = \frac{(1.64 + 2.58)^2 \times \left(0.49^2 + \frac{0.37^2}{3}\right)}{0.3^2} = 56.54 \approx 57$$

and

$$n_2 = \frac{(1.64 + 2.58)^2 \times \left(3 \times 0.49^2 + 0.37^2\right)}{0.3^2} = 169.63 \approx 170$$

Based on this assumption, the researcher must select 57 smoking mothers and 170 non-smoking mothers.

Example 6.10: Let us assume that the blood pressure of individuals over 50 years old is expected to be twice as high as that of younger individuals under 50 years old. Our project aims to estimate the mean blood pressure in each age group. We need to determine how many samples are required for each group if we conduct a two-sided test with a 5% significance level and 80% power.

Solution: To determine the sample sizes using the appropriate equations, we assume a mean difference of $\mu_1 - \mu_2 = 10 \; mmHg$, standard deviations: $\sigma_1 = 19.2 \; and \; \sigma_2 = 14.4$, an allocation ratio of k = 2, a significance level α = 0.05 (with a corresponding value of 1.96), and a power of $1-\beta$ = 0.80 (with a corresponding value of 0.84).

The relevant formulas for unequal allocation (Equations 6.6 and 6.7) are

$$n_1 = \frac{\left(\sigma_1^2 + \frac{\sigma_2^2}{K}\right)(z_{1-\frac{\alpha}{2}} + z_{1-\beta})^2}{(\mu_2 - \mu_1)^2} = \frac{(1.96 + 0.84)^2 \times \left(19.2^2 + \frac{14.4^2}{2}\right)}{10^2} = 37.03 \approx 37$$

and

$$n_2 = \frac{\left(K.\, \sigma_1^2 + \sigma_2^2\right)(z_{1-\frac{\alpha}{2}} + z_{1-\beta})^2}{(\mu_2 - \mu_1)^2} = \frac{(1.96 + 0.84)^2 \times \left(2 \times 19.2^2 + 14.4^2\right)}{\times 10^2} = 74.06 \approx 72$$

or we can multiply n_1 by k to obtain n_2: $n_2 = K \times n_1 = 2 \times 37.03 = 74.06$.

Based on these assumptions, the researcher must select 37 participants under the age of 50 and 74 participants over the age 50.

The relevant formulas for unequal allocation (Equations 6.6 and 6.7) are

$$n_1 = \frac{\left(\sigma_1^2 + \frac{\sigma_2^2}{K}\right)(z_{1-\frac{\alpha}{2}} + z_{1-\beta})^2}{(\mu_2 - \mu_1)^2} = \frac{(1.96+0.84)^2 \times \left(19.2^2 + \frac{14.4^2}{2}\right)}{10^2} = 37.03 \approx 37$$

and

$$n_2 = \frac{\left(K.\, \sigma_1^2 + \sigma_2^2\right)(z_{1-\frac{\alpha}{2}} + z_{1-\beta})^2}{(\mu_2 - \mu_1)^2} = \frac{(1.96+0.84)^2 \times \left(2 \times 19.2^2 + 14.4^2\right)}{\times 10^2} = 74.06 \approx 72$$

or we can multiply n_1 by k to obtain n_2: $n_2 = K \times n_1 = 2 \times 37.03 = 74.06$ 50 years old and 74 participants over 50 years old.

> **Example 6.11:** A group of eight non-pregnant, premenopausal women aged 35–39 who use oral contraceptives (OC) has an average systolic blood pressure (SBP) of 132.86 mmHg with a standard deviation of 15.34 mmHg. Another group of 21 non-pregnant, premenopausal women in the same age range who do not use OCs has an average SBP of 127.44 mmHg with a standard deviation of 18.23 mmHg. These SBP data for OC and non-OC users serve as a preliminary study to estimate parameters for a larger study. Assuming a normal distribution of blood pressure for both groups, we want to test whether the mean SBP for OC users (μ_1) is equal to the mean SBP for non-OC users (μ_2). We anticipate having twice as many non-OC users in the larger study. We will calculate the required sample size for a two-sided test with a 5% significance level and 80% power (derived from Rosner, p. 308).

Solution: With $\mu_1 = 132.86,\ \sigma_1 = 15.34,\ \mu_2 = 127.44,\ \sigma_2 = 18.23\ and\ k = 2,$ to achieve 80% power with a two-sided test at α = 0.05, the required number of OC users can be calculated using Equation 6.6 as follows:

$$n_1 = \frac{\left(\sigma_1^2 + \frac{\sigma_2^2}{K}\right)(z_{1-\frac{\alpha}{2}} + z_{1-\beta})^2}{(\mu_2 - \mu_1)^2} = \frac{\left(15.34 + \frac{18.23}{2}\right)(1.96+0.84)^2}{(132.86 - 127.44)^2} = 107.1 \approx 108$$

For non-OC users:

$$n_2 = k \times n_1 = 2 \times 108 = 216$$

If the variances in the two groups are assumed to be equal, then the smallest total sample size needed for a given α and β is obtained using the equal-sample-size allocation rule in Equation 6.4. Therefore, when the variances are equal, the two groups should be balanced to optimise statistical power.

6.8 Sample Size for Estimating Standard Deviation

Determining the sample size necessary to estimate the standard deviation is more complex than calculating sample sizes for means and proportions. For normally distributed populations, researchers often refer to summary tables rather than relying on a specific formula. However, a straightforward formula can be used to calculate the sample size required to estimate a population standard deviation σ (Triola et al., 2006, p. 324):

$$n = 0.50 \times \left(\frac{z_{1-\frac{\alpha}{2}}}{d} \right)^2 \tag{6.10}$$

In this equation, $z_{1-\frac{\alpha}{2}}$ corresponds to the z-value associated with the desired confidence level, and d represents the decimal form of the acceptable percentage error.

> **Example 6.12:** To illustrate, let us determine how many samples are required to estimate the standard deviation of a population with 95% confidence, ensuring that the sample standard deviation s is within 15% of the true value of σ.

Solution: Using $z_{1-\frac{\alpha}{2}} = 1.96$ for a 95% confidence level and $d = 0.15$, we calculate the required sample size as follows:

$$n = 0.50 \times \left(\frac{z_{1-\frac{\alpha}{2}}}{d} \right)^2 = 0.50 \times \left(\frac{1.96}{0.15} \right)^2 = 85.37 \approx 86$$

Thus, a sample size of 86 is required.

> **Example 6.13:** Next, consider the scenario in which we need to estimate the standard deviation (σ) of all IQ scores for individuals exposed to lead. We want to achieve 99% confidence that our estimate is within 5%

of the true value of σ. We will assume that the population follows a normal distribution.

Solution: For a 99% confidence level, the corresponding z-value is 2.58. Given that $d = 0.05$, the sample size can be calculated as follows:

$$n = 0.50 \times \left(\frac{z_{1-\frac{\alpha}{2}}}{d} \right)^2 = 0.50 \times \left(\frac{2.58}{0.05} \right)^2 = 1331.28 \approx 1332$$

Therefore, we should obtain a simple random sample of 1,332 IQ scores from the population of subjects who have been exposed to lead.

6.9 Sample Size for Ratio Estimators

In various studies, the goal is to estimate the ratio of two variables that vary from unit to unit. For instance, one might examine the ratio of bilirubin levels in jaundiced babies in neonatal intensive care to their birth weights, or the ratio of acres of wheat to total acres on a farm (Samawi & Siam, 2003). Additionally, the prevalence of cocaine use in South London has been estimated using this method (Gossop et al., 1994). This approach is also employed to enhance the precision of estimating population means or totals by leveraging the correlation between an auxiliary variable X and the variable of interest Y (Bhuyan, 2021, p. 408; Latpate et al., 2021, p. 26; Scheaffer et al., 2011, p. 170).

TIP

The ratio estimator involves the relationship between two variables, x and y. When each sampled element can be observed and information about the total of x is available, we can estimate the total of y by multiplying the known total of x by the ratio of the two variables. This ratio can be estimated using the sample means of both variables derived from the observed sampled elements.

This technique, known as the *ratio estimation procedure*, is commonly used for estimating population totals or means. Ratio estimation involves incorporating an auxiliary variable x_i that is closely related to the outcome variable Y to improve the estimate of a given population parameter. Although the outcome variable may be costly or difficult to measure, the auxiliary information is often easier and more economical to obtain.

The formula for ratio estimation is straightforward: divide the known ratio by the sample ratio, and then multiply the result by the sample mean or total. This process allows researchers to make population inferences based on sample data. Ratio estimation is a valuable statistical tool for producing accurate predictions about a population without the need to survey every individual.

TIP

When the variance of r is unknown due to a lack of prior information or expert judgment, determining the appropriate sample size can be challenging. In such cases, the most effective approach is to conduct a pilot study to estimate the variance of r.

The ratio estimator of the population mean μ_y is given by

$$r = \frac{\sum y_i}{\sum x_i} = \frac{\bar{y}}{\bar{x}} = \frac{\mu_y}{\mu_x} \qquad \mu_y = r \cdot \mu_x$$

The variance of the estimated ratio can be calculated using the following equation (Thompson, 2012, p. 95):

$$\hat{\sigma}_r^2 = \frac{\sum_{i=1}^{n} (y_i - rx_i)^2}{n-1} = \frac{\sum_{i=1}^{n} y_i^2 + r^2 \sum_{i=1}^{n} x_i^2 - 2r \sum_{i=1}^{n} x_i y_i}{n-1} \tag{6.12}$$

To determine the sample size needed to estimate the ratio r with a specified margin of error d, the following formula is used:

$$n_o = \frac{z^2 . \sigma_r^2}{d^2} \tag{6.13}$$

However, when the variance of r is unknown from previous studies or expert judgment, determining the appropriate sample size becomes more

TABLE 6.2

Sick Leave Hours for a Sample of Nine Employees from Two Sources

	Systolic Blood Pressure		
Employee	**Last Year (x)**	**Current Year (y)**	$x.y$
1	12	13	156
2	24	25	600
3	15	15	225
4	30	32	960
5	32	36	1152
6	26	24	624
7	10	12	120
8	15	16	240
9	0	2	0
Sum	164	175	4077
Sum of squares	3870	4319	–

challenging. In such situations, conducting a pilot study to estimate the variance of r is often the only practical approach.

> **Example 6.14:** An organisation with 1,000 employees aims to estimate changes in sick leave hours compared to the previous year. The only available data are the organisation's employment records, which indicate that all employees took a total of 16,300 sick leave hours last year. Due to limited information, the organisation conducted a small study involving nine employees to analyse their sick leave hours, and the results are summarised in Table 6.2. How many employees need to participate in the sample to estimate the ratio of $\frac{Y}{X}$ with a significance level of 0.05 and a margin of error of 0.01 hours?

Note: A margin of error is expressed as $B = 1.96\frac{S}{\sqrt{n}}$ (Scheaffer et al., 2011, p. 83).

Solution: To estimate the ratio r using the sampled data from Table 6.2, we calculate:

$$r = \frac{\sum_{i=1}^{10} y_i}{\sum_{i=1}^{10} x_i} = \frac{175}{164} = 1.067$$

Next, we estimate the variance of r using Equation 6.12. We first calculate the following:

$$\text{Sum of squares of x: } \sum x_i^2$$

$$\text{Sum of squares of y: } \Sigma y_i^2$$

$$\text{Sum of products of x and y: } \Sigma x_i \cdot y_i$$

Using the values provided in the table:

$$\hat{\sigma}_r^2 = \frac{\sum_{i=1}^{n}(y_i - r.\, x_i)^2}{n-1} = \frac{\sum_{i=1}^{n} y_i^2 + r^2 \sum_{i=1}^{n} x_i^2 - 2r \sum_{i=1}^{n} x_i.\, y_i}{n-1}$$

Calculating gives

$$\hat{\sigma}_r^2 = \frac{4319 + \left(1.067^2 \times 3870\right) - \left(2 \times 1.067 \times 4077\right)}{9-1} = \frac{24.634}{8} = 3.079$$

The estimation error is set at 0.01 hours per employee. To estimate the sample size for the population mean, we multiply the desired margin of error by the mean (Scheaffer et al., 2011, p. 180).

$$d = d_0 \times \mu_x \tag{6.14}$$

For this example:

$$d = d_0 \times \mu_x = 0.01 \times 16.30 = 0.163$$

The sample size required to estimate the population mean is calculated as follows:

$$n_o = \frac{z^2 . \sigma_r^2}{d^2} = \frac{(1.96^2 \times 3.079)}{(0.16.3)^2} = 445.23 \approx 446$$

Since the sampling fraction ($\frac{n_0}{N} = \frac{446}{1000} > 0.05$), we must apply the finite population correction (FPC).

Therefore, the final sample size is

$$n = \frac{N \times n_0}{N + n_0} = \frac{1000 \times 446}{1000 + 446} = 308.44 \approx 309$$

The required sample size for this study is 309 employees.

TABLE 6.3

Systolic Blood Pressure for a Sample of 11 Participants from Two Sources

	Systolic Blood Pressure		
Employee	**Last Year (x)**	**Current Year (y)**	$x.y$
1	108	129	13932
2	136	107	14552
3	122	132	16104
4	115	102	11730
5	143	95	13585
6	107	111	11877
7	103	96	9888
8	119	94	11186
9	130	117	15210
10	119	92	10948
11	118	91	10738
Sum	1320	1166	139750
Mean	120	106	–
Sum of squares	159922	125750	–

Exercise 6.14: A research study on the effects of exercise on blood pressure aims to estimate changes in systolic blood pressure compared to last year. The study has access to the medical records of 1,000 participants, all of whom had an average systolic blood pressure of 120 mmHg last year. A small pilot study involving 11 participants was conducted to analyse their blood pressure after exercise, and the results are summarised in Table 6.3. How many additional participants need to be included in the study to estimate the ratio of $\frac{Y}{X}$ with a significance level of 0.05 and a margin of error of 10 mmHg?

Solution: We are estimating the ratio r using the sampled data provided in Table 6.3:

$$r = \frac{\bar{y}}{\bar{x}} = \frac{106}{120} = 0.883$$

To estimate the variance of r using Equation 6.12, we first calculate the following:

$$\text{Sum of squares of } x\text{: } \sum x_i^2$$

$$\text{Sum of squares of } y\text{: } \sum y_i^2$$

$$\text{Sum of products of } x \text{ and } y\text{: } \sum x_i \cdot y_i$$

Using these values, the variance of r is calculated as

$$\hat{\sigma}_r^2 = \frac{\sum_{i=1}^{n}(y_i - rx_i)^2}{n-1} = \frac{\sum_{i=1}^{n} y_i^2 + r^2\sum_{i=1}^{n} x_i^2 - 2r\sum_{i=1}^{n} x_i y_i}{n-1}$$

Substituting the values, we have

$$\hat{\sigma}_r^2 = \frac{125750 + (0.883^2 \times 159922) - (2 \times 0.883 \times 139750)}{11-1}$$

Calculating this gives

$$\hat{\sigma}_r^2 = \frac{17615.924}{10} = 1761.6$$

The estimation error is set at 10 mmHg. To estimate the required sample size for the population mean, we need to calculate:

$$n_o = \frac{z^2 . \sigma_r^2}{d^2} = \frac{1.96^2 \times 1761.6}{10^2} = 67.67 \cong 68$$

Therefore, the study requires approximately 68 additional participants to achieve the desired level of precision in estimating the ratio of systolic blood pressure changes.

Example 6.15: A health expert is trying to estimate the average number of patients with a newly emerged disease in the state (μ_y) to ensure proper drug and equipment supply. Given the state's large size, with 350 districts, it is impractical to count all patients, and there is an increased risk of disease transmission. The expert can obtain necessary information and population data for different regional areas from the provincial statistics centre to calculate the average population (μ_x). By selecting a sample of n districts and counting the number of patients in each, the expert can use the ratio estimation method to estimate the actual mean number of patients (μ_y). How many districts need to be included in the sample to estimate μ_y with a 0.05 significance level and a margin of error of 100 people?

Solution: Since there is no prior information available on the number of newly emerging patients, it is recommended that a pilot study be conducted to estimate the variance of the ratio of the actual number of patients to the

TABLE 6.4

Number of Patients and Population for Eight Areas from Two Sources

	Number of Patients		
Centre	**Population (x)**	**Patients (y)**	$x.y$
1	25	23	575
2	15	14	210
3	22	20	440
4	24	25	600
5	13	12	156
6	18	18	324
7	35	30	1050
8	30	27	810
Total	182	169	4165
SS	4528	3847	–

population data provided by the state statistical centre. To achieve this, eight regions are selected, and the total number of patients (y) is determined.

Additionally, the population under coverage (in thousands) (x) for each region is provided by the State Statistical Center. The results are summarised in Table 6.4.

The ratio r is calculated as follows:

$$\mathbf{r} = \frac{\sum y_i}{\sum x_i} = \frac{\mathbf{182}}{\mathbf{169}} = \mathbf{1.077}$$

To estimate the variance of r, we use the following formula:

$$\hat{\sigma}_r^2 = \frac{\sum_{i=1}^{n} (y_i - rx_i)^2}{n-1} = \frac{\sum_{i=1}^{n} y_i^2 + r^2 \sum_{i=1}^{n} x_i^2 - 2r \sum_{i=1}^{n} x_i y_i}{n-1}$$

Substituting the values gives

$$\hat{\sigma}_r^2 = \frac{4528 + (1.077^2 \times 3847) - (2 \times 1.077 \times 4165)}{8-1}$$

Calculating these yields

$$\hat{\sigma}_r^2 = \frac{18.837}{7} = 2.69$$

The sample size required to estimate the population mean is calculated as follows:

$$n_o = \frac{z^2.\sigma_r^2}{d^2} = \frac{1.96^2 \times 2.69}{1} = 10.34 \cong 11$$

Since the sampling fraction is less than 5%, the finite population correction (FPC) can be ignored. Therefore, the expert needs to include 11 districts in the sample to accurately estimate the average number of patients with the newly emerged disease.

References

Bhuyan, K. (2021). *Design of experiments and sampling methods.* New Central Book Agency.

Chow, S.-C., Shao, J., Wang, H., & Lokhnygina, Y. (2017). *Sample size calculations in clinical research.* Chapman and Hall and CRC Press.

Gossop, M., Strang, J., Griffiths, P., Powis, B., & Taylor, C. (1994). A ratio estimation method for determining the prevalence of cocaine use. *The British Journal of Psychiatry, 164*(5), 676–679.

Julious, S., & Campbell, M. J. (1998). Sample size calculations for paired or matched ordinal data. *Statistics in Medicine, 17*(14), 1635–1642.

Latpate, R., Kshirsagar, J., Gupta, V. K., & Chandra, G. (2021). *Advanced sampling methods.* Springer.

Malone, H. E., Nicholl, H., & Coyne, I. (2016). Fundamentals of estimating sample size. *Nurse Researcher, 23*(5), 21–25.

Rosner, B. A. (2006). *Fundamentals of biostatistics* (Vol. 6). Thomson-Brooks.

Samawi, H. M., & Siam, M. I. (2003). Ratio estimation using stratified ranked set sample. *Metron – International Journal of Statistics, 61*(1), 75–90.

Scheaffer, R. L., Mendenhall III, W., Ott, R. L., & Gerow, K. G. (2011). *Elementary survey sampling.* Cengage Learning.

Thompson, S. K. (2012). *Sampling* (Vol. 755). John Wiley & Sons.

Triola, M. M., Triola, M. F., & Roy, J. A. (2006). *Biostatistics for the biological and health sciences.* Pearson Addison-Wesley Boston.

7

Sample Size for Disease Proportions in Clinical Research

7.1 Introduction

In certain situations, researchers may wish to estimate the proportion, rate, ratio, prevalence or percentage of units in a population that possess a specific characteristic or fall into a defined category. When measuring a characteristic that represents the presence or absence of a dichotomous attribute, it is often desirable to estimate the proportion of elementary units in the population that exhibit this attribute. Commonly, census or survey results are expressed as proportions, such as the number of unemployed individuals, the percentage of immigrants in a population, or the proportion of urban residents. This classification may be obtained directly through simple "yes" or "no" questions or indirectly through the categorisation and tabulation of responses to quantitative questions. For example, by asking participants their ages and then tabulating the responses, we can determine the percentage of the population aged 60 years and over.

If the attribute is denoted by x and X represents the total number of elementary units in the population that possess this attribute, then the population proportion is denoted by P and defined as $P = \frac{X}{N}$, which can be estimated by the sample proportion $p = \frac{x}{n}$.

In statistical analysis, the binomial distribution is frequently used to estimate a proportion p, with its variance given by $p(1-p)$. Consequently, the appropriate test for comparing two independent proportions, or for comparing a single observed proportion with a specified value, is the z-test (Cochran & Inc, 1977, p. 50; Levy & Lemeshow, 2013, p. 14; Lwanga et al., 1991; Malone et al., 2016, p. 4).

In this chapter, we outline the methodology for determining the required sample size for each of the scenarios mentioned above and provide illustrative examples.

DOI: 10.1201/9781003749783-7

7.2 Sample Size for Estimating a Proportion with Constant Precision

When the goal of a study is to estimate a proportion, ratio, prevalence rate, incidence rate, or percentage in a population (p), we can utilise the fact that the variance of a proportion, which follows a binomial distribution, is equal to $p(1-p)$. Similar to the method for calculating sample size for the mean discussed in Chapter 6, and ignoring the finite population correction (FPC), the required minimum sample size can be calculated using the following formula:

$$n = z_{1-\alpha/2}^2 \times \frac{p(1-p)}{d^2} \tag{7.1}$$

In this formula, P represents an estimate of the proportion or ratio of the attribute in the reference population, which can be obtained from similar studies, previous research, or expert opinion. However, these formulas depend on the unknown population proportion p.

When the population proportion p is uncertain and could take a wide range of values, it is advisable to choose a value close to 0.5. Selecting a value near 0.5 will yield the largest required sample size, because $p(1-p)$ reaches its maximum at $p = 0.5$. Therefore, if an estimate of p is unavailable prior to the survey, or if the researcher is uncertain about the value of P in the population or expects it to fall within a range, it is recommended to adopt a conservative estimate closest to 0.5 for P in the formula. This approach ensures that the sample size will be sufficient, regardless of the actual value of the true proportion.

TIP

If the researcher is uncertain about the population proportion P or expects it to fall within a range of values, it is recommended to use a conservative estimate closest to 0.5 for P in the formula.

The quantity $p(1-p)$, and consequently the value of n required by the formula, reaches its maximum when $p = 1/2$ (Lemeshow et al., 1988, p. 2; Thompson, 2012, p. 60). However, an approximate estimate of P is generally sufficient for planning purposes. The following table and figure illustrate that $p(1-p)$ decreases as the value of p deviates further from 0.5.

p	0.1	0.2	0.3	0.4	0.5	0.6	0.7	0.8	0.9
P(1-p)	0.09	0.16	0.21	0.24	0.25	0.24	0.21	0.16	0.09

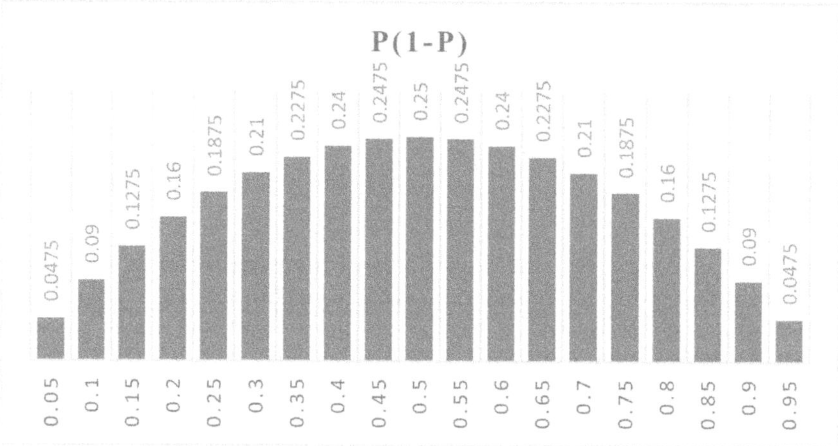

The maximum acceptable estimation error, or precision, is denoted by $d = |p - P|$, where P is the true proportion in the population and p is the proportion anticipated by the researcher for the sample. This difference is taken into account in practice to define d and ensure sufficient accuracy in the estimation process.

> **Example 7.1:** A public opinion polling organisation aims to estimate the percentage of residents in a small town with a population of 11,000 who will vote in the upcoming election. How many samples are needed for this survey to estimate the proportion of voters with a 5% significance level and a precision of 4%? In the last election, neighbouring towns reported voter turnout rates ranging from 35% to 60%.

Solution: Given that the voter turnout rate varies between 35% and 60%, we choose $p = 0.50$ to ensure the largest required sample size and therefore the most precise estimation.

$$n_0 = \frac{(z_{1-\frac{\alpha}{2}})^2\, p(1-p)}{d^2} = \frac{(1.96)^2 \times 0.5 \times (1-0.5)}{0.04^2} = 600.25 \approx 601$$

The finite population correction (FPC) is applied because it is greater than 0.05

$$FPC = \frac{601}{11000} = 0.055 > 0.05$$

The corrected sample size is

$$n = \frac{N \times n_0}{N + n_0} = \frac{11000 \times 601}{11000 + 601} = 569.86 \approx 570$$

Example 7.2: An immunologist is planning to determine the percentage of children who have received full vaccinations. What sample size should be used to ensure that 95% of the estimate is within 10% of the actual rate? The researcher lacks prior information about vaccination coverage.

Solution: In the absence of prior information regarding vaccination coverage, the most conservative approach is to use $p = 0.5$. This choice maximises $p(1-p)$ and ensures the largest required sample size, providing the most precise estimation.

The sample size can be calculated using the standard formula for estimating a proportion:

$$n = \frac{z_{1-\alpha/2}^2 \, p(1-p)}{d^2} = 1.96^2 \times \frac{0.5 \times (1-0.5)}{(0.10)^2} = 96.04 \approx 97$$

Example 7.3: What should the sample size be in Example 7.2 if we want to reduce the estimation error to 5%? Can you explain why the sample size has increased?

Solution: By reducing the estimation error from $d = 0.10$ to $d = 0.05$ in the denominator of the sample size formula, the resulting fraction quadruples. This occurs because the denominator is squared in the formula. Consequently, the new sample size should be approximately four times the original, as shown below:

$$n_0 = 1.96^2 \times \frac{0.5 \times (1-0.5)}{(0.05)^2} = 384.16 \approx 385$$

The increase in sample size occurs because reducing the margin of error requires more observations to maintain the same level of confidence. Specifically, halving the estimation error (from 10% to 5%) increases the sample size by a factor of four due to the square of the denominator in the formula.

To facilitate the calculation of sample size when estimating a population proportion, the second term of Formula 7.1, $p(1-p)/d^2$, is computed for various margins of error ranging from 1% to 40%, and for different proportions up to 50%. This information is presented in Table 7.1.

TABLE 7.1

The Second Term of the Sample Size Calculation, $\frac{p(1-p)}{d^2}$, for Estimating a Population Proportion with a Constant Estimation Error (Specified Precision), Excluding the Terms Corresponding to Confidence Level and Statistical Power

d												
0.40	0.33	0.30	0.25	0.20	0.15	0.10	0.05	0.04	0.03	0.02	0.01	*p*
–	–	–	–	–	–	–	19	29.7	52.8	118.8	475	0.05
–	–	–	–	–	–	9	36	56.3	100	225	900	0.10
–	–	–	–	–	5.7	12.8	51	79.7	141.7	318.8	1275	0.15
–	–	–	–	4.0	7.1	16	64	100	177.8	400	1600	0.20
–	–	–	3	4.7	8.3	18.8	75	117.2	208.3	468.8	1875	0.25
–	–	2.3	3.4	5.3	9.3	21	84	131.3	233.3	525	2100	0.30
–	2.1	2.5	3.6	5.7	10.1	22.8	91	142.2	252.8	568.8	2275	0.35
1.5	2.2	2.7	3.8	6.0	10.7	24	96	150	266.7	600	2400	0.40
1.5	2.3	2.8	4.0	6.2	11.0	24.8	99	154.7	275	618.8	2475	0.45
1.6	2.3	2.8	4.0	6.3	11.1	25	100	156.3	277.8	625	2500	0.50

Note: When dealing with proportions greater than 0.50, it is advisable to use the complementary value $(1-p)$. For instance, if the proportion is $p = 0.70$, the complementary proportion $1-0.70 = 0.30$ should be used in the calculation. To calculate the sample size for your study, first locate the cell in Table 7.1 that corresponds to your selected proportion and margin of error. Next, multiply this value by the squared critical value corresponding to the desired confidence level.

For example, to determine the required sample size for Example 7.1, multiply $1.96^2 = 3.84$ by 156.3:

$$1.96^2 \times 156.3 = 3.8416 \times 156.3 = 600.44 \approx 601$$

Thus, the required sample size is approximately 601.

7.3 Sample Size for Estimating a Proportion with Relative Precision

It is important to note that the precision of estimation can sometimes be defined as *relative precision*, expressed as a fraction or percentage of the proportion p. In this case, the estimation error ε is defined as a function of the actual population proportion:

$$d = \varepsilon \times p$$

For instance, the proportion in the population is required to fall within 10% of the true value, rather than reflecting an absolute difference of 10% from the actual proportion or the mean ± 10%.

By substituting $d = \varepsilon \times p$ into the standard sample size formula, the proportion p in the numerator cancels with one factor of p in the denominator, yielding:

$$n = \left(z_{1-\frac{\alpha}{2}}\right)^2 \times \frac{p(1-p)}{d^2} = \left(z_{1-\frac{\alpha}{2}}\right)^2 \times \frac{p(1-p)}{(\varepsilon . p)^2} = \left(z_{1-\frac{\alpha}{2}}\right)^2 \times \frac{(1-p)}{\varepsilon^2 . p}$$

Thus, the sample size formula for relative precision becomes (Indrayan & Holt, 2016, p. 548; Levy & Lemeshow, 2013, p. 73; Lwanga et al., 1991, p. 2):

$$n = \left(z_{1-\frac{\alpha}{2}}\right)^2 \times \frac{(1-P)}{\varepsilon^2 . P} \tag{7.2}$$

It is important to remember that when the margin of error or precision is expressed as a *function or percentage of the proportion*, the calculated sample size will always be maximised if the smallest proportion in the expected range is selected. This ensures a sufficiently large and conservative sample. The rationale is that the complementary term $(1-p)$ in the numerator becomes larger when p is smaller, as shown:

TIP

Relative precision is calculated by subtracting the estimate from the true value and dividing the result by the true value, providing a measure of the accuracy of the estimation.

$$\frac{p(1-p)}{d^2} = \frac{p(1-p)}{(\varepsilon \times p)^2} = \frac{1-p}{\varepsilon^2 \times p}$$

Example 7.4: A study has been planned to estimate the prevalence of pulmonary tuberculosis (TB) in Kermanshah Province. Currently, no data on TB prevalence in the province exist, and comparable studies from other provinces are not available. However, experts predict that the prevalence is unlikely to be lower than 3 per thousand (0.003). If the objective is to estimate the prevalence with a precision equal to one-quarter of the true prevalence, how many residents should be included in the study?

Solution: Because there is no existing information about TB prevalence in the province, the minimum predicted prevalence ($p = 0.003$) is used for the sample-size calculation. The desired precision (d) is one-quarter of the true proportion:

$$d = \frac{p}{4} = \frac{0.003}{4} = 0.00075.$$

Using a 5% significance level ($Z = 1.96$) and assuming a large reference population (so that finite population correction can be ignored), the required sample size is calculated using Equation 7.2:

$$n = \left(z_{1-\frac{\alpha}{2}}\right)^2 \times \frac{(1-P)}{\varepsilon^2 . P} = (1.96)^2 \times \frac{(1-0.003)}{\left(\frac{1}{4}\right)^2 \times 0.003} = 20427$$

Therefore, at least 20,427 residents should be included in the study to estimate the prevalence of TB in Kermanshah Province with 95% confidence and a precision equal to one-quarter of the true prevalence (i.e., from 2.25 to 3.75 per thousand).

TIP

In sample size calculations for a proportion, when relative precision is used and p lies within a given range, the smallest value of p should be used to ensure a conservatively large sample size. This is because, in this case, the term $\left[\frac{1-p}{p}\right]$ is maximised, resulting in a larger required sample size.

Example 7.5: The objective of this study is to determine the proportion of pregnant women who seek prenatal care during the first trimester of pregnancy. How many participants are required to estimate this proportion with 95% confidence and within 5% of the true proportion? It is anticipated that the percentage of women seeking this care will fall between 25% and 40%.

Solution: The expected proportion in this population ranges from 25% to 40%. To calculate the sample size conservatively, we choose the smallest proportion value ($p = 0.25$), which ensures a larger sample size. Using a confidence level of 95% ($z_{1-\frac{\alpha}{2}} = 1.96$) and a desired estimation error of $\varepsilon = 0.05$, the required sample size is calculated as follows:

$$n = (z_{1-\frac{\alpha}{2}})^2 \times \frac{(1-P)}{\varepsilon^2 . P} = (1.96)^2 \times \frac{(1-0.25)}{0.05^2 \times 0.25} = 4607$$

If we choose $p = 0.40$, the sample size is

$$n = (z_{1-\frac{\alpha}{2}})^2 \times \frac{(1-P)}{\varepsilon^2 . P} = (1.96)^2 \times \frac{(1-0.40)}{0.05^2 \times 0.40} = 2305$$

This demonstrates that using a smaller anticipated proportion yields a larger required sample size, which is a conservative approach.

To provide a clearer understanding and assist readers, we calculated the second term of the sample size formula:

$$\frac{1-p}{\varepsilon^2 p}$$

for common proportions ranging from 0.05 to 0.80, with relative precision (ε) expressed as fractions from 0.01 to 0.40. The results are summarised in Table 7.2, which excludes the multiplicative term for the confidence level Z^2.

In Table 7.2, the term $\left[\frac{(1-p)}{\varepsilon^2 \times p}\right]$ is calculated for various proportions and relative errors, with estimation errors (ε) ranging from 0.01 to 0.40.

It is important to note that when the expected value of p is 0, 1, or very close to these extremes, the formula above (Equation 7.2) should not be used. In such cases, the alternative method described by Machin et al. should be applied (Machin et al., 2018, p. 139).

7.4 Sample Size for Equality Test of a Population Proportion with a Constant Proportion

Suppose we want to conduct a hypothesis test for $H_0 : p = p_0$ versus $H_1 : p \neq p_0$. To perform a two-sided test with a significance level α and a power of $1-\beta$ for the specific alternative hypothesis $H_1 : p = p_a$, we can calculate the required sample size. In this scenario, p_0 represents the success rate or proportion under H_0, while p_a is the medically significant value of the population proportion under H_A. The study aims to test the equality of proportions against a known or reference proportion.

The null hypothesis is $H_0 : p = p_0$, and the alternative hypothesis is $H_A : p \neq p_0$, specifically $H_A : p = p_a$. The number of subjects needed in a single group to detect the proposed difference $d = p_0 - p_a$, given a significance level α and a power of $1-\beta$, can be calculated using the following formula (Rosner, 2006, p. 257):

$$n = \frac{p_0 \cdot (1 - p_0)\left(z_{1-\frac{\alpha}{2}} + z_{1-\beta}\sqrt{\frac{p_a \cdot (1-p_a)}{p_o \cdot (1-p_o)}}\right)^2}{(p_a - p_o)^2} \tag{7.3a}$$

There is an equivalent equation for calculating the sample size when testing the equality of a proportion with a reference proportion. This equation can be found in Chow et al. (2017, p. 76; Indrayan & Holt, 2016, p. 555; Machin et al., 2018, p. 44):

$$n = \frac{\left(Z_{1-\frac{\alpha}{2}} \cdot \sqrt{p_o(1-p_o)} + Z_{1-\beta}\sqrt{p_a(1-p_a)}\right)^2}{(p_o - p_a)^2} \tag{7.3b}$$

TABLE 7.2

Second Term of the Sample Size Calculation $\left[\dfrac{(1-p)}{\varepsilon^2 \times p}\right]$ for Common Proportions, with a Relative Estimation Error (Determined Precision)

ε												
0.40	**0.33**	**0.30**	**0.25**	**0.20**	**0.15**	**0.10**	**0.05**	**0.04**	**0.03**	**0.02**	**0.01**	p
118.8	171.3	211.1	304	475	844.4	1900	7600	11875	21111	47500	190000	**0.05**
56.3	81.2	100	144	225	400	900	3600	5625	10000	22500	90000	**0.10**
35.4	51.1	63	90.7	141.7	251.9	566.7	2267	3542	6296	14167	56667	**0.15**
25	36.1	44.4	64	100	177.8	400	1600	2500	4444	10000	40000	**0.20**
18.8	27.1	33.3	48	75	133.3	300	1200	1875	3333	7500	30000	**0.25**
14.6	21	25.9	37.3	58.3	103.7	233.3	933	1458	2593	5833	23333	**0.30**
11.6	16.7	20.6	29.7	46.4	82.5	185.7	743	1161	2063	4643	18571	**0.35**
9.4	13.5	16.7	24	37.5	66.7	150	600	938	1667	3750	15000	**0.40**
7.6	11	13.6	19.6	30.6	54.3	122.2	489	764	1358	3056	12222	**0.45**
6.3	9	11.1	16	25	44.4	100	400	625	1111	2500	10000	**0.50**
5.1	7.4	9.1	13.1	20.5	36.4	81.8	327	511	909	2045	8182	**0.55**
4.2	6	7.4	10.7	16.7	29.6	66.7	267	417	741	1667	6667	**0.60**
3.4	4.9	6	8.6	13.5	23.9	53.8	215	337	598	1346	5385	**0.65**
2.7	3.9	4.8	6.9	10.7	19	42.9	171	268	476	1071	4286	**0.70**
2.1	3	3.7	5.3	8.3	14.8	33.3	133	208	370	833	3333	**0.75**
1.6	2.3	2.8	4	6.3	11.1	25	100	156	278	625	2500	**0.80**

Note: The table does not include the factor corresponding to power or significance level.

Example 7.6: Let us assume that the prevalence rate of breast cancer among individuals over 50 years old in the population is 2.5%. Research indicates that women with a family history of breast cancer have a 6% risk of developing the disease. We want to determine how many women aged over 50 should participate in the study to achieve 85% power using a two-sided significance test with $\alpha = 0.05$.

Solution: The given data are $p_0 = 0.025$, $p_a = 0.06$, $\alpha = 0.05$, and $1-\beta = 0.85$. Using the corresponding values from the standard normal distribution, which are $z_{1-\alpha/2} = 1.96$ and $z_{1-\beta} = 1.04$, we can substitute them into Equation 7.3a. The sample size is calculated as:

$$n = \frac{p_0 \cdot (1-p_0)\left(z_{1-\frac{\alpha}{2}} + z_{1-\beta}\sqrt{\frac{p_a \cdot (1-p_a)}{p_o \cdot (1-p_o)}}\right)^2}{(p_a - p_o)^2}$$

Substituting the values:

$$n = \frac{0.025 \times 0.975\left(1.96 + 1.04\sqrt{\frac{0.06 \times 0.94}{0.025 \times 0.975}}\right)^2}{(0.06 - 0.025)^2}$$

Calculating this gives

$$n = \frac{0.024375 \times 3.5420}{0.001225} = 249.63 \approx 250$$

Using Equation 7.3b also yields the same sample size:

$$n = \frac{\left(Z_{1-\frac{\alpha}{2}} \cdot \sqrt{p_o(1-p_o)} + Z_{1-\beta}\sqrt{p_a(1-p_a)}\right)^2}{(p_o - p_a)^2}$$

Substituting the values:

$$n = \frac{\left(1.96\sqrt{0.025(1-0.025)} + 1.04\sqrt{0.06(1-0.06)}\right)^2}{(0.06 - 0.025)^2}$$

Calculating these terms:

$$n = \frac{0.3058}{0.001225} = 249.63 \approx 250$$

Therefore, 250 women with a family history of breast cancer must participate to achieve 85% power for detecting a significant difference using a two-sided test with $\alpha = 0.05$, assuming that the true rate of breast cancer among women with a family history is 2.4 times higher than that of a typical woman over 50 years old.

> **Example 7.7:** Previous studies have reported a 70% success rate for a surgical operation used to treat a specific type of heart disease. A new treatment claims to have a comparable success rate. Another hospital, which lacks sufficient personnel and equipment for surgery, has decided to use the new treatment method for their patients if its success rate is equal to that of the usual treatment within a margin of error of 5%.

How many patients must be included in their study to ensure that the new treatment has an equal success rate, with 80% power and a significance level of 5%?

Solution: In this two-tailed test, the alternative hypothesis is $H_A : p = 0.65$. Given that the success rate under the null hypothesis is 70%, we have $p_0 = 0.70$ and $p_a = 0.65$. The researcher aims to detect at most a 5% difference in the success rate from the null hypothesis.

An 80% test power corresponds to a z-score of 0.84, and a two-sided significance level of $\alpha = 0.05$ corresponds to $z_{1-\alpha/2} = 1.96$. Substituting these values into the sample size formula:

$$n = \frac{\left[1.96\sqrt{0.70(1-0.70)} + 0.84\sqrt{0.65(1-0.65)}\right]^2}{(0.70-0.65)^2}$$

Calculating this gives:

$$n = \frac{1.2988}{0.0025} = 674.79 \approx 675$$

Therefore, 675 patients must be included in the study to ensure that the new treatment has an equal success rate, with 80% power and a significance level of 5%.

Since the success rate under the null hypothesis is 70%, we again have $p_0 = 0.70$ and $p_a = 0.65$. The researcher is looking to detect at most a 5% difference in the success rate from the null hypothesis; therefore, $p_a = 0.65$. An 80% power corresponds to a z-score of 0.84, and a two-sided significance level of 5% corresponds to $z_{1-\alpha/2} = 1.96$. Substituting these values into Equation 7.3b, the sample size is calculated as follows:

$$n = \frac{\left[1.96 \times \sqrt{0.70(1-0.70)} + 0.84 \times \sqrt{0.65(1-0.65)}\right]^2}{(0.70-0.65)^2}$$

Performing the calculation:

$$n = \frac{1.2988}{0.0025} = 674.79 \cong 675$$

Thus, using Equation 7.3b also yields the same required sample size.

> **Example 7.8:** The national proportion of pregnant women seeking prenatal care during the first trimester is 65%. A local health department aims to compare its success in providing similar care services with the national level. They seek to establish equality, allowing for a threshold of up to a 5% difference from the national rate. Any difference greater than 5% (i.e., below 60%) would not be considered equal. Thus, the alternative hypothesis is $H_A : p < 0.60$. How many pregnant women should be included in the local study to compare its success rate and potentially reject the equality of prenatal care services relative to the national level?

Solution: This test is one-tailed since the alternative hypothesis is $H_A : p < 0.60$. We substitute the following values: $p_0 = 0.65$, $p_a = 0.60$, and $d = 0.05$. A power of 0.85 corresponds to a z-score of 1.04, while a value of 1.645 is used for the 5% one-tailed significance level. These values are substituted into Equations 7.3a or 7.3b to determine the required sample size.

The sample size is calculated using Equations 7.3a:

$$n = \frac{p_0.(1-p_0)\left(z_{1-\frac{\alpha}{2}} + z_{1-\beta}\sqrt{\frac{p_a.(1-p_a)}{p_o.(1-p_o)}}\right)^2}{(p_a - p_o)^2}$$

Substituting the values, we have

$$n = \frac{0.65 \times 0.35\left(1.645 + 1.04\sqrt{\frac{0.60 \times 0.40}{0.65 \times 0.35}}\right)^2}{(0.65 - 0.60)^2}$$

Calculating this gives

$$n = \frac{0.2275 \times 2.7132}{0.0025} = 246.9 \approx 247$$

To enhance understanding and assist readers, we also use Equation 7.3b for testing the equality of a population proportion. This equation is particularly suitable for proportions typically ranging from 0.05 to 0.60, as shown in Table 7.3.

TABLE 7.3

Sample Size Calculation for a Two-Tailed Test of Proportion with 80% Power and 5% Significance Level

p_0												
0.70	0.60	0.50	0.45	0.40	0.35	0.30	0.25	0.20	0.15	0.10	0.05	p_a
*	5	7	9	11	14	19	27	42	78	238	–	0.05
*	6	10	13	17	23	34	54	108	363	–	185	0.10
5	8	14	19	26	39	64	132	470	–	316	53	0.15
7	11	20	28	43	72	153	562	–	430	86	26	0.20
8	15	29	45	78	169	637	–	527	114	41	16	0.25
11	21	47	83	181	697	–	609	137	53	24	11	0.30
14	30	85	190	741	–	675	157	63	31	16	8	0.35
20	48	194	770	–	726	172	71	36	20	12	6	0.40
28	85	782	–	760	183	77	41	24	14	9	5	0.45
44	191	–	779	191	82	44	26	17	11	7	*	0.50
172	–	194	86	48	30	20	13	9	7	*	*	0.60
–	181	47	30	21	15	11	8	6	*	*	*	0.70

**Sample size less than 5.*

7.5 Sample Size for Confidence Intervals for One Proportion

This procedure calculates the sample size needed to achieve a specified margin of error (*E*) for a single population proportion. The margin of error, E, represents the difference between the sample proportion ($\hat{p}$) and the population proportion $\left(E = \hat{p} - p\right)$. The margin of error (*E*) for a confidence interval of a single population proportion is defined as follows:

In this equation, *z* is the *z*-score such that the area under the standard normal distribution between −*z* and +*z* corresponds to the desired confidence level. We can rearrange this equation to solve for *n* (Lohr, 2021, p. 48; Machin et al., 2018, p. 139; Navidi & Monk, 2013, p. 393):

$$n = \left(\frac{z}{E}\right)^2 \times p \times (1 - p) \tag{7.4}$$

This formula indicates that the sample size (n) is influenced by the margin of error (E), the estimated proportion $(\hat{p})$, and the significance level. Therefore, to determine the sample size (n), we need values for z, E, and p.

> **Example 7.9:** Some parents believe that learning a specific type of music can positively impact academic performance. To evaluate this belief, determine the sample size required to obtain a 95% confidence interval for the population proportion with a margin of error of 0.05.

Solution: The specified confidence level is 95%, which corresponds to a z-value of $z_{1-\alpha/2} = 1.96$. Since we do not have an available value for $\hat{p}$, we use the conservative estimate of 0.50 to produce the maximum required sample size. The desired margin of error is $E = 0.05$.

Substituting these values into the formula gives

$$n = 0.5 \times 0.5 \left(\frac{z_{1-\frac{\alpha}{2}}}{E}\right)^2 = 0.25\left(\frac{1.96}{0.05}\right)^2 = 384.16 \cong 385$$

We estimate that a sample of 385 parents is required to obtain a 95% confidence interval with a margin of error of 0.05.

> **Example 7.10:** Let us consider a scenario in which we want to use random sampling with a 95% confidence level to estimate the proportion of participants in the upcoming national presidential election who plan to vote. Our goal is to ensure that the estimate is within 3% of the true voter proportion. How many individuals should be sampled?

Solution: Because no prior information about the anticipated proportion is available, we use $p = 0.50$ to obtain the maximum possible sample size:

$$n = 0.5 \times 0.5 \left(\frac{z_{1-\frac{\alpha}{2}}}{E} \right)^2 = 0.25 \left(\frac{1.96}{0.03} \right)^2 = 1067.11 \approx 1068$$

Most public opinion polls typically use a sample size of approximately 1,100, which is obtained by rounding the value from Example 7.10 to the nearest hundred. It is important to note that the population size in such surveys is usually much larger than the sample size, allowing us to ignore the finite population correction (FPC). For very large populations, the precision of an opinion poll depends primarily on the sample size rather than on the proportion of the population that is sampled (Lohr, 2021, p. 48).

> **Example 7.11:** The Regional Health Organisation aims to estimate the prevalence of tuberculosis (TB) in children under 5 years of age within its coverage area. They need to determine the sample size required to estimate TB prevalence with 5% Type I error and confidence limits that are no more than 4% from the true prevalence rate. The researchers do not expect the actual prevalence of TB to exceed 20%. How many children should be included in the sample?

Solution: A 5% Type I error (significance level) corresponds to a z-value of 1.96, and we will use the maximum expected prevalence rate of 20% for the calculation. Given that the margin of error is E = 0.04, the required sample size can be computed as follows:

$$n = p(1-p)\left(\frac{z_{1-\alpha/2}}{E} \right)^2 = 0.2 \times 0.8 \left(\frac{z_{1-\frac{\alpha}{2}}}{E} \right)^2 = 0.16 \left(\frac{1.96}{0.04} \right)^2 = 384.16 \cong 385$$

Therefore, 385 children must be included in the sample to estimate TB prevalence with 5% Type I error and a margin of error of ±4%, assuming the true prevalence rate does not exceed 20%.

7.6 Sample Size Determination to Compare Two Independent Proportions

Comparing proportions in two independent populations – similar to comparing means between two groups – is a common objective in descriptive and analytical studies. Let p_1 and p_2 represent the expected proportions or disease rates in the two populations, and let $d = p_1 - p_2$ denote the estimation error. The required sample size for each group to compare the difference between two population proportions, at a specified significance level α and power $1-\beta$ for a two-tailed test, can be calculated using the following equation:

$$n_1 = n_2 = \frac{\left[Z_{1-\frac{\alpha}{2}} \cdot \sqrt{2\overline{p}(1-\overline{p})} + Z_{1-\beta} \cdot \sqrt{p_1(1-p_1)+p_2(1-p_2)}\right]^2}{(p_1-p_2)^2} \tag{7.5a}$$

The absolute precision or estimation error is defined as the detectable difference between the two population proportions ($d = p_1 - p_2$), where $\overline{p}$ is the average of the two proportions:

$$\overline{p} = \frac{p_1 + p_2}{2}.$$

Since the expressions under the square roots tend to remain relatively stable for reasonable values of the proportions, this equation is often simplified (Julious, p. 11) to:

$$n_1 = n_2 = \left(Z_{1-\frac{\alpha}{2}} + Z_{1-\beta}\right)^2 \times \frac{(p_1(1-p_1)+p_2(1-p_2))}{(p_1-p_2)^2} \tag{7.5b}$$

Example 7.12: How many participants should a researcher include in a study to detect the difference in the proportion of Alzheimer's disease among women compared to men over 65 years of age, with a power of 85% and a significance level of 0.05? Previous research indicates that among 890 men over age 65, 90 developed Alzheimer's disease, whereas among 1,222 women over age 65, 220 developed the disease.

Solution: The proportion for men is approximately $p_1 = 0.10$ (90/890), and for women it is approximately $p_2 = 0.18$(220/1222), yielding an average proportion $\overline{p} = \frac{p_1 + p_2}{2} = 0.14$. The z-value corresponding to a 5% significance level (two-tailed) is $Z_{1-\alpha/2} = 1.96$, and the z-value corresponding to a power of 85% is $Z_{1-\beta} = 1.04$. Using Equation 7.5a:

$$n = \frac{\left[Z_{1-\frac{\alpha}{2}} \cdot \sqrt{2\overline{P}(1-\overline{P})} + Z_{1-\beta} \cdot \sqrt{P_1(1-P_1)+P_2(1-P_2)}\right]^2}{(P_1-P_2)^2}$$

$$n = \frac{\left[1.96\sqrt{2 \times 0.14(1-0.14)} + 1.04\sqrt{0.10(1-0.10)+0.18(1-0.18)}\right]^2}{(0.18-0.10)^2}$$

Substituting the values:

$$n = \frac{\left[1.96.\sqrt{2 \times 0.14(1-0.14)} + 1.04.\sqrt{0.10(1-0.10)+0.18(1-0.18)}\right]^2}{(0.18-0.10)^2}$$

Calculating this gives

$$n = \frac{2.1572}{(0.08)^2} == 337.52 \cong 380$$

Approximately 338 participants per group. Therefore, 338 men and 338 women should be included in the study to detect the difference in Alzheimer's disease prevalence with 85% power and a 5% significance level.

> **Example 7.13:** There are two surgical methods to treat a specific type of disease: the standard method and a new method. The proportion of patients who experience problems after undergoing these two methods is 5% and 15%, respectively. If a researcher wants to determine, with 90% probability (power) and a significance level of 5%, whether the number of problems associated with the second surgical method is higher than with the first, how many samples should be chosen in each group?

Solution: This hypothesis test should be conducted as a *one-tailed test,* with the alternative hypothesis $H_A : P_1 - P_2 < 0$. The test has a power of 90%, corresponding to a z-value of 1.28, and a one-tailed significance level of 5%, corresponding to a z-value of 1.64.

The average proportion is calculated as

$$\bar{p} = \frac{P_1 + P_2}{2} = \frac{0.15+0.05}{2} = 0.10, \; p_2 = 0.05 \; and \; p_1 = 0.15$$

The required sample size for each group is given by

$$n = \frac{\left[1.28\sqrt{0.15 \times 0.85 + 0.05 \times 0.95} + 1.64\sqrt{2 \times 0.10 \times 0.90}\right]^2}{(0.15-0.05)^2} = 151.6 \approx 152$$

At least 152 samples per group are necessary to detect a significant difference in the proportion of patients experiencing problems with these two surgical methods, with 90% power and a significance level of 0.05.

Table 7.4 presents the calculated sample sizes based on Formula 7.5b for two-tailed equality testing of proportions in two populations. The common proportions range from 0.05 to 0.60.

TABLE 7.4

Sample Size Calculation for a Two-Tailed Test Comparing a Proportion to a Reference Proportion with 80% Power and a 5% Significance Level

P1												
0.70	0.60	0.50	0.45	0.40	0.35	0.30	0.25	0.20	0.15	0.10	0.05	P2
5	8	12	15	19	24	33	47	73	138	432	–	0.05
7	11	17	22	29	40	59	97	196	683	–	432	0.10
9	15	25	33	47	70	118	247	902	–	683	138	0.15
12	20	36	52	79	136	291	1090	–	902	196	73	0.20
16	28	55	86	149	326	1247	–	1090	247	97	47	0.25
21	40	91	160	353	1372	–	1247	291	118	59	33	0.30
28	59	167	373	1467	–	1373	326	136	70	40	24	0.35
40	95	385	1529	–	1467	353	149	78	47	29	19	0.40
58	170	1561	–	1529	373	160	86	52	33	22	15	0.45
91	385	–	1561	385	167	91	55	36	25	17	12	0.50
353	–	385	170	95	59	40	28	20	15	11	8	0.60
–	353	91	58	40	28	21	16	12	9	7	5	0.70

For example, if we assume $p_2 = 0.05$ *and* $p_1 = 0.15$, the required sample size is calculated as follows:

$$n_1 = (1.96 + 0.84)^2 \times \frac{[0.05(0.95) + 0.15(0.85)]}{(0.15 - 0.05)^2} = 137.2 \approx 138$$

Similarly, if we assume $p_2 = 0.15$ *and* $p_1 = 0.20$, the required sample size is:

$$n_1 = (2.8)^2 \times \frac{[0.15(0.85) + 0.20(0.80)]}{(0.20 - 0.15)^2} = 901.6 \approx 902$$

7.7 Sample Size Determination to Estimate the Difference between Two Proportions

In some studies, researchers aim to estimate the difference between two population proportions with absolute precision. This difference is referred to as the *risk difference (RD)*, denoted as $|p_1 - p_2|$, which reflects the absolute difference in risk between the two groups. However, instead of knowing the exact difference, an interval is established on both sides of the actual difference.

The following formula is used when a researcher wants to determine the sample size required to calculate the risk difference between two populations. It is important to note that, although this involves proportions and two populations, the *power of the test is not included* in the sample size calculation. Therefore, the sample size needed to estimate this difference can be calculated using the following formula (Lwanga et al., 1991, p. 9):

$$n = Z^2_{1-\frac{\alpha}{2}} \times \frac{[p_1(1-p_1) + p_2(1-p_2)]}{d^2} \tag{7.6}$$

where p_1 and p_2 are the expected proportions in the two populations, and d is the absolute precision required on both sides of the difference in proportions. If no information is available for either p_1, p_2, or both, it is recommended to use the conservative value of 0.5 to maximise the required sample size.

Example 7.14: An epidemiologist is interested in conducting a large study to estimate the difference in schistosomiasis risk between workers in an irrigation project and those not employed on the project. The goal is to determine the sample size needed from each group to estimate the *risk* difference within 5 percentage points of the actual difference, with

95% confidence. A pilot study in each area revealed disease rates of 40% and 32%, respectively.

Solution: The provided information includes $p_1 = 0.40$, $p_2 = 0.32$, $d = 0.05$, and a 5% significance level corresponding to $Z = 1.96$. Plugging these values into the sample size formula for estimating a risk difference:

$$n = \frac{Z^2_{1-\frac{\alpha}{2}} \times \left[p_1(1-p_1)+p_2(1-p_2)\right]}{d^2} = \frac{(1.96)^2 \times \left[0.40(1-0.40)+0.32(1-0.32)\right]}{(0.05)^2}$$

$$n = Z^2_{1-\frac{\alpha}{2}} \times \frac{\left[p_1(1-p_1)+p_2(1-p_2)\right]}{d^2} = (1.96)^2 \times \frac{\left[0.40(1-0.40)+0.32(1-0.32)\right]}{(0.05)^2}$$

Calculating this gives

$$n = (1.96)^2 \times \frac{0.4576}{0.0025} = 703.17 \cong 704$$

The required sample size from each group is approximately 704 participants.

Example 7.15: How many people should be included in the sample from each of the two groups to estimate a *risk difference* within 5 percentage points of the actual difference, with 95% confidence, especially when the proportions in these groups cannot be reasonably predicted?

Solution: Since there is no available information about the two population proportions (p_1 and p_2), the most appropriate assumption is $p_1 = 0.50$ and $p_2 = 0.50$. With an absolute precision of 5% and a 95% confidence level corresponding to $Z = 1.96$, the required sample size is:

$$n = Z^2_{1-\frac{\alpha}{2}} \times \frac{\left[p_1(1-p_1)+p_2(1-p_2)\right]}{d^2}$$

$$= (1.96)^2 \times \frac{\left[0.50(1-0.50)+0.50(1-0.50)\right]}{(0.05)^2}$$

$$= (1.96)^2 \times \frac{0.50}{0.0025} = 768.32 \cong 769$$

The calculated sample size is based on Equation 7.6 for a two-tailed estimation of the difference between two population proportions with a specified absolute precision. Sample sizes are calculated for different values of V ranging from 0.01 to 0.50, and various levels of precision are provided in Table 7.5.

TABLE 7.5

Sample Size Calculation for Estimating the Difference Between Two Population Proportions with a Specified Absolute Precision at a 5% Significance Level

$V = p_1(1-p_1)+p_2(1-p_2)$												
0.50	**0.45**	**0.40**	**0.35**	**0.30**	**0.25**	**0.20**	**0.15**	**0.10**	**0.05**	**0.03**	**0.01**	***d***
19209	17288	15367	13446	11525	9604	7684	5763	3842	1921	1153	**385**	**0.01**
4802	4322	3842	3362	2882	2401	1921	1441	961	481	289	97	**0.02**
2135	1921	1708	1494	1281	1068	854	641	427	214	129	43	**0.03**
1201	1081	961	841	721	601	481	361	241	121	73	25	**0.04**
769	692	615	538	461	385	308	231	154	77	47	16	**0.05**
193	173	154	135	116	97	77	58	39	20	12	4	**0.10**
86	77	69	60	52	43	35	26	18	9	6	*	**0.15**
49	44	39	34	29	25	20	15	10	5	*	*	**0.20**
31	28	25	22	19	16	13	10	7	4	*	*	**0.25**
22	20	18	15	13	11	9	7	5	*	*	*	**0.30**
16	15	13	11	10	8	7	5	*	*	*	*	**0.35**
13	11	10	9	8	7	5	4	*	*	*	*	**0.40**
10	9	8	7	6	5	4	*	*	*	*	*	**0.45**
8	7	7	6	5	4	4	*	*	*	*	*	**0.50**

**Sample size less than 4.*

7.8 Sample Size Determination to Compare Two Small Proportions

In situations where the underlying rate is extremely low, the previously mentioned methods may not be suitable. For phenomena such as diseases with rare incidences, the arcsine formula, as demonstrated by Lemeshow et al., provides the most accurate results for sample size calculation (Lemeshow et al., 1988, p. 15).

The sample size can be calculated using either of the following formulas:

$$n = \frac{(Z_{1-\frac{\alpha}{2}} + Z_{1-\beta})^2}{2(\arcsin\sqrt{p_2} - \arcsin\sqrt{p_1})^2} \tag{7.7a}$$

or

$$n = \frac{(Z_{1-\frac{\alpha}{2}} + Z_{1-\beta})^2}{0.00061(\arcsin\sqrt{p_2} - \arcsin\sqrt{p_1})^2} \tag{7.7b}$$

The *arcsine function* is the inverse of the sine function, meaning that they cancel each other out in composition (i.e., $sine\, x \times arcsine\, x = 1$).

> **Example 7.16:** Two communities will be selected to participate in a study evaluating the widespread use of a new screening programme for the early identification of a specific type of cancer. In one community, all adults over the age of 35 will undergo the screening programme, while no screening will take place in the second community. The annual incidence rate of this type of cancer is 50 per 100,000 (0.0005) in the unscreened population. A decrease in the rate to 20 per 100,000 (0.0002) would justify the widespread implementation of the screening programme. To achieve an 80% probability of detecting a decrease of this magnitude, how many adults should be followed in each of the two communities if a hypothesis test is conducted at the 5% significance level?

Solution: The relevant information includes $p_1 = 0.0002$ and $p_2 = 0.0005$. The power $1-\beta = 0.80$ corresponds to $Z_{1-\beta} = 0.84$, and for a one-tailed test at $\alpha = 0.05$, $Z_{1-\alpha} = 1.645$, since researchers are only interested in a decrease to 0.0002. Plugging these values into Equation 7.7 will yield the required sample size.

Using Equation 7.7a:

$$n = \frac{(Z_{1-\alpha} + Z_{1-\beta})^2}{2(\arcsin\sqrt{p_2} - \arcsin\sqrt{p_1})^2} = \frac{(1.645 + 0.84)^2}{2(\arcsin\sqrt{0.0005} - \arcsin\sqrt{0.0002})^2}$$

$$= \frac{(1.96 + 0.84)^2}{2(0.02236254 - 0.01414261)^2} = \frac{6.175225}{0.000135135} = 45697$$

Using Equation 7.7b:

$$n = \frac{(0.84 + 1.645)^2}{0.00061\left(\arcsin\sqrt{0.0005} - \arcsin\sqrt{0.0002}\right)^2}$$

$$= \frac{6.175225}{0.00061(1.28128 - 0.810312)^2} = \frac{6.175225}{0.000135305} = 45640$$

Using either arcsine-based formula, the required sample size in each community is approximately 45,650 adults to detect the expected decrease in incidence with 80% power and a one-tailed 5% significance level.

If you need to use the sample sizes provided in Table 7.6 for a *one-tailed test* with a 5% significance level and 80% power, simply multiply the sample sizes in the table by 0.788. This coefficient is derived from the square of the sum of the z-scores for the one-tailed significance level and the desired power, that is, $(1.645 + 0.84)^2$.

7.9 Sample Size Determination for Independence of Matched Pairs (Discordant Probabilities)

To illustrate discordant probabilities in a matched pairs setup, we refer to the McNemar test, as shown in Table 7.7. This test assesses the statistical significance of the association between two attributes when pairs of observations are collected from the same group of subjects.

In such tables, the outcomes in cells **a** and **d** are the same, referred to as concordant pairs, while the outcomes in cells **b** and **c** differ, termed discordant pairs. Thus, a concordant pair is defined as a matched pair where the outcomes are identical for both members, whereas a discordant pair is one where the outcomes differ. In this context, p_{11} and p_{00} represent concordant probabilities, while p_{01} and p_{10} represent discordant probabilities (Indrayan & Holt, 2016, p. 555; Machin et al., 2018, p. 120; Rosner, 2006, p. 407).

Different authors present various formats for the sample size equation. For instance, Machin et al. (2018, p. 120) provide the following formula:

$$n_{Pairs} = \frac{\left[z_{1-\frac{\alpha}{2}}(\psi + 1) + z_{1-\beta}\sqrt{(\psi + 1)^2 - p_{Dis} \times (\psi - 1)^2}\right]^2}{p_{Dis} \times (\psi - 1)^2}$$

where: $\psi = \dfrac{p_{10}}{p_{01}}$, $p_{Dis} = p_{10} + p_{01}$

TABLE 7.6

Sample Size Calculation for One-Tailed Test of a Small Proportion with 80% Power and a 5% Significance Level

0.0500	0.0450	0.0400	0.0350	0.0300	0.0250	0.0200	0.0150	0.0100	0.075	0.0050	0.0025	0.0010	P2
105	119	137	160	194	243	323	472	835	1292	2559	11588	–	**0.0010**
128	147	172	206	255	332	465	741	1559	2912	9106	–	11588	**0.0025**
164	192	230	285	368	507	775	1449	4536	15426	–	9106	2559	**0.0050**
204	243	299	381	514	755	1288	3013	21649	–	15426	2912	1292	**0.0075**
250	303	383	506	718	1142	2252	7665	–	21649	4536	1559	835	**0.0100**
372	474	635	917	1490	3026	10730	–	7665	3013	1449	741	472	**0.0150**
561	760	1109	1830	3785	13753	–	10730	2252	1289	775	465	323	**0.0200**
881	1298	2163	4532	16740	–	13753	3026	1142	755	507	332	243	**0.0250**
1482	2491	5270	19693	–	16740	3785	1490	718	514	368	255	194	**0.0300**
2815	5999	22614	–	19693	4532	1830	917	506	381	285	296	160	**0.0350**
6719	25502	–	22614	5270	2163	1109	635	383	299	230	172	137	**0.0400**
28358	–	25502	5999	2490	1298	760	474	304	243	192	147	119	**0.0450**
–	28358	6719	2815	1482	881	561	372	250	204	164	128	105	**0.0500**

TABLE 7.7

Probabilities in a Matched Pairs Setup

		First Clinician		
		Positive Outcome	**Negative Outcome**	**Total**
	Positive Outcome	$a(p_{11})$	$b(p_{10})$	$a+b(p_{1.})$
Second Clinician	Negative Outcome	$c(p_{01})$	$d(p_{00})$	$c+d(p_{0.})$
	Total	$a+c(p_{.1})$	$b+d(p_{.0})$	

Indrayan and Holt (Indray2016, p. 555) offer a different formula based on the null hypothesis $H_0 : p_{10} = p_{01}$ (i.e., the probabilities of discordance for both types are equal) with a two-sided alternative $H_1 : p_{10} \neq p_{01}$:

$$n = \frac{\left(Z_{1-\frac{\alpha}{2}} \cdot \sqrt{p_{10} + p_{01}} + Z_{1-\beta} \cdot \sqrt{p_{10} + p_{01} - (p_{10} - p_{01})} \right)^2}{(P_{01} - P_{10})^2}$$

Rosner (2006, p. 407) proposes a two-tailed equation, which is considered more realistic and straightforward:

$$n = \frac{p_0 q_0 \left(Z_{1-\frac{\alpha}{2}} + Z_{1-\beta} \cdot \sqrt{\frac{p_1 q_1}{p_0 q_0}} \right)^2}{(p_1 - p_0)^2} \tag{7.8}$$

where: $H_0 : p = p_0$, $H_1 : p \neq p_0$ indicating $H_1 : p = p_1$.

To apply this formula for *McNemar's test*, set $p_0 = 1 - p_0 = 0.5$ and $p_1 = p_A$, representing the proportion of discordant pairs of type A, and let $n = n_D$ denote the number of discordant pairs. Upon substitution, the sample size formula becomes:

$$n = \frac{\left(Z_{1-\frac{\alpha}{2}} + 2Z_{1-\beta} \cdot \sqrt{p_A q_A} \right)^2}{4p_D(p_1 - 0.5)^2}$$

TABLE 7.8

A2x2 Contingency Table with Matched Pairs as the Sampling Unit (Based on 560 Matched Pairs)

		Treatment B		
		Survive	**Die**	**Total**
Treatment A	Survive	459	15	474
	Die	5	81	86
	Total	464	96	560

Example 7.17: Suppose the goal of the study is to compare two different chemotherapy regimens (A and B), with cancer recurrence or death as the outcome measure over a five-year period. The study will utilise a *matched-pairs design*, where patients are matched based on their age and disease stage. One patient in each pair is assigned to treatment A, while the other receives treatment B. Previous research indicates that patients in matched pairs respond similarly to treatments in 82% of cases. This suggests that both patients will either die or experience a recurrence within five years, or both will survive without recurrence after five years.

Additionally, among matched pairs with a response difference, it is estimated that in 65% of the pairs, the treatment A patient will either die or have a recurrence within five years, while the treatment B patient will not; conversely, in 35% of the pairs, the treatment B patient will die or have a recurrence within five years, while the treatment A patient will not.

The question is: How many participants (or matched pairs) need to be enrolled in the study to achieve an 85% chance of detecting a significant difference using a two-sided test with a type I error of 0.05 (Rosner, 2006, p. 408)?

Solution: Given that $\alpha = 0.05$, $\beta = 0.15$, $p_D = 1 - 0.82 = 0.18$, $p_A = 0.65$, and $q_A = 0.35$, the required number of pairs can be calculated as follows:

$$n = \frac{\left(Z_{1-\frac{\alpha}{2}} + 2Z_{1-\beta}.\sqrt{p_A q_A}\right)^2}{4p_D(p_1 - 0.5)^2}$$

Substituting the values:

$$= \frac{\left(1.96 + 2(1.04)\sqrt{0.65 \times 0.35}\right)^2}{4 \times 0.18(0.65 - 0.5)^2} = \frac{8.715}{0.0162} = 538 \textit{ matched pairs}$$

Thus, the total number of individuals required is

$$2n = 2 \times 538 = 1076 \textit{ individuals}$$

Therefore, 1076 individuals in 538 matched pairs must be enrolled. This will yield approximately $0.18 \times 538 \approx 97$ discordant pairs.

For the convenience of users, sample sizes for specific cases of p_1 and p_2 for two-tailed tests are provided in Table 7.5.

7.10 Sample Size Determination for Equivalence Studies

Unbalanced or imbalanced sample sizes – referring to unequal allocation of participants across different groups or treatment conditions – are common in research studies. This situation arises when the number of participants in the groups is not equal due to various practical or methodological factors. Unequal allocation may be preferable for reasons such as differences in relative costs and available resources, the desire for more precise estimates in one group, variability differences across groups, or other considerations that necessitate selecting unequal sample sizes from two populations. Additionally, if one treatment exhibits greater variation (i.e., lower precision) in outcome response than the other, the statistical power for comparing treatments can be maximised through unequal allocation.

In such cases, the allocation ratio should reflect the known standard deviations, expressed as $k = \sigma_2 / \sigma_1$.

The treatment with lower precision (larger standard deviation) should receive a larger number of participants, resulting in unequal allocation. This approach helps mitigate heterogeneity by increasing the sample size for treatments with greater dispersion. Unequal allocation may also be desirable when one therapy is substantially more expensive than the other, as budget limitations may restrict the number of patients assigned to the costlier treatment. Ethical considerations – such as minimising exposure to potential adverse effects – may likewise justify unequal sample sizes.

Consider a scenario involving a standard treatment (treatment 1) and an experimental treatment (treatment 2), where p_1 and p_2 denote the treatment success rates in groups 1 and 2, respectively. The treatments are considered equivalent if the upper bound of the $(1-\alpha)\times 100\%$ confidence interval for $p_1 - p_2$ is less than or equal to δ. Suppose that the success rate in one group is expected to be k times the success rate in the other group, where $k \neq 1$, and that

$$n_2 = k n_1.$$

To establish equivalence with probability $1-\beta$ using a two-sided significance test at level α, the required sample sizes for the two treatment groups can be computed using the following formulas (Chow et al., 2017, p. 77; Fleiss et al., 2013, p. 76; Rosner, 2006, p. 712):

$$n_1 = \left(z_{1-\frac{\alpha}{2}} + z_{1-\beta}\right)^2 \frac{\left(p_1(1-p_1) + \frac{p_2(1-p_2)}{k}\right)}{\left(\delta - (p_1 - p_2)\right)^2} \tag{7.9a}$$

An alternative set of formulas for calculating the sample size for unequal groups – which yields similar results – is as follows (Fleiss et al., 2013, p. 76; Lemeshow et al., 1988, p. 9; Rosner, 2006, p. 404):

$$n_1 = \frac{\left[z_{1-\frac{\alpha}{2}}\sqrt{\bar{p}.\bar{q}.(k+1)} + z_{1-\beta}\sqrt{k.p_1.q_1 + p_2.q_2}\right]^2}{k(p_2 - p_1)^2} \tag{7.9b}$$

$$n_1 = \frac{\left[z_{1-\frac{\alpha}{2}}\sqrt{\bar{p}.\bar{q}.\left(\frac{1}{k+1}\right)} + z_{1-\beta}\sqrt{p_1.q_1 + \frac{p_2.q_2}{k}}\right]^2}{(p_2 - p_1)^2} \tag{7.9c}$$

Here, $\bar{p}$ is the weighted average of the two proportions:

$$\bar{p} = \frac{p_1 + K.p_2}{1+K}, \quad \bar{q} = 1 - \bar{p}.$$

The corresponding sample size for group 2 is

$$n_2 = \left(z_{1-\frac{\alpha}{2}} + z_{1-\beta}\right)^2 \times \frac{\left[k.p_1(1-p_1) + p_2(1-p_2)\right]}{\left[\delta - (p_1 - p_2)\right]^2} \tag{7.10}$$

or simply

$$n_2 = k\,n_1.$$

Example 7.18: It is believed that the risk of lung cancer among workers exposed to oil mist is twice as high as that for workers in other sectors. To detect the difference in lung cancer rates between these groups with 90% probability at a significance level of 0.05, how many workers should be selected from each sector? Previous studies indicate a lung cancer rate of 0.33 for workers exposed to oil mist and 0.20 for those in other sectors.

Solution: Assuming a two-tailed test, the critical values are 1.28 for 90% power $(z_{1-\beta})$and 1.96 for a 5% significance level $(z_{1-\alpha/2})$. Let the proportions be $p_1 = 0.33$ and $p_2 = 0.20$. Given that $k = 2$ (where $n_2 = k.n_1$), the required sample size for the first group is computed using:

$$n_1 = \frac{\left(z_{1-\frac{\alpha}{2}} + z_{1-\beta}\right)^2\left[p_1(1-p_1) + \frac{p_2(1-p_2)}{k}\right]}{\left(\delta - (p_1 - p_2)\right)^2}$$

Substituting the values:

$$n_1 = \frac{(1.96+1.28)^2\left[0.33(1-0.33)+\dfrac{0.20(1-0.20)}{2}\right]}{\left(0-(0.33-0.20)\right)^2}$$

Computing this gives

$$n_1 = \frac{10.4976\times 0.3011}{0.0169} = 187.03 \cong 188$$

For the second group:

$$n_2 = \frac{\left(z_{1-\frac{\alpha}{2}}+z_{1-\beta}\right)^2\left[k.p_1(1-p_1)+p_2(1-p_2)\right]}{\left[\delta-(p_1-p_2)\right]^2}$$

Substituting the values:

$$n_2 = \frac{(1.96+1.28)^2\left[2\times 0.33(1-0.33)+0.20(1-0.20)\right]}{\left[0-(0.33-0.20)\right]^2}$$

Calculating this gives:

$$n_2 = \frac{10.4976\times 0.6022}{0.0169} = 374.06 \cong 375$$

Thus, the required sample size can also be calculated using Equation 7.9b:

$$\bar{p} = \frac{\mathrm{p}_1+\mathrm{K.p}_2}{1+\mathrm{K}} = \frac{0.33+2\times 0.20}{1+2} = \frac{0.73}{3} = 0.2433$$

Using this in the formula:

$$n_1 = \frac{\left[z_{1-\frac{\alpha}{2}}\sqrt{\bar{p}.\bar{q}.(k+1)}+z_{1-\beta}\sqrt{k.p_1.\,q_1+p_2.\,q_2}\right]^2}{k(p_2-p_1)^2}$$

Substituting the values:

$$n_1 = \frac{\left[1.96\times\sqrt{0.2433\times 0.7567\times(1+2)}+1.28\times\sqrt{2\times 0.33\times 0.67+0.20\times 0.80}\right]^2}{2(0.33-0.20)^2}$$

Calculating this gives

$$n_1 = \frac{(1.4566 + 0.9933)^2}{0.0338} = 177.57 \cong 178$$

Example 7.19: In Example 7.13, if the number of applicants for the common and standard surgical method is four times that of the new surgical method, how many samples should be taken from each group?

Solution: Assuming a two-tailed test with a critical value of 1.28 for 90% power and 1.96 for a 5% significance level, we have $p_1 = 0.15$ and $p_2 = 0.05$ with k = 4 and $n_2 = k.n_1$. The required sample size for each group can be calculated as follows:

$$n_1 = \frac{\left(z_{1-\frac{\alpha}{2}} + z_{1-\beta}\right)^2 \left(p_1(1-p_1) + \frac{p_2(1-p_2)}{k}\right)}{\left(\delta - (p_1 - p_2)\right)^2}$$

Substituting the values:

$$n_1 = \frac{(1.96 + 1.28)^2 \left(0.15(1-0.15) + \frac{0.05(1-0.05)}{4}\right)}{\left(0 - (0.15 - 0.05)\right)^2}$$

Calculating this gives:

$$n_1 = \frac{10.4976 \times 0.13938}{0.01} = 146.31 \cong 147$$

Using Equation 7.9b, we can also calculate the sample size as follows:

$$\bar{p} = \frac{p_1 + K.p_2}{1+K} = \frac{0.15 + 4 \times 0.05}{1+4} = 0.07$$

Then:

$$n_1 = \frac{\left[z_{1-\frac{\alpha}{2}}\sqrt{\bar{p}.\bar{q}.(k+1)} + z_{1-\beta}\sqrt{k.p_1.\,q_1 + p_2.\,q_2}\right]^2}{k(p_2 - p_1)^2}$$

Substituting the values:

$$n_1 = \frac{\left[1.96 \times \sqrt{0.07 \times 0.93.(1+4)} + 1.28 \times \sqrt{4 \times 0.15 \times 0.85 + 0.05 \times 0.95}\right]^2}{4(0.15 - 0.05)^2}$$

Calculating this gives

$$n_1 = \frac{(1.11823 + 0.95572)^2}{0.04} = 107.53 \cong 108$$

> **Example 7.20:** Suppose we want to compare the rates of social participation among children with cerebral palsy (CP) who attend an occupational therapy clinic (hypothesised proportion $p_1 = 0.40$) and those who do not attend (hypothesised proportion $p_2 = 0.25$). The significance level is set at 0.01, and the power at $1 - \beta = 0.90$. Given that recruitment of clinic attendees is easier than that of non-attendees, the investigator decides to study half as many non-attendees as attendees, resulting in $k = 0.5$. How many samples must we take from each group?

Solution: For this scenario, the power $1 - \beta = 0.90$ corresponds to a critical value of 1.28, and the significance level $\alpha = 0.01$ corresponds to a critical value of 2.33 for a two-tailed test. We can calculate the required sample size for clinic attendees using Equation 7.9b as follows:

$$\bar{p} = \frac{p_1 + K.p_2}{1 + K} = \frac{0.40 + 0.5 \times 0.25}{1 + 0.5} = \frac{0.525}{1.5} = 0.35$$

Then:

$$n_1 = \frac{\left[z_{1-\frac{\alpha}{2}} \sqrt{\bar{p}.\bar{q}.(k+1)} + z_{1-\beta} \sqrt{k.p_1.\, q_1 + p_2.\, q_2} \right]^2}{k(p_2 - p_1)^2}$$

Substituting the values:

$$n_1 = \frac{\left[1\,.96\sqrt{0.35 \times 0.65(1 + 0.50)} + 1.28\sqrt{(0.5 \times 0.40 \times 0.60) + 0.25 \times 0.75} \right]^2}{0.5(0.40 - 0.25)^2}$$

Calculating this gives

$$n_1 = \frac{(1.145 + 0.7098)^2}{0.5 \times 0.0225} = 305.80 \cong 306$$

Finally, since the sample size for non-attendees is half that of attendees:

$$n_2 = \frac{n_1}{2} = \frac{306}{2} = 153$$

Conclusion: 306 clinic attendees and 153 non-attendees are required to achieve the desired power and significance level.

7.11 Sample Size for Estimating Several Proportions Simultaneously

The sample sizes for simultaneously estimating several proportions – that is, k proportions that sum to 1 – are based on the normal approximation along with Bonferroni's inequality. This inequality states that the probability that any one or more of the estimates deviates from the corresponding true value by more than d is less than or equal to the sum of the k individual probabilities of deviating from them.

The theorem presented by Fitzpatrick and Scott (1987) and Thompson (2012) demonstrates that the worst-case scenario, where the population values demand the largest sample size, occurs when some m of the proportions in the population are equal and the remainder are zero. The value of m depends on α; for instance, when $\alpha = 0.01$, $m = 2$, and when $\alpha = 0.05$, $m = 3$. The sample size does not depend on the number k of categories in the population as long as $k \geq m$. These sample sizes are considered "conservative" because they may be larger than necessary to achieve the desired precision (Fitzpatrick & Scott, 1987; Thompson, 2012).

The worst-case population is characterised by a combination of k proportions that maximises the likelihood of obtaining a sample in which at least one sample proportion significantly deviates from its corresponding population proportion. Since the proportions must sum to 1, not all population proportions can equal $\frac{1}{k}$. This situation typically arises when the population is nearly evenly distributed among two or three health conditions. The specific worst-case scenario depends on the chosen α-level but remains independent of the number k of categories in the population.

To determine the sample size for this scenario, Thompson presents the following equation (Thompson, 2012, p. 43):

$$n = \max\left(\frac{z^2_{\frac{1}{m}} \times \left(1 - \frac{1}{m}\right)}{d^2}\right) \tag{7.11}$$

Calculating the above equation may be challenging; therefore, Thompson provides Table 7.9 for n_0 in terms of various d and α.

Depending on the population size and finite-population correction factors (FPC), the sample size can be adjusted using the following equation:

$$n = \frac{1}{\frac{1}{N} + \frac{1}{n_0}}$$

TABLE 7.9

Sample Size n_0 for Simultaneously Estimating Several Proportions within Distance d of the True Values at Confidence Level $1 - \alpha$

α	$d_2 \times n_0$	n_0 **with** $d = 0.05$	m
0.50	0.44129	177	4
0.40	0.50729	203	4
0.30	0.60123	241	3
0.20	0.74739	299	3
0.10	1.00635	403	3
0.05	1.27359	510	3
0.025	1.55963	624	2
0.02	1.65872	664	2
0.01	1.96986	788	2
0.005	2.28514	915	2
0.001	3.02892	1212	2
0.0005	3.33530	1342	2
0.0001	4.11209	1645	2

where N is the population size and n_0 is the initial sample size calculated without considering the finite population.

> **Example 7.21:** Suppose a public health researcher wants to collect a sample of individuals to estimate the prevalence/proportion of different health conditions (such as diabetes, hypertension, and obesity) in a community. She aims to be at least 95% confident that all of the estimates are simultaneously within 0.05 of the true population proportions. However, she does not have prior knowledge of the population proportions and is uncertain about the exact number of health conditions to consider. How large a sample size should she take?

Solution: The required sample size can be obtained from Table 7.9. For this example, the researcher has chosen $d = 0.05$ and $\alpha = 0.05$. In the row of the table corresponding to $\alpha = 0.05$, the entry 1.27359 for $d^2 n_0$ is divided by $d^2 = 0.05^2$ to determine the sufficient sample size:

$$n_0 = \frac{1.27359}{0.05^2} = 510$$

This sample size ensures that all estimates will simultaneously be as close as desired to their respective population proportions. It is adequate whether the population is divided into 3 health conditions or 15.

The sample size n_0 from Table 7.9 for estimating multinomial proportions is appropriate when the population size N is large relative to the sample size n, allowing us to ignore finite-population correction (FPC) factors in the variances. When the population size N is small, a smaller sample size n will suffice to meet the same precision criteria for d and α.

For example, if the population size is $N = 1000$ and the goal is for each estimated proportion to be simultaneously within $d = 0.05$ of the true value with a probability of $1 - \alpha = 0.95$, the adjusted sample size is calculated using the FPC formula:

$$n = \frac{1}{\frac{1}{N} + \frac{1}{n_0}} = \frac{1}{\frac{1}{1000} + \frac{1}{510}} = 338$$

Therefore, the final sample size required to estimate the prevalence/ proportion of different health conditions is 338 individuals.

References

Chow, S.-C., Shao, J., Wang, H., & Lokhnygina, Y. (2017). *Sample size calculations in clinical research*. Chapman and Hall and CRC Press.

Cochran, W. G. (1977). *Sampling techniques*. John Wiley & Sons, Inc.

Fitzpatrick, S., & Scott, A. J. (1987). Quick simultaneous confidence intervals for multinomial proportions. *Journal of the American Statistical Association, 82*(399), 875–878.

Fleiss, J. L., Levin, B., & Paik, M. C. (2013). *Statistical methods for rates and proportions*. John Wiley & Sons.

Indrayan, A., & Holt, M. P. (2016). *Concise encyclopedia of biostatistics for medical professionals*. Chapman and Hall and CRC Press.

Lemeshow, S., Hosmer Jr, D. W., & Klar, J. (1988). Sample size requirements for studies estimating odds ratios or relative risks. *Statistics in Medicine, 7*(7), 759–764.

Levy, P. S., & Lemeshow, S. (2013). *Sampling of populations: Methods and applications*. John Wiley & Sons.

Lohr, S. L. (2021). *Sampling: Design and analysis*. Chapman and Hall and CRC Press.

Lwanga, S. K., & Lemeshow, S. (1991). *Sample size determination in health studies: A practical manual/SK Lwanga and S. Lemeshow*. World Health Organization.

Machin, D., Campbell, M. J., Tan, S. B., & Tan, S. H. (2018). *Sample sizes for clinical, laboratory and epidemiology studies*. John Wiley & Sons.

Malone, H. E., Nicholl, H., & Coyne, I. (2016). Fundamentals of estimating sample size. *Nurse Researcher, 23*(5), 21–25.

Navidi, W. C., & Monk, B. J. (2013). *Elementary statistics*. McGraw-Hill Education.

Rosner, B. A. (2006). *Fundamentals of biostatistics* (Vol. 6). Thomson-Brooks.

Thompson, S. K. (2012). *Sampling* (Vol. 755). John Wiley & Sons.

8

Sample Size Estimation for Epidemiological Studies

8.1 Introduction

Sample size is a critical component and the initial practical step in designing a clinical trial; however, it is frequently the most neglected aspect of clinical research studies. The question of how many subjects are needed often arises during the planning phase of research projects, particularly in clinical and epidemiological studies focused on human health. Unfortunately, this question is often inadequately addressed in proposals, as it requires both statistical reasoning and informed estimation. Moreover, economic factors significantly influence clinical research, as experiments, interventions, treatments, and drugs incur substantial costs. An undersized study can lead to wasted resources by failing to produce meaningful results, whereas an oversized study unnecessarily consumes additional resources.

The odds ratio (OR) in case–control studies and the relative risk (RR) in prospective studies, such as cohort studies, are two of the most commonly analysed parameters in medical and health research. Given their importance, the beginning of this chapter is dedicated to determining the sample size for estimating and testing hypotheses involving odds ratios (OR) and relative risks (RR). Subsequently, the chapter explores various epidemiological study designs and different types of health measurements.

For a foundational understanding of sample size determination, refer to Chapters 1 and 4 for an overview of the key principles. The procedures and requirements for estimation (confidence intervals) differ from those for hypothesis testing. If the goal is estimation, it is essential to specify the confidence level $(1 - \alpha)$ and the desired precision around both the relative risk (RR) and the odds ratio (OR), typically expressed as a proportion of these measures. Additionally, the anticipated RR, OR, or the expected probability of disease (or exposure) in the respective groups must be defined.

Conversely, if the objective is hypothesis testing, specifying relative precision is unnecessary. Instead, the significance level must be established in place of the confidence level. In a hypothesis-testing framework, it is also

DOI: 10.1201/9781003749783-8

crucial to specify the statistical power (1 – β) and the minimum detectable difference (Indrayan & Holt, 2016, p. 552).

While α and β are often determined externally, selecting appropriate values for effect size in these calculations is vital. Achieving this requires a thorough literature review to identify studies conducted in similar contexts, ensuring that the estimates are plausible for your research. The choice of the minimal effect size to be detected should be both reasonable and meaningful, ensuring that the study is practically significant and feasible. Factors such as time, cost, and participant recruitment must be considered alongside power and the minimal detectable difference.

8.2 Case–Control Studies

Case–control studies offer a straightforward approach to investigating the causes of diseases, particularly rare ones. These studies involve individuals diagnosed with a specific disease or outcome of interest, alongside a control group of unaffected individuals. Subjects are selected based on the presence of the disease, with the affected group referred to as "cases" and the healthy group as "controls". Both groups are then examined for exposure to potential risk factors, either in the past or present. The study subjects can be organised into a standard 2 × 2 table, as illustrated in Table 8.1.

TIP

The exposure-odds ratio is calculated by dividing the odds of exposure among diseased subjects by the odds of exposure among nondiseased subjects (Rosner, 2006, p. 641).

Case–control studies compare the occurrence of potential causes between cases (individuals with the disease) and controls (those without the disease).

TABLE 8.1

Classification of Study Subjects Based on Exposure to a Risk Factor and Disease Presence

Unexposed	Exposed	
b	a	Patient **(Cases)**
d	c	Impatient **(Controls)**

While disease status is observed at a single point in time, exposure data reflect a prior time frame. These studies are often classified as retrospective because investigators examine past exposures in relation to current disease status (Bonita et al., 2006, p. 44). Although case–control studies are theoretically a subset of cohort studies, their structure can be complex. Cases and controls can originate from primary or secondary study bases. A primary study base must ensure that all eligible cases are identified and that non-cases have an equal chance of selection. This relationship implies that if a case had not been diagnosed, they might have been selected as a control (Boslaugh, 2007, p. 1011).

The odds ratio (OR) is used to compare the likelihood of an event occurring in the exposed group versus the unexposed group. It is commonly applied in case–control studies to assess the strength of the association between a risk factor and a specific outcome. The odds ratio is calculated by dividing the odds of the event occurring in the exposed group by the odds of the event occurring in the unexposed group. Mathematically, the OR is expressed as:

$$OR = \frac{a \times d}{b \times c}$$

where a, b, c, and d represent the cell counts in a standard 2 × 2 contingency table. An odds ratio greater than 1 indicates that the event is more likely to occur in the exposed group, whereas an odds ratio less than 1 suggests that the event is less likely to occur in the exposed group.

8.3 Sample Size Needed to Estimate OR

To estimate the odds ratio (OR) with a specified level of relative precision, the minimum required sample size can be determined using the following equation:

$$n = \left[\frac{z_{1-\frac{\alpha}{2}}}{Ln(1-\varepsilon)}\right]^2 \times \left[\frac{1}{p_1(1-p_1)} + \frac{1}{p_2(1-p_2)}\right] \tag{8.1}$$

In this equation, ε represents the relative precision, indicating the expected difference between the estimated odds ratio from the sample and the true odds ratio in the population, expressed as a proportion of the true OR. The probabilities p_1 and p_2 represent the expected probabilities of exposure in the case and control groups, respectively, and can be derived from Table 8.1 as follows:

$$p_1 = \frac{a}{a+b} \quad and \quad p_2 = \frac{c}{c+d}$$

Typically, one of the two probabilities, p_1 or p_2, is provided along with the OR. Consequently, the other probability can be calculated using the following equation:

$$p_1 = \frac{OR \times p_2}{OR \times p_2 + (1 - p_2)} \tag{8.2}$$

$$p_2 = \frac{p_1}{OR \times p_1 + (1 - p_1)} \tag{8.3}$$

TIP

The required sample sizes for estimating the odds ratio (OR) for common proportions and OR values ranging from 1 to 5.0, using a 5% significance level and 20% relative precision, are presented in Table 8.2. If the OR is equal to or greater than 1, both OR and p_2 must be specified. Conversely, if the OR is less than 1, use the column value corresponding to $\frac{1}{RR}$ and the row value corresponding to p_1.

Example 8.1: In a community, fear of falling is a significant concern among the elderly population. Experts estimate that approximately 40% of older adults have a history of falls, having experienced at least one fall in the past. A case–control study is proposed to investigate the association between fear of falling and exposure to falls among the elderly. To estimate the odds ratio (OR) within 30% of its anticipated value of OR = 1.5, we need to determine the required sample size for both the control and case groups.

Solution: The expected probability of falling in the control group (those without fear) is assumed to be equal to the exposure rate in the overall population, giving $p_2 = 0.40$. The expected probability of falling in the case group (those with fear) is unknown and can be calculated using Equation 8.2:

$$p_1 = \frac{p_2 \times OR}{OR \times p_2 + (1 - p_2)} = \frac{0.40 \times 1.5}{1.5 \times 0.40 + (1 - 0.4)} = 0.50$$

We assume a relative precision of $\varepsilon = 0.30$, an anticipated odds ratio of OR = 1.5, and a significance level of 5%. The required sample size is calculated using Equation 8.1:

$$n = \left[\frac{1.96}{Ln(1-0.30)} \right]^2 \times \left[\frac{1}{0.5(1-0.5)} + \frac{1}{0.40(1-0.40)} \right] = 246.6 \approx 247$$

This indicates that a sample size of 247 is required for each group.

Example 8.2: Chronic obstructive pulmonary disease (COPD) represents a significant public health issue, particularly among the elderly. It is estimated that approximately 15% of individuals over the age of 65 are affected by COPD. A case–control study is being designed to explore the relationship between exposure to secondhand smoke and the development of COPD. The researchers aim to estimate the odds ratio (OR) within 20% of its expected value of OR = 2.0. Assuming equal numbers of cases and controls, we must determine the sample size required for each group to achieve this level of precision.

Solution: The expected probability of COPD in the control group is assumed to be equal to the exposure rate in the overall population, giving $p_2 = 0.15$. The expected probability of COPD in the case group is unknown and can be calculated using Equation 8.2:

$$p_1 = \frac{p_2 \times OR}{OR \times p_2 + (1-p_2)} = \frac{0.15 \times 2.0}{2.0 \times 0.15 + (1-0.15)} = 0.261$$

We assume a relative precision of ε = 0.20, with an anticipated odds ratio of OR = 2.0, and a significance level of 5%. The required sample size can be calculated using Equation 8.1:

$$n = \left[\frac{1.96}{Ln(1-0.20)} \right]^2 \times \left[\frac{1}{0.261(1-0.261)} + \frac{1}{0.15(1-0.15)} \right] = 1005.11 \approx 1006$$

Thus, a sample size of 1006 is required for each group.

8.4 Sample Size for Hypothesis Testing of the Odds Ratio (OR)

The most common hypothesis test for the odds ratio (OR) evaluates whether there is no effect due to the exposure variable. This involves testing the null hypothesis, which posits that the proportion of exposed individuals is the same in both groups: cases (patients) and controls (non-patients). Under the null hypothesis, the odds ratio is assumed to be 1 ($H_0 : OR = 1$), indicating that the proportion of exposed individuals among the cases is equal to that among the controls. In other words, the null hypothesis asserts that the two proportions are equal.

TABLE 8.2

Required Sample Sizes for Estimating the Odds Ratio (OR), with a 5% Significance Level and 20% Relative Precision, extracted from Lemeshow et al. (1988, p. 154)

	OR										
p_2	1.00	1.25	1.50	1.75	2.00	2.50	3.00	3.50	4.00	4.50	5.00
0.01	15587	14059	13041	12314	11768	11005	10496	10133	9860	9649	9479
0.02	7873	7117	6614	6254	5984	5607	5356	5177	5042	4938	4855
0.03	5303	4805	4473	4236	4058	3810	3645	3527	3439	3371	3317
0.04	4019	3649	3403	3228	3096	2913	2791	2704	2640	2590	2550
0.05	3249	2957	2762	2624	2520	2376	2280	2212	2162	2123	2093
0.10	1715	1578	1488	1424	1376	1311	1269	1240	1220	1205	1194
0.15	1211	1127	1072	1034	1006	969	946	932	924	918	915
0.20	965	908	872	847	830	809	798	793	791	792	795
0.25	823	784	759	744	733	723	721	722	727	733	741
0.30	735	708	692	683	678	677	681	689	699	711	724
0.35	679	660	652	649	649	655	666	680	696	713	730
0.40	643	633	631	632	637	651	669	689	711	733	757
0.45	624	621	624	631	640	662	687	714	743	772	801
0.50	618	622	631	643	656	687	721	755	791	828	865
0.55	624	635	650	668	687	728	770	815	859	905	951
0.60	643	662	684	708	733	786	841	896	952	1008	1065
0.70	735	774	814	856	899	985	1073	1162	1251	1340	1429
0.80	965	1038	1113	1188	1264	1416	1569	1723	1876	2030	2184
0.90	1715	1887	2059	2232	2405	2751	3098	3445	3792	4139	4486

In contrast, the alternative hypothesis suggests that the odds ratio differs from 1 ($H_A : OR \neq 1$). The required sample size for this hypothesis test can be calculated using the following formula:

$$n = \left[\frac{Z_{1-\frac{\alpha}{2}} \cdot \sqrt{2\bar{p}(1-\bar{p})} + Z_{1-\beta} \cdot \sqrt{p_1(1-p_1) + p_2(1-p_2)}}{(p_1 - p_2)} \right]^2 \tag{8.4}$$

where

$$\bar{p} = \frac{(p_1 + p_2)}{2},$$

and the null and alternative hypotheses are $H_0 : OR = 1$ and $H_A : OR \neq 1$.

It is important to note that some references, such as Lemeshow et al. (1988, p. 19), modify the formula by substituting $2p_2(1-p_2)$. They argue that the population typically contains a larger number of non-cases (controls) than cases and that the exposure rate among controls is generally known with high precision. Under the null hypothesis, this exposure rate applies to cases as well. Therefore, it is reasonable to use p_2 as the population proportion for each group.

The use of $2\bar{p}(1-\bar{p})$ in the earlier formula reflects uncertainty about the common exposure proportion for the two groups. If the exposure rate among controls is not known with certainty, then $2\bar{p}(1-\bar{p})$ should be used instead. The modified formula is:

$$n = \left[\frac{Z_{1-\frac{\alpha}{2}} \cdot \sqrt{2p_2(1-p_2)} + Z_{1-\beta} \cdot \sqrt{p_1(1-p_1) + p_2(1-p_2)}}{(p_1 - p_2)} \right]^2 \tag{8.5}$$

> **Example 8.3:** The influence of falls on the fear of falling among the elderly remains unclear. A study is designed to compare the frequency distribution of falls in individuals with a fear of falling (cases) versus those without such fear (controls). Current data suggest that approximately 30% of the control group, consisting of individuals without a fear of falling, have no history of falls. The researcher aims to identify a significant difference in the odds ratio from 1, with a significance level of 5% and a power of 80%. Assuming that the expected difference corresponds to an odds ratio of 2, the required sample size for each group (cases and controls) must be determined.

Solution: The odds ratio will be tested under the null hypothesis $H_0 : OR = 1$, and the alternative hypothesis $H_A : OR \neq 1$, implying a two-tailed test. The expected odds ratio is OR = 2. The expected probability of falling for individuals without fear is $p_2 = 0.30$, while the expected probability for individuals with fear is unknown and can be calculated using Equation 8.2:

$$p_1 = \frac{p_2 \times OR}{OR \times p_2 + (1 - p_2)} = \frac{0.30 \times 2.0}{2.0 \times 0.30 + (1 - 0.3)} = 0.46$$

Given a power of 80% and a significance level of 5%, the required sample size is calculated using Equation 8.5:

$$n = \left[\frac{Z_{1-\frac{\alpha}{2}} \cdot \sqrt{2p_2(1-p_2)} + Z_{1-\beta} \cdot \sqrt{p_1(1-p_1) + p_2(1-p_2)}}{(p_1 - p_2)} \right]^2$$

Substituting the values:

$$n = \left[\frac{1.96 . \sqrt{2 \times 0.3(1-0.3)} + 0.84 . \sqrt{0.3(1-0.3) + 0.46(1-0.46)}}{(0.46 - 0.3)} \right]^2 = 130$$

Thus, the required sample size for each group (cases and controls) is 130 participants.

> **Example 8.4:** The impact of antibiotic resistance in urinary tract infections (UTIs) is a growing concern in healthcare. A study was conducted to compare the frequency of antibiotic resistance in individuals with recurrent UTIs (cases) versus those with no history of UTIs (controls). Preliminary data suggest that 20% of the control group shows no resistance to common antibiotics. The researchers aim to detect a significant difference in the odds ratio (OR) from 1, with a significance level of 5% and 90% power for the test. If the expected odds ratio for antibiotic resistance between the two groups is 3, the required sample size for each group (controls and cases) must be determined.

Solution: The odds ratio will be tested under the null hypothesis $H_0 : OR = 1$ and the alternative hypothesis $H_A : OR \neq 1$, implying a two-tailed test. The expected odds ratio is OR = 3. The expected probability of antibiotic resistance among individuals without a history of UTIs is $p_2 = 0.20$. The expected probability among individuals with recurrent UTIs is unknown and can be calculated using Equation 8.2:

$$p_1 = \frac{p_2 \times OR}{OR \times p_2 + (1 - p_2)} = \frac{0.20 \times 3.0}{3.0 \times 0.20 + (1 - 0.20)} = 0.429$$

Given a significance level of 5% and 90% power, the required sample size is calculated using Equation 8.5:

$$n = \left[\frac{Z_{1-\frac{\alpha}{2}} \cdot \sqrt{2p_2(1-p_2)} + Z_{1-\beta} \cdot \sqrt{p_1(1-p_1) + p_2(1-p_2)}}{(p_1 - p_2)} \right]^2$$

Substituting the values:

$$n = \left[\frac{1.96 \times \sqrt{2 \times 0.2(1-0.2)} + 1.28 \times \sqrt{0.429(1-0.429) + 0.2(1-0.2)}}{(0.429 - 0.20)} \right]^2 = 70.80 \approx 71$$

Thus, the required sample size for each group (cases and controls) is 71 participants.

The required sample sizes for hypothesis testing of OR = 1 for common proportions and various odds ratios ranging from 1.25 to 5, with a significance level of 5% and 90% power in a two-sided alternative test, are presented in Table 8.3. If OR ≥ 1, both the OR and p_2 must be known. However, if OR < 1, the column value corresponding to $\frac{1}{OR}$ and the row value corresponding to p_1 should be used.

8.5 Cohort Studies

Cohort studies, also referred to as follow-up or incidence studies, begin with a group of disease-free individuals who are categorised according to their exposure to a potential disease-causing factor. Key variables are identified and measured, and the cohort is followed over time to observe the development of new disease cases in both exposed and unexposed groups. Cohort studies are longitudinal by design.

Although cohort studies are often called prospective studies, this terminology can be misleading, as it refers to the timing of data collection rather than the exposure–effect relationship. Both prospective and retrospective cohort studies can be conducted. These studies provide reliable information on causation and allow for the direct measurement of disease risk. However, they can be complex and may require long follow-up periods due to the time lag between exposure and disease onset.

TIP

The relative risk (RR) can be expressed as the ratio of the probability of disease occurring among exposed subjects (p_1) to the probability of disease occurring among unexposed subjects (p_2).

TABLE 8.3

Required Sample Sizes for Hypothesis Testing of the Odds Ratio, Assuming a Two-Sided Test with a 5% Significance Level and 80% Power (Lemeshow et al., 1988, p. 165)

	OR									
p_2	**1.25**	**1.50**	**1.75**	**2.00**	**2.50**	**3.00**	**3.50**	**4.00**	**4.50**	**5.0**
0.01	26421	6858	3157	1836	868	516	348	254	195	156
0.02	13400	3492	1614	942	448	269	182	134	103	83
0.03	9063	2371	1100	644	309	186	127	94	73	59
0.04	6896	1811	843	496	239	145	100	74	58	47
0.05	5598	1476	690	407	198	121	83	62	49	40
0.10	3016	810	386	231	116	73	52	39	32	26
0.15	2172	595	288	175	90	58	42	33	27	23
0.20	1766	492	242	150	79	52	39	31	26	22
0.25	1537	436	218	137	74	50	38	30	26	22
0.30	1400	404	205	130	72	50	38	31	26	23
0.35	1318	387	199	128	73	51	39	32	28	25
0.40	1273	380	198	129	75	53	42	35	30	27
0.45	1259	381	202	133	78	56	45	38	33	30
0.50	1270	391	209	139	84	61	49	42	37	33
0.55	1307	408	221	149	91	67	54	47	42	38
0.60	1373	435	239	162	100	75	61	53	48	44
0.70	1629	531	298	206	131	100	83	73	66	61
0.80	2216	742	425	300	196	152	128	113	103	96
0.90	4083	1403	820	586	392	309	264	236	216	203

The feasibility of conducting cohort studies is influenced by challenges in accurately measuring individual exposures. If the disease is rare in both exposed and unexposed groups, assembling a sufficiently large study population may be difficult. Cohort studies, which begin with healthy individuals, allow for the examination of multiple outcomes, including those that are not possible to study in case–control designs.

Relative risk (RR), also known as the risk ratio, is defined as the ratio of the probability (risk) of disease occurring among exposed individuals to the probability of disease occurring among unexposed individuals (Bonita et al., 2006, p. 35). Using the notation presented in Table 8.1, relative risk can be calculated as follows (Equation 8.6):

$$RR = \frac{p_1}{p_2} = \frac{\text{Risk in exposed}}{\text{Risk in unexposed}} = \frac{a/(a+c)}{b/(b+d)} = \frac{a(b+d)}{b(a+c)} \tag{8.6}$$

where p_1 is the probability of disease in the exposed group and p_2 is the probability of disease in the unexposed group.

8.6 Sample Size Needed to Estimate Relative Risk (RR)

The required sample size for estimating the relative risk (RR) with a relative precision of ε can be calculated using Equation 8.7 (Lemeshow et al., 1988, p. 21):

$$n = Z^2_{1-\frac{\alpha}{2}} \times \frac{\left[\frac{(1-p_1)}{p_1} + \frac{(1-p_2)}{p_2}\right]}{\left[Ln(1-\varepsilon)\right]^2} \tag{8.7}$$

where

- p_1 and p_2 are the expected probabilities of outcomes occurring in the exposed and unexposed groups, respectively.
- ε represents the relative precision of the estimate.

Typically, one of the two probabilities, p_1 *or* p_2, is provided along with the anticipated relative risk (RR). The other probability can then be calculated using the following relationship:

$$p_2 = \frac{p_1}{RR} \quad or \quad p_1 = RR \times p_2 \tag{8.8}$$

Example 8.5: In a cohort study, an outcome is observed in 24% of the unexposed group. How many participants would be needed in both the exposed and unexposed study groups to estimate the relative risk within 15% of the true value? The true value is believed to be approximately 2.2, with a significance level of 5%.

Solution: The anticipated probability of the outcome in the unexposed group is $p_2 = 0.24$, the anticipated relative risk is RR = 2.2, and the relative precision is ε = 0.15. The expected probability of the outcome in the exposed group can be calculated as:

$$p_1 = p_2 \times RR = 0.24 \times 2.2 = 0.528$$

The required sample size for each group can be determined using Equation 8.7:

$$n = Z^2_{1-\frac{\alpha}{2}} \times \frac{\left[\frac{(1-p_1)}{p_1} + \frac{(1-p_2)}{p_2}\right]}{\left[Ln(1-\varepsilon)\right]^2}$$

Calculating this gives:

$$n = 1.96^2 \times \frac{\left[\frac{(1-0.528)}{0.528} + \frac{(1-0.24)}{0.24}\right]}{\left[Ln(1-0.15)\right]^2} = 3.8416 \times \frac{15.6075}{0.0264} = 591.53 \approx 592$$

To estimate the relative risk within 15% of the true value, a sample size of 592 participants is required for each of the two exposure groups.

Example 8.6: A health researcher is planning a study to investigate the potential association between a specific lung disease and exposure to a recently identified air pollutant. The researcher aims to estimate the relative risk within 50% of the true value (believed to be around 2) with 95% confidence in two groups: exposed and not exposed. If the disease affects 20% of individuals not exposed to the air pollutant, what sample size would be required in each group?

We can calculate the expected probability of disease among the exposed group, and the required sample size in each group can be obtained by substituting the provided information into Equation 8.7.

Solution: The information provided includes the anticipated probability of disease among the unexposed group ($p_2 = 0.20$), the anticipated relative risk (RR = 2), and the relative precision (ε = 0.50). The expected probability of disease among the exposed group is:

$$p_1 = p_2 \times RR = 0.20 \times 2 = 0.40$$

The required sample size in each group can be calculated using Equation 8.7:

$$n = Z^2_{1-\frac{\alpha}{2}} \times \frac{\left[\frac{(1-p_1)}{p_1} + \frac{(1-p_2)}{p_2}\right]}{\left[Ln(1-\varepsilon)\right]^2}$$

Substituting the values:

$$n = 1.96^2 \times \frac{\left[\frac{(1-0.40)}{0.40} + \frac{(1-0.20)}{0.20}\right]}{\left[Ln(1-0.50)\right]^2} = 43.97 \approx 44$$

Thus, 44 participants are required in each group.

The necessary sample size for estimating the relative risk (RR) for common proportions and various RR values ranging from 1 to 5, with a 5% significance level and 20% relative precision, is presented in Table 8.4. When RR ≥ 1, both RR and p_2 must be known. However, if RR < 1, refer to the column value corresponding to $\frac{1}{RR}$ and the row value corresponding to p_1.

8.7 Sample Size for Hypothesis Testing of Relative Risk (RR)

Similar to hypothesis testing for the odds ratio, the most common hypothesis test for the relative risk (RR) posits that the proportion of individuals who develop the disease in the exposed group (p_1) is equal to the proportion who develop the disease in the unexposed group (p_2). This can be expressed as the null hypothesis $H_0 : RR = 1$, which implies the probability of developing the disease is identical in both groups. Thus, this null hypothesis is equivalent to the general null hypothesis of equality of two proportions discussed in Chapter 7, stated as $H_0 : p_1 = p_2$.

As with other hypothesis tests, the alternative hypothesis may be one-sided ($H_A : RR > 1$ or $H_A : RR < 1$) or two-sided ($H_A : RR \neq 1$). These alternatives may also be expressed in terms of the corresponding disease probabilities for the two groups as $H_A : p_1 > p_2$, $H_A : p_1 < p_2$ or $H_A : p_1 \neq p_2$.

The required sample size for testing the null hypothesis $H_0 : RR = 1$ is analogous to the sample size needed for testing the equality of two independent proportions ($H_0 : p_1 = p_2$). In most applications, the values of $RR\,and\,p_2$ are provided, allowing the computation of $p_1 = RR \times p_2$. The necessary

TABLE 8.4

The Required Sample Size for Estimating the Relative Risk (RR) with a 5% Significance Level and 20% Relative Precision, extracted from Lemeshow et al. (1988, p. 171)

	RR										
p_2	1.00	1.25	1.50	1.75	2.00	2.50	3.00	3.50	4.00	4.50	5.00
0.01	26387	23722	21945	20676	19724	18391	17503	16868	16392	16022	15726
0.02	13061	11728	10840	10205	9729	9063	8618	8301	8063	7878	7730
0.03	8618	7730	7138	6715	6397	5953	5657	5445	5287	5163	5065
0.04	6397	5731	5287	4969	4731	4398	4176	4018	3899	3806	3732
0.05	5065	4532	4176	3922	3732	3465	3288	3161	3066	2992	2932
0.10	2399	2133	1955	1828	1733	1600	1511	1447	1400	1363	1333
0.15	1511	1333	1215	1130	1067	978	919	876	845	820	800
0.20	1067	933	845	781	733	667	622	591	567	548	534
0.25	800	693	622	572	534	480	445	419	400	–	–
0.30	622	534	474	432	400	356	326	–	–	–	–
0.35	495	419	369	332	305	267	–	–	–	–	–
0.40	400	334	289	258	234	200	–	–	–	–	–
0.45	326	267	228	199	178	–	–	–	–	–	–
0.50	267	214	178	153	134	–	–	–	–	–	–
0.55	219	170	138	115	–	–	–	–	–	–	–
0.60	178	134	104	–	–	–	–	–	–	–	–
0.70	115	77	–	–	–	–	–	–	–	–	–
0.80	67	34	–	–	–	–	–	–	–	–	–
0.90	30	–	–	–	–	–	–	–	–	–	–

sample size for a two-sided test can be obtained from the following formula (Lemeshow et al., 1988, p. 22; Lwanga et al., 1991, p. 60):

$$n = \left[\frac{Z_{1-\frac{\alpha}{2}} \cdot \sqrt{2\bar{p}(1-\bar{p})} + Z_{1-\beta} \cdot \sqrt{p_1(1-p_1) + p_2(1-p_2)}}{(p_1 - p_2)} \right]^2 \tag{8.9}$$

In this hypothesis test, the average proportion is defined as:

$$\bar{p} = \frac{p_1 + p_2}{2} = \frac{p_{2(RR+1)}}{2},$$

corresponding to the null and alternative hypotheses $H_0 : RR = 1$ and $\mathrm{H_A} : RR \neq 1$.

> **Example 8.7:** A medical research centre intends to conduct a cohort study to determine whether there is an increased risk of developing hypertension among individuals who consume high levels of salt compared to those who consume low levels of salt. The researcher plans to follow two groups: one with high salt consumption (exposed group) and one with low salt consumption (unexposed group). The hypothesised relative risk (RR) of developing hypertension is 1.8 for the high salt consumption group compared to the low salt consumption group. The significance level is set at $\alpha = 0.05$, and the power is set at 80% ($1 - \beta = 0.80$) to detect the hypothesised effect if it exists. The prevalence of hypertension in the low salt consumption group (unexposed group) is known to be 10%. The researcher plans to enrol equal numbers of participants in both groups (ratio of unexposed to exposed, $r = 1$). How many samples are required for each group in this cohort study?

Solution: The significance level of 5% corresponds to $Z_{1-\frac{\alpha}{2}} = 1.96$, and the power of 80% corresponds to $Z_{1-\beta} = 0.84$. The values:

$$p_2 = 0.12,\ RR = 1.8$$

$$p_1 = RR \times p_2 = 1.8 \times 0.10 = 0.18$$

Calculating the average proportion:

$$\bar{p} = \frac{p_1 + p_2}{2} = \frac{0.10 + 0.18}{2} = 0.14$$

Using Equation 8.9:

$$n = \left[\frac{Z_{1-\frac{\alpha}{2}} \cdot \sqrt{2\bar{p}(1-\bar{p})} + Z_{1-\beta} \cdot \sqrt{p_1(1-p_1) + p_2(1-p_2)}}{(p_1 - p_2)} \right]^2$$

Substituting the values:

$$n=\left[\frac{1.96.\sqrt{2\times0.14\times0.86}+0.84.\sqrt{0.18\times0.82+0.10\times0.90}}{(0.18-0.10)}\right]^2$$

$$=\left(\frac{1.3713}{0.08}\right)^2=293.82\approx294$$

Rounding up to the nearest whole number, the researcher needs to enrol approximately 294 individuals in each group (high salt consumption and low salt consumption) for this cohort study.

Example 8.8 (Clinical Trial on Cancer Treatments): A clinical trial is currently underway to compare the efficacy of two cancer treatments. Participants enrolled in the trial will be randomly assigned to receive either Treatment A or Treatment B. Over a five-year period, researchers will monitor the participants to determine the recurrence of their cancer. The primary objective of this trial is to assess whether Treatment A, a novel therapeutic approach, is superior to Treatment B in reducing the likelihood of cancer recurrence. If Treatment A demonstrates a 50% reduction in recurrence risk, it is expected to become the preferred treatment option. Currently, approximately 35% of patients receiving Treatment B experience a recurrence of their disease.

The critical question is: What sample size is required for each treatment group to achieve 90% power to reject the null hypothesis (H_0: RR = 1) if it is indeed false, while maintaining a 5% significance level?

Solution: The available information includes:

- Null hypothesis: $H_0: RR=1$
- Alternative hypothesis: $H_A: RR\neq1$
- Significance level of 5%: $Z_{1-\frac{\alpha}{2}}=1.96$
- Power of 90%: $Z_{1-\beta}=1.28$
- Expected recurrence risk for Treatment B: $p_2=0.35$
- Expected recurrence risk for Treatment A given a 50% reduction (RR = 0.50)
- $p_1=0.175$

This leads to the average proportion as follows:

$$\bar{p}=\frac{p_1+p_2}{2}=\frac{0.35+0.175}{2}=0.2625$$

The required sample size for each group is calculated using Equation 8.9:

$$n = \frac{\left[Z_{1-\frac{\alpha}{2}} \cdot \sqrt{2\bar{p}\left(1-\bar{p}\right)} + Z_{1-\beta} \cdot \sqrt{p_1\left(1-p_1\right)+p_2\left(1-p_2\right)} \right]^2}{\left[p_1 - p_2\right]^2}$$

Substituting the values:

$$n = \frac{\left[1.96.\sqrt{2 \times 0.2625 \times 0.7375} + 1.28.\sqrt{0.35 \times 0.65 + 0.175 \times 0.825}\right]^2}{\left[0.350 - 0.175\right]^2}$$

Calculating this gives:

$$n = \frac{\left[1.96 \cdot 0.3874 + 1.28 \cdot 0.22875\right]^2}{\left(0.175\right)^2} = 65.31 \approx 66$$

Rounding up to the nearest whole number, a sample size of 66 participants is required in each treatment group.

The required sample sizes for hypothesis testing of RR = 1 for common proportions and various relative risks ranging from 1 to 5, with a 5% significance level and 90% power in a two-sided alternative test, are provided in Table 8.5. If the value of RR is equal to or greater than 1, both RR and p_2 must be known. Conversely, if RR is less than 1, use the column value corresponding to $\frac{1}{RR}$ and the row value corresponding to p_1.

8.8 Incidence Rate

The incidence rate is a vital metric in epidemiology that quantifies the frequency of new disease cases within a population over a specified period of time. It is calculated by dividing the number of new cases by the total number of individuals at risk in the population during that period. This rate is often expressed per 1,000, 10,000, or 100,000 persons, providing a measure of the risk or probability that an individual in the population will develop the disease.

As a critical tool for public health officials, the incidence rate allows for the assessment of disease distribution and patterns, the identification of high-risk groups, and the monitoring of the impact of control measures. By analysing changes in the incidence rate over time, researchers can evaluate the effectiveness of interventions and policies aimed at reducing disease occurrence. Furthermore, the incidence rate aids in the allocation of healthcare resources and in planning public health campaigns, ultimately contributing to improved disease prevention and control within communities.

TABLE 8.5

Required Sample Size for Hypothesis Testing of Relative Risk (RR) with a 5% Significance Level and an 80% Power of the Test for a Two-Sided Alternative Hypothesis, extracted from Lemeshow et al. (1988, p. 186)

	RR										
p_2	1.00	1.25	1.50	1.75	2.00	2.50	3.00	3.50	4.00	4.50	5.00
0.01	27946	7752	3785	2319	1606	943	644	481	379	311	–
0.02	13814	3827	1866	1142	789	462	315	234	184	151	–
0.03	9103	2518	1226	749	517	302	205	152	119	97	–
0.04	6747	1864	906	553	381	222	150	111	87	70	–
0.05	5334	1471	714	435	299	174	117	86	67	54	–
0.10	2508	686	330	200	136	77	51	37	28	22	–
0.15	1566	425	202	121	82	45	29	20	15	11	–
0.20	1095	294	138	82	54	29	18	12	8	6	–
0.25	812	215	100	58	38	20	12	7	–	–	–
0.30	623	163	74	42	27	13	7	–	–	–	–
0.35	489	125	56	31	19	9	–	–	–	–	–
0.40	388	97	42	23	14	–	–	–	–	–	–
0.45	309	76	31	16	–	–	–	–	–	–	–
0.50	247	58	23	11	–	–	–	–	–	–	–
0.55	195	44	16	–	–	–	–	–	–	–	–
0.60	152	32	11	–	–	–	–	–	–	–	–
0.70	85	–	–	–	–	–	–	–	–	–	–
0.80	35	–	–	–	–	–	–	–	–	–	–

TIP

It is essential to distinguish clearly between incidence and prevalence. *Incidence* refers to the number of new cases of a disease or event that occur within a specified period and provides an estimate of the risk of developing the disease in a population during that time. It can also be used to compare disease risk across different populations or time periods. In contrast, *prevalence* represents the total number of existing cases of a disease or event at a particular point in time.

Formally, the incidence rate is defined as the number of new cases of a disease or event that occur in a population at risk per unit of time. It is typically expressed as a fraction, with the number of new cases in the numerator and the population at risk in the denominator, often standardised to populations of 1,000, 10,000, or 100,000 individuals. The formula for the incidence rate is:

$$\text{Incidence rate} = \frac{\text{Number of new events in a specified period}}{\text{Number of persons exposed to risk during this period}} \times 10^{n}$$

In this formula, the denominator may also be expressed in person-years, person-months, or other units of time, depending on the study design and the length of follow-up.

8.8.1 Sample Size Determination to Estimate Incidence Rate

As previously explained, the incidence rate is typically considered a type of proportion (Rothman et al., 2008, p. 39). The required sample size for estimating this rate is presented in Chapter 7 through Equation 7.2, which incorporates relative precision:

$$n = \left(z_{1-\frac{\alpha}{2}}\right)^2 \times \frac{(1-P)}{\varepsilon^2.P}$$

In this equation, if there is no prior expectation of the incidence rate, it is advisable to assume $p = 0.50$ to obtain a more conservative (i.e., larger) sample size estimate. Under this assumption, $1-p$ also equals 0.50, allowing both terms (p and $1-p$) both to cancel out in the calculation. Thus, to estimate the incidence rate of an event with $100(1 - \alpha)\%$ confidence in a single group, the required sample size can be derived using Equation 8.10 (Indrayan & Holt, 2016, p. 562; Lemeshow et al., 1988, p. 30):

$$n = \left(\frac{z_{1-\frac{\alpha}{2}}}{\varepsilon} \right)^2 \tag{8.10}$$

where ε represents the desired relative precision, expressed as a fraction of the anticipated incidence.

> **Example 8.9:** What is the required sample size of patients that a researcher should follow to estimate the incidence rate of a disease within 15% of its true value with 95% confidence?

Solution: By substituting $\varepsilon = 0.15$ and $z_{1-\frac{\alpha}{2}} = 1.96$, which corresponds to a 95% confidence level, into Equation 8.9, the required sample size can be determined as follow:

$$n = \left(\frac{z_{1-\frac{\alpha}{2}}}{\varepsilon} \right)^2 = \left(\frac{1.96}{0.15} \right)^2 = 170.74 \approx 171$$

Thus, the researcher will need to follow **171 individuals** until the "success" time (i.e., the event of interest) is observed for each participant. Alternatively, a sample size of 171 can be obtained directly from Table 8.6.

Table 8.6 presents sample sizes required to estimate the incidence rate with specified relative precisions at three significance levels: 90%, 95%, and 99%, for user convenience.

8.8.2 Sample Size Determination to Test the Equality of an Incidence Rate Against a Specific Value

To test the null hypothesis that the incidence rate of an event – expressed as the probability of events per a specified number of individuals over a given time unit – is equal to a particular value p_0 (i.e., $H_0 : p = p_0$), a z-test statistic is used. This is evaluated against the alternative hypothesis that the incidence rate differs from p_0 (i.e., $H_A : p \neq p_0$). The sample size required for this two-tailed test, given a desired power of $(1-\beta)$ and an α% significance level, can be calculated using Equation 8.11:

$$n = \frac{(Z_{1-\frac{\alpha}{2}} \cdot p_o + Z_{1-\beta} \cdot p_a)^2}{(p_0 - p_a)^2} \tag{8.11}$$

In this equation,

- p_0 represents the expected incidence rate under the null hypothesis,

- p_a is the specific incidence rate under the alternative hypothesis,
- ε denotes the required relative precision expressed as a fraction of the anticipated incidence.

TABLE 8.6

Required Sample Size to Estimate the Incidence Rate within ε Percent with 99%, 95%, or 90% Confidence Level

	Confidence Level		
ε	99%	95%	90%
0.01	66358	38417	27061
0.02	16590	9605	6766
0.03	7374	4269	3007
0.04	4148	2402	1692
0.05	2655	1537	1083
0.06	1844	1068	752
0.07	1355	785	553
0.08	1037	601	423
0.09	820	475	335
0.10	664	385	271
0.12	461	267	188
0.14	339	197	139
0.15	295	171	121
0.16	260	151	106
0.18	205	119	84
0.20	166	97	68
0.22	138	80	56
0.24	116	67	47
0.25	107	62	44
0.26	99	57	41
0.28	85	50	35
0.30	74	43	31
0.333	60	35	25
0.35	55	32	23
0.38	46	27	19
0.40	42	25	17
0.42	38	22	16
0.44	35	20	14
0.46	32	19	13
0.48	29	17	12
0.50	27	16	11

Example 8.10: A specific coronavirus strain has been identified, with initial studies suggesting an incidence rate of 20% among those exposed to

the virus in a specific setting. Public health authorities aim to verify this incidence rate through a more comprehensive study. They plan to test the hypothesis that the true incidence rate is 20% ($H_0 : p = 0.20$) against the alternative hypothesis that it differs from 20% ($H_A : p \neq 0.20$) by ±0.05, with a desired power of 80% and a two-sided significance level set at 0.05. What is the minimum sample size required?

Solution: To calculate the minimum sample size, we use Equation 8.11 for a two-sided test. Considering the incidence rates $p_0 = 0.20$ *and* $p_a = 0.15$ *or* 0.25, along with a desired power of 0.80 ($Z_{1-\beta} = 0.84$) and a significance level of 0.05 ($Z_{1-\frac{\alpha}{2}} = 1.96$), we proceed as follows:

1. Assuming $p_o = 0.15$:

$$n = \frac{(Z_{1-\frac{\alpha}{2}}.p_o + Z_{1-\beta}.p_a)^2}{(p_0 - p_a)^2} = \frac{(1.96 \times 0.20 + 0.84 \times 0.15)^2}{(0.20 - 0.15)^2} = 107.33 \approx 108$$

2. Assuming $p_o = 0.25$:

$$n = \frac{(Z_{1-\frac{\alpha}{2}}.p_o + Z_{1-\beta}.p_a)^2}{(p_0 - p_a)^2} = \frac{(1.96 \times 0.20 + 0.84 \times 0.25)^2}{(0.20 - 0.25)^2} = 145.2 \approx 146$$

Thus, a total of 146 subjects would need to be followed up. These results could also be obtained from Table 8.7 by selecting the larger number in the column labelled 0.20 and the rows labelled 0.15 and 0.25.

Example 8.11: In a similar context, public health authorities aim to verify the incidence rate of 20% against the alternative hypothesis that it may be greater than 20%, specifically testing for an incidence rate of 30%. With a desired power of 80% and a significance level set at 0.05, what is the minimum sample size required?

Solution: For this example, we will use Equation 8.11 for a one-sided test. Given $p_0 = 0.20$ *and* $p_a = 0.30$, along with a desired power of 0.80 (equivalent to $Z_{1-\beta} = 0.84$ and a one-sided significance level of 0.05 (equivalent to $Z_{1-\frac{\alpha}{2}} = 1.645$), we calculate:

$$n = \frac{(Z_{1-\alpha}.p_o + Z_{1-\beta}.p_a)^2}{(p_0 - p_a)^2} = \frac{(1.645 \times 0.20 + 0.84 \times 0.30)^2}{(0.20 - 0.30)^2} = 33.76 \approx 34$$

Since Table 8.7 is based on a two-sided test, it cannot be used for this one-sided test.

Table 8.7 Sample Sizes for Estimating the Incidence Rate with Specified Relative Precisions at Three Significance Levels: 90%, 95%, and 99%, for User Convenience. Derived from Lemeshow et al. (1988, p. 220)

TABLE 8.7

Sample Sizes for Estimating the Incidence Rate with Specified Relative Precisions at Three Significance Levels: 90%, 95%, and 99%, for User Convenience. Derived from Lemeshow et al. (1988, p. 220)

	p_0												
p_a	**0.05**	**0.10**	**0.15**	**0.20**	**0.25**	**0.30**	**0.35**	**0.40**	**0.45**	**0.50**	**0.60**	**0.70**	**0.80**
0.05	–	23	12	9	8	7	6	6	6	6	5	5	5
0.10	14	–	58	23	15	12	10	9	8	8	7	6	6
0.15	6	42	–	108	38	23	17	14	12	10	9	8	7
0.20	<	14	86	–	174	58	33	23	18	15	12	10	9
0.25	<	8	26	146	–	256	81	44	30	23	16	13	11
0.30	<	6	14	42	221	–	353	108	58	38	23	17	14
0.35	<	<	9	21	62	312	–	466	139	73	35	23	18
0.40	<	<	7	14	31	86	419	–	595	174	58	33	23
0.45	<	<	6	10	19	42	114	541	–	739	108	50	31
0.50	<	<	5	8	14	26	55	146	680	–	256	81	44
0.60	<	<	<	6	9	14	23	42	86	221	–	353	108
0.70	<	<	<	<	6	9	14	21	35	62	312	–	466
0.80	<	<	<	<	<	7	10	14	20	31	86	419	–

8.8.3 Hypothesis Testing for Incidence Rates in Two Populations

Some studies are designed to test and compare the hypothesis of equal incidence rates of a phenomenon in two populations. In these studies, one sample is selected from each population and followed over time until a final conclusion can be drawn, which involves observing the trait of interest for a specified or unspecified duration.

The primary objective of such a cohort study is to test the hypothesis that the true incidence rates of a disorder or characteristic are equal in two groups of individuals. Typically, the null hypothesis is stated as:

$$H_0: p_1 = p_2 \text{ or, } H_0: p_1 - p_2 = 0,$$

and the alternative hypothesis as:

$$H_A: p_1 \neq p_2 \text{ or } H_A: p_1 - p_2 \neq 0.$$

The sample size required to test the incidence rates in two populations is determined using Equation 8.12b (Lemeshow et al.,1988, p. 229):

$$n = \frac{\left[Z_{1-\frac{\alpha}{2}} \times \sqrt{2.\bar{p}^2} + Z_{1-\beta}\sqrt{\left(p_1^2 + p_2^2\right)}\right]^2}{\left[p_1 - p_2\right]^2} \tag{8.12}$$

where

p_1 and p_2 are the expected incidence rates in the two populations, and

$\bar{p} = \frac{p_1 + p_2}{2}$ is the average of the two incidence rates.

> **Example 8.12**: A study is being conducted to compare the incidence of hearing impairment between workers in a noisy industry and those in a quieter industry. The noisy industry has an estimated annual incidence rate of 25%, while the quieter industry is expected to have a rate closer to the national average of about 10%. The study will follow participants until hearing impairment occurs or for the duration of their lives. How many individuals should be included in each group to detect a difference in incidence rates with 80% power and a 5% significance level?

Solution: This is a two-tailed test because the alternative hypothesis is:

$$H_A: p_1 - p_2 \neq 0$$

where $p_1 = 0.25$, $p_2 = 0.10$, and the average incidence rate is:

$$\bar{p} = \frac{p_1 + p_2}{2} = 0.175$$

The test has 80% power ($Z_{1-\beta} = 0.84$) and a 5% significance level ($Z_{1-\frac{\alpha}{2}} = 1.96$).
Using Equation 8.12:

$$n = \frac{\left[Z_{1-\frac{\alpha}{2}} \times \sqrt{2.\bar{p}^2} + Z_{1-\beta}\sqrt{\left(p_1^2 + p_2^2\right)}\right]^2}{\left[p_1 - p_2\right]^2}$$

Plugging in the values:

$$n = \frac{\left[1.96 \times \sqrt{2 \times (0.175)^2} + 0.84\sqrt{\left(0.25^2 + 0.10^2\right)}\right]^2}{\left[0.25 - 0.10\right]^2} = 23.45 \approx 24$$

This value can be obtained from Table 8.6. Consequently, a minimum of 24 subjects must be monitored in each group until hearing impairment occurs.

> **Example 8.13:** A research project has been designed to investigate the impact of exposure to a chemical on respiratory health among workers. The goal is to compare the occurrence of respiratory issues between workers exposed to the chemical and those who are not. The exposed group consists of workers who handle the chemical directly, whereas the unexposed group comprises workers in a different department where the chemical is not used. Historical data suggest that the exposed group has a 26% incidence rate, while the unexposed group is expected to have a 10% rate based on national averages. To detect the effect of chemical exposure on respiratory health with 90% power and a 5% significance level, how many individuals should be followed in each group?

Solution: This test is also a two-tailed test, with $p_1 = 0.26$, $p_2 = 0.10$, and

$$\bar{p} = \frac{p_1 + p_2}{2} = 0.18$$

The test has 90% power, corresponding to $Z_{1-\beta} = 1.28$, and a 5% significance level, corresponding to $Z_{1-\frac{\alpha}{2}} = 1.96$. Substituting these values into Equation 8.12 gives:

$$n = \frac{\left[Z_{1-\frac{\alpha}{2}} \times \sqrt{2.\bar{p}^2} + Z_{1-\beta}\sqrt{\left(p_1^2 + p_2^2\right)}\right]^2}{\left[p_1 - p_2\right]^2}$$

Plugging in the values:

$$n = \frac{\left[1.96 \times \sqrt{2 \times (0.18)^2} + 1.28\sqrt{\left(0.26^2 + 0.10^2\right)}\right]^2}{\left[0.26 - 0.10\right]^2}$$

Calculating this gives:

$$n = \frac{[0.8555]^2}{[0.16]^2} = 28.59 \approx 29$$

Thus, at least 29 subjects are needed in each group.

For user convenience, Table 8.9 provides sample sizes for testing the equality of incidence rates between two populations at a significance level of 5% and a power of 80%.

If a researcher intends to use unequal sample sizes from two populations, denoted as n_1 and n_2, where $n_2 = k.n_1$, the sample size can be calculated using Equation 8.13 as follows (Lemeshow et al., 1988, p. 33):

$$n_1 = \frac{\left[Z_{1-\frac{\alpha}{2}} \times \sqrt{(1+k).\bar{p}^2} + Z_{1-\beta}\sqrt{\left(kp_1^2 + p_2^2\right)}\right]^2}{k\left[p_1 - p_2\right]^2} \tag{8.13}$$

In this equation, p_1 and p_2 represent the expected incidence rates in the two populations, and $\bar{p} = \frac{p_1 + kp_2}{1+k}$ is the weighted average of the two incidence rates.

Example 8.14: Building on the information provided in Example 8.13, consider a scenario in which the researcher wishes to use unequal sample sizes, with twice as many participants in the unexposed group (n_2) compared to the exposed group (n_1). The sample size in each department can be calculated as follows.

Solution: The methodology remains consistent with Example 8.13, except that k = 2, and the average incidence rate is calculated as:

$$\bar{p} = \frac{p_1 + 2p_2}{1+k} = \frac{0.26 + 2 \times 0.10}{1+2} = 0.1533$$

Using Equation 8.13, the required sample size is:

$$n_1 = \frac{\left[Z_{1-\frac{\alpha}{2}} \times \sqrt{(1+k).\bar{p}^2} + Z_{1-\beta}\sqrt{\left(kp_1^2 + p_2^2\right)}\right]^2}{k\left[p_1 - p_2\right]^2}$$

Substituting the relevant values:

$$n_1 = \frac{\left[1.96 \times \sqrt{(1+2).0.1533^2} + 1.28\sqrt{\left(2 \times 0.26^2 + 0.10^2\right)}\right]^2}{2[0.26 - 0.10]^2} = \frac{(1.00817)^2}{0.0512} = 19.69 \approx 20$$

TABLE 8.8

Necessary Sample Size for Testing the Equality of Incidence Densities. The significance level is 5%, power is 80%, and the alternative hypothesis is two-sided. This information is derived from Lemeshow et al. (1988, p. 229)

	p_1												
p_2	**0.05**	**0.10**	**0.15**	**0.20**	**0.25**	**0.30**	**0.35**	**0.40**	**0.45**	**0.50**	**0.60**	**0.70**	**0.80**
0.05	–	37	17	13	10	9	9	8	8	7	7	7	7
0.10	37	–	100	37	23	17	14	13	11	10	9	9	8
0.15	17	100	–	194	64	37	26	21	17	15	13	11	10
0.20	13	37	194	–	320	100	54	37	28	23	17	14	13
0.25	10	23	64	320	–	477	143	75	50	37	25	19	16
0.30	9	17	37	100	477	–	665	194	100	64	37	26	21
0.35	9	14	26	54	143	665	–	885	253	128	58	37	27
0.40	8	13	21	37	75	194	885	–	1136	320	100	54	37
0.45	8	11	17	28	50	100	253	1136	–	1419	194	85	52
0.50	7	10	15	23	37	64	128	320	1419	–	477	143	75
0.60	7	9	13	17	25	37	58	100	194	477	–	665	194
0.70	7	9	11	14	19	26	37	54	85	143	665	–	885
0.80	7	8	10	13	16	21	27	37	52	75	194	885	–

Thus, the sample size for the unexposed group is calculated as:

$$n_2 = k.n_1 = 2 \times 20 = 40$$

Finally, this study requires enrolling 20 participants in the exposed group and 40 participants in the unexposed group.

Additional Remark: In some studies, researchers may choose to end the study at a predetermined time point, even if not all subjects have reached the planned endpoint. In such cases, these observations are considered *censored*. The study begins on a designated start date, allows patients to enrol throughout the study period, and terminates enrolment and follow-up after T years. This approach helps control the overall duration of the study; however, researchers must also consider how to handle the censored observations that are likely to occur. This requires modifications to the value of p. While the mathematical adjustments are not detailed in this book, the modified sample size equation is presented in Equation 8.14:

$$n = \frac{\left[Z_{1-\frac{\alpha}{2}} \times \sqrt{2f(\bar{p})} + Z_{1-\beta}\sqrt{f(p_1) + f(p_2)} \right]^2}{\left[p_1 - p_2 \right]^2} \tag{8.14}$$

where $f(p)$ is defined in Equation 8.15.

$$f(p) = \frac{T \cdot p^3}{T.p - 1 + e^{-T.p}} \tag{8.15}$$

To obtain $f(p_1), f(p_2) \, and \, f(\bar{p})$, the values of $p_1, p_2 \, and \, \bar{p}$ must be substituted into Equation 8.15. Once these values are computed, the required sample size for follow-up studies with planned endpoints can be determined using Equation 8.14.

> **Example 8.15:** Based on the insights gained from Example 8.13, consider a scenario in which the study is constrained to conclude within 5 years. The researcher aims to test the hypothesis $H_0 : p_1 = p_2 = 0.15$ against the alternative hypothesis $H_A : p_1 = 0.26 \, and \, p_2 = 0.10$, with a significance level of 0.05 and a power of 0.80. The objective is to determine the number of individuals that should be monitored in each department.

Solution: The choice of $\bar{p}$ depends on the null hypothesis; here we first set $\bar{p} = 0.15$. Using $p_1 = 0.26, p_2 = 0.10, \, \bar{p} = 0.15 \, and \, T = 5$ into Equation 8.15 for $f(p)$, we calculate $f(p_1), f(p_2) \, and \, f(\bar{p})$ as follows:

$$f(p_1) = \frac{T \cdot p^3}{Tp - 1 + e^{-Tp}} = \frac{5 \times 0.26^3}{5 \times 0.26 - 1 + e^{-5 \times 0.26}} = \frac{0.08788}{0.5725} = 0.1535$$

$$f(p_2) = \frac{T \cdot p^3}{Tp - 1 + e^{-Tp}} = \frac{5 \times 0.10^3}{5 \times 0.10 - 1 + e^{-5 \times 0.10}} = \frac{0.005}{0.1065} = 0.04693$$

$$f(\bar{p}) = \frac{T \cdot p^3}{Tp - 1 + e^{-Tp}} = \frac{5 \times 0.15^3}{5 \times 0.15 - 1 + e^{-5 \times 0.15}} = \frac{0.016875}{0.4724} = 0.0357$$

The sample size can then be calculated using the following equation:

$$n = \frac{\left[Z_{1-\frac{\alpha}{2}} \times \sqrt{2 f(\bar{p})} + Z_{1-\beta} \sqrt{f(p_1) + f(p_2)} \right]^2}{\left[p_1 - p_2 \right]^2}$$

Substituting the values:

$$n = \frac{\left[1.96 \times \sqrt{2 \times 0.0357} + 1.28 \sqrt{0.1535 + 0.04693} \right]^2}{\left[0.26 - 0.10 \right]^2} = 46.93 \approx 47$$

If we choose $\bar{p} = 0.15$ based on the null hypothesis, the sample size is smaller (approximately 47). If we choose $\bar{p} = 0.18$, the sample size increases to approximately 64.

The choice of $\bar{p}$ directly impacts the sample size calculation and depends on whether one wants to be conservative and aligned with the null hypothesis (using $\bar{p} = 0.15$) or reflect a more realistic scenario based on expected incidence rates (using $\bar{p} = 0.18$).

Example 8.16: In this example, we consider a researcher from Example 8.12, who previously identified an incidence rate of hearing impairment of 25% in a noisy industry compared to approximately 10% in a quieter industry, which aligns with the national average. The researcher plans to conduct a follow-up study on hearing impairment over a period of 3 years. The objective is to determine the necessary sample size for each group to detect a difference in incidence rates with 80% power and a significance level of 5%.

Solution: The relevant parameters are as follows:

- $p_1 = 0.25$ (incidence rate in the noisy industry),
- $p_2 = 0.10$(incidence rate in the quieter industry),
- $\bar{p} = 0.175$ (average incidence rate), and
- $T = 3$ (duration of the study in years).

We will substitute these values into the equation to calculate $f(p_1), f(p_2) \, and \, f(\bar{p})$ and ultimately determine the required sample size for each group.

$$f(p_1) = \frac{T \cdot p^3}{Tp - 1 + e^{-Tp}} = \frac{3 \times 0.25^3}{3 \times 0.25 - 1 + e^{-3 \times 0.25}} = \frac{0.046875}{0.2224} = 0.2108$$

$$f(p_2) = \frac{T \cdot p^3}{Tp - 1 + e^{-Tp}} = \frac{3 \times 0.10^3}{3 \times 0.10 - 1 + e^{-3 \times 0.10}} = \frac{0.003}{0.0408} = 0.0735$$

$$f(\bar{p}) = \frac{T \cdot p^3}{Tp - 1 + e^{-Tp}} = \frac{3 \times 0.175^3}{3 \times 0.175 - 1 + e^{-3 \times 0.175}} = \frac{0.01608}{0.1166} = 0.1379$$

The sample size can then be calculated using the following equation:

$$n = \frac{\left[Z_{1-\frac{\alpha}{2}} \times \sqrt{2f(\bar{p})} + Z_{1-\beta} \sqrt{f(p_1) + f(p_2)} \right]^2}{\left[p_1 - p_2 \right]^2}$$

Substituting the values:

$$n = \frac{\left[1.96 \times \sqrt{2 \times 0.1379} + 1.28 \sqrt{0.2108 + 0.0735} \right]^2}{\left[0.25 - 0.10 \right]^2}$$

Calculating further:

$$n = \frac{\left[1.96 \times 0.5252 + 1.28 \times 0.5332 \right]^2}{\left[0.25 - 0.10 \right]^2} = 130.24 \approx 131$$

Thus, the required sample size for each group should be approximately **131** individuals.

8.9 Prevalence Rates

Prevalence studies are a specific type of epidemiological research in which a representative sample is selected from the population to estimate the proportion of individuals with a particular condition at a given point in time. This condition may relate to exposure or disease and is typically expressed as a proportion, referred to as prevalence. This measure provides an immediate snapshot of the number of individuals with the condition relative to the total number of eligible individuals in the population.

It is important to distinguish prevalence from incidence, which measures the number of new cases occurring in the population within a defined time period. Prevalence may be higher or lower than incidence, depending on the duration of the condition and the rates at which new cases arise or existing cases exit the population. Therefore, prevalence and incidence should not be used interchangeably (Lemeshow et al., 1988, p. 71).

TIP

The goal of prevalence studies is to obtain an accurate proportion from a sample that can be generalised to the larger population; therefore, using sample size formulas for proportions is essential to determine the number of participants needed to estimate prevalence rates effectively.

Prevalence itself is inherently a proportion, representing the fraction of individuals in a population who exhibit a specific characteristic or condition at a given time. When estimating prevalence, the goal is to derive an accurate proportion from the sample that can be generalised to the larger population. Consequently, sample size formulas for proportions can be used to calculate the number of participants needed to estimate prevalence rates effectively.

Statistical considerations for sample size calculations when estimating proportions are directly applicable to prevalence studies. These considerations include the desired precision of the estimate (margin of error), the confidence level, and any design effects if the sampling method is more complex than simple random sampling. Therefore, it is unnecessary to develop separate methods for sample size determination specifically for estimating prevalence or for hypothesis testing related to prevalence. For a more detailed discussion on calculating sample size, refer to Chapter 7 (Daniel & Cross, 2018; Lemeshow et al., 1988, p. 71).

For example, Example 7.4 determines the sample size required to estimate the prevalence of pulmonary tuberculosis (TB) in Kermanshah province using the standard formula for estimating a proportion.

8.10 Sample Sizes for Sensitivity and Specificity

Sensitivity and specificity are critical measures used to evaluate the accuracy of a diagnostic test relative to a gold standard. Determining an adequate sample size is essential for precisely estimating the validity of a diagnostic test and for testing statistical significance. To achieve accurate estimates with a desired level of precision, formulas similar to those used for proportions are employed, but they must be adjusted according to the prevalence of the disease.

For situations in which both the diagnostic test and the gold standard yield dichotomous outcomes, the sample size formulas are as follows (Indrayan & Holt, 2016, p. 558):

$$n_{Sen} = \frac{z^2_{1-\frac{\alpha}{2}} \times Sen\ (1 - Sen)}{L^2 \times Prevaalence} \tag{8.16}$$

$$n_{Sp} = \frac{z^2_{1-\frac{\alpha}{2}} \times Sp(1 - Sp)}{L^2 \times (1 - Prevaalence)} \tag{8.17}$$

where

- Sen = anticipated sensitivity,
- SP = anticipated specificity,
- $(1 - \alpha)$ confidence level, and
- L = absolute precision desired on either side (half-width of the confidence interval) of sensitivity or specificity.

For example, consider a disease with a prevalence of 8% in the target population. To accurately estimate the sensitivity of a diagnostic test, the sample must include a sufficient number of individuals who actually have the disease (true positives). Since only 8% of the population is expected to be disease-positive, the calculated sample size for sensitivity must be divided by 0.08. This adjustment ensures that enough disease-positive individuals are included to achieve the desired precision in the sensitivity estimate.

Similarly, to estimate specificity, the sample must include a sufficient number of disease-negative individuals (true negatives). Because 92% of the population is expected to be disease-negative (1 – 0.08 = 0.92), the sample size for specificity must be divided by 0.92. By making these prevalence-based adjustments, the study ensures that both disease-positive and disease-negative subgroups are adequately represented, allowing for precise and reliable estimates of sensitivity and specificity.

> **Example 8.17:** A diagnostic test is being evaluated for detecting a rare disease with a prevalence of 8% in the target population. The anticipated sensitivity of the test is 85%, and the anticipated specificity is 90%. The researcher wants to estimate both sensitivity and specificity with an absolute precision of ±10% at a 95% confidence level. What is the minimum total sample size required to achieve this?

Solution: We first calculate the number of disease-positive individuals needed to estimate sensitivity, using the formula for estimating a proportion and substituting the values of Sen = 0.85, L = 0.10 and $Z_{1-\frac{\alpha}{2}} = 1.96$:

$$n_{positive} = \frac{Z^2_{1-\frac{\alpha}{2}} \cdot Sen \cdot (1 - Sen)}{L^2} = \frac{1.96^2 \times 0.85 \times (1 - 0.85)}{0.10^2} \approx 49$$

This means 49 disease-positive individuals are required to estimate sensitivity with the desired precision.

Since the disease prevalence is 8%, only 8% of the population will be disease-positive. Therefore, the total sample size should be adjusted by dividing by 0.08 as below:

$$N_{total} = \frac{n_{positive}}{prevalence} = \frac{49}{0.08} \approx 613$$

Next, we calculate the number of disease-negative individuals needed to estimate specificity using the formula for estimating a proportion. Here, Sp = 0.90, $L = 0.10$, and $Z_1 - \alpha/2 = 1.96$:

$$n_{negative} = \frac{Z^2_{1-\frac{\alpha}{2}} \cdot Sp \cdot (1 - Sp)}{L^2} = \frac{1.96^2 \times 0.90 \times (1 - 0.90)}{0.10^2} \approx 35$$

This means 35 disease-negative individuals are required to estimate specificity with the desired precision.

Since 92% of the population is disease-negative $(1 - 0.08 = 0.92)$, the total sample size should be adjusted by dividing by 0.92:

$$N_{total} = \frac{n_{negaive}}{prevalence} = \frac{35}{0.92} \approx 38$$

Therefore, to estimate both sensitivity and specificity with ±10% precision at a 95% confidence level:

- The number of disease-positive individuals required is 49 → total population needed ≈ 613.
- The number of disease-negative individuals required is 35 → total population needed ≈ 38.

Because we must satisfy both criteria simultaneously, the total sample size should be the larger of the two totals. Therefore, the minimum total sample size required is approximately 613 participants.

8.11 Lot Quality Assurance Sampling

Lot quality assurance sampling (LQAS) is a statistical method used to evaluate the quality of a production lot by inspecting a sample of items. Developed in the 1920s, LQAS is widely employed in manufacturing to ensure that quality standards are met for the entire lot before distribution. This method analyses data from a small sample to facilitate industrial quality control. By randomly selecting items and assessing their quality, companies can make informed decisions about accepting or rejecting the entire lot, thereby minimising the risk of distributing defective products and ensuring that customers receive high-quality items.

In the health sector, LQAS is similarly utilised to assess health programmes. Adapted in the mid-1980s for this purpose, its use was further promoted by a 1991 World Health Organization (WHO) report on epidemiological and statistical methods for rapid monitoring of health programmes. Health events, such as disease prevalence, are monitored using quantified indices and measures. By analysing sample data, LQAS helps determine whether a population has been immunised against a disease based on established standards or thresholds.

The null hypothesis in LQAS posits that the proportion of individuals exhibiting a specific characteristic is equal to a predetermined value. In a one-sided test, this null hypothesis can only be rejected if the sample meets a specified standard. A "threshold value" is calculated to establish a decision rule: if the number of sampled individuals with the characteristic falls below the threshold, the null hypothesis is rejected and the lot is accepted. Conversely, if the threshold is exceeded, the lot is rejected.

TIP

LQAS survey problems involve one-sided tests. This means that the null hypothesis $H_0 : p = p_0$ is tested against the alternative hypothesis $H_A : p_0 > p_a$, where p_a is specified (Lemeshow et al., 1988, p. 27).

LQAS methodology offers several advantages, including simplicity in sampling procedures and analyses, rapid utilisation of findings by local managers and health workers, and the ability to aggregate data from individual supervision areas to estimate coverage for the entire programme catchment area. A small sample is sufficient to determine whether a supervision area meets the average coverage of the catchment area or a predetermined target.

The required sample size for LQAS studies, applicable to both finite and infinite populations, is calculated using Equations 8.18 and 8.19:

$$\frac{\sum_{x=0}^{d^*} MC_x^{(N-M)} C_{(n-x)}^{M}}{C_n^N} < \alpha \tag{8.18}$$

$$\sum_{x=0}^{d^*} C_x^n P^x (1-P)^{n-x} < \alpha \tag{8.19}$$

where $M = N.p$, α represents the significance level, p is the anticipated population prevalence, and C_n^x denotes the number of combinations of x from n.

Solving these inequalities can be challenging and time-consuming. To facilitate the process, necessary sample sizes for LQAS have been compiled for various proportions and population sizes ranging from 200 to 25,000, as well as for infinite populations. This compilation is based on information from Lwanga (pp. 63–68) and is summarised in Table 8.10, which outlines the sample size calculations for LQAS with a 95% confidence level and 90% power of the test.

TABLE 8.9

Sample Size Calculation for LQAS for Selected Proportions with a 95% Confidence Interval and 90% Power of the Test (extracted from Lwanga et al., 1991, pp. 63–69)

		p							
N	*d*	0.90	0.70	0.50	0.40	0.30	0.20	0.10	0.05
200	*d* = 0	2	2	4	0	7	10	20	41
	d = 1	3	5	8	10	14	21	42	77
	d = 2	5	7	11	14	19	28	54	98
	d = 3	6	9	13	17	23	34	66	116
	d = 4	7	10	16	20	27	41	77	132
1000	*d* = 0	2	2	4	0	7	11	22	44
	d = 1	3	5	8	10	14	22	45	90
	d = 2	5	7	11	14	19	29	60	118
	d = 3	6	9	13	17	24	36	74	145
	d = 4	7	10	16	21	28	43	87	170
2000	*d* = 0	2	2	4	0	7	11	22	45
	d = 1	3	5	8	10	14	22	46	92
	d = 2	5	7	11	14	19	30	61	122
	d = 3	6	9	13	17	24	37	75	150
	d = 4	7	10	16	21	28	43	88	176

(Continued)

TABLE 8.9 (CONTINUED)

Sample Size Calculation for LQAS for Selected Proportions with a 95% Confidence Interval and 90% Power of the Test (extracted from Lwanga et al., 1991, pp. 63–69)

		p							
N	*d*	0.90	0.70	0.50	0.40	0.30	0.20	0.10	0.05
	$d = 0$	2	2	4	0	7	11	22	45
	$d = 1$	3	5	8	10	14	22	46	93
	$d = 2$	5	7	11	14	19	30	61	122
	$d = 3$	6	9	13	17	24	37	75	150
2500	$d = 4$	7	10	16	21	28	43	89	177
	$d = 0$	2	2	4	0	7	11	22	45
	$d = 1$	3	5	8	10	14	22	46	93
	$d = 2$	5	7	11	14	19	30	61	123
	$d = 3$	6	9	13	17	24	37	75	152
5000	$d = 4$	7	10	16	21	28	43	89	179
	$d = 0$	2	2	4	0	7	11	22	45
	$d = 1$	3	5	8	10	14	22	46	93
	$d = 2$	5	7	11	14	19	30	61	123
	$d = 3$	6	9	13	17	24	37	75	152
10000	$d = 4$	7	10	16	21	28	44	89	180
	$d = 0$	2	3	5	0	9	14	29	59
	$d = 1$	3	5	8	10	14	22	46	93
	$d = 2$	5	7	11	14	19	30	62	124
	$d = 3$	6	9	13	17	24	37	76	153
25000	$d = 4$	7	10	16	21	28	44	90	181
	$d = 0$	2	3	5	0	9	14	29	59
	$d = 1$	3	5	8	10	14	22	46	94
	$d = 2$	5	7	11	14	19	30	62	125
	$d = 3$	6	9	13	17	24	37	76	155
Infinity	$d = 4$	7	10	16	21	28	44	90	181

Table 8.9 is used when a researcher has the following information:

- The population size (N),
- The number of individuals exhibiting a particular characteristic (d), and
- The prevalence of that characteristic in the population (p).

This information enables the researcher to determine the required sample size such that, if the number of individuals with the specified characteristic does not exceed d, the population can be accepted as not surpassing a predefined threshold.

> **Example 8.18:** In a college with 2,000 students, how many students should be examined to conclude, with 95% confidence and 90% power, that the prevalence of influenza in the college is no more than 10% if no more than three students are found to have the flu?

Solution: The expected population prevalence of influenza is 10%. Given a population size of 2,000 and a maximum of three flu cases in the sample, with a confidence level of 95% and a power of 90%, Table 8.10 indicates that a sample size of 75 randomly selected students is required.

> **Example 8.19:** The health department aims to determine whether the COVID-19 unvaccinated rate among citizens in a city of 10,000 people is 20%. They need to ascertain how many citizens should be surveyed to conclude, with 95% confidence and 90% power, that the unvaccinated rate is no more than 25% if no more than four unvaccinated individuals are identified.

Solution: With a population size of 10,000 and an expected unvaccinated rate of 20%, along with a maximum of four unvaccinated cases in the sample and a confidence level of 95%, Table 8.10 indicates that a sample size of 89 randomly selected citizens is required.

8.11.1 Another Perspective on LQAS

From a different viewpoint, some studies utilising lot quality assurance sampling (LQAS) aim to determine the number of subjects exhibiting a specific characteristic (denoted as "d") that must be observed in a sample (denoted as "n") drawn from a given population. This assessment helps evaluate whether the population meets a particular standard, a process referred to as the "decision rule for rejecting a lot".

In simpler terms, researchers focus on testing a specific "lot" (the sampled population) to determine if it meets established criteria. In these tests, the null hypothesis posits that the proportion of individuals with a certain characteristic in the population (p_0) is equal to a specified value (p_a). These one-sided tests are designed such that the sample is accepted only if it meets the predetermined standard; otherwise, the null hypothesis can be rejected.

To facilitate this, a "threshold value" of individuals with the characteristic (d^*) is calculated as the basis for the decision rule. If the observed number of individuals with this characteristic does not exceed the threshold, the null hypothesis is rejected, indicating that the lot is accepted. Conversely, if the observed number exceeds the threshold, there is insufficient reason to reject the null hypothesis, resulting in the rejection of the lot.

The necessary sample size (n) and the required threshold (d^*) are determined using the following equations:

$$n = \frac{\left(Z_{1-\alpha}\sqrt{p_o(1-p_o)} + Z_{1-\beta}\sqrt{p_a(1-p_a)}\right)^2}{(p_o - p_a)^2} \tag{8.20}$$

$$d^* = n.p_o - Z_{1-\alpha}\sqrt{n \cdot p_o(1-p_o)} \tag{8.21}$$

It is important to note that the calculated value of d* from the above equation should always be rounded down to the nearest integer. For example, both 5.8 and 5.1 would be rounded to 5.

> **Example 8.20:** A hospital manager aims to ensure that hand hygiene compliance among healthcare workers reaches at least 90%. However, they suspect that the actual compliance rate may be as low as 70%. To monitor this compliance, they decide to employ lot quality assurance sampling (LQAS). The manager needs to determine the appropriate number of healthcare worker observations to sample, as well as the maximum acceptable number of non-compliant observations in the sample, in order to test the programme's performance target at a 5% significance level with 80% power.

Solution: In this example, the compliance rate under the null hypothesis is $p_0 = 0.90$, and under the alterhypothesis, it is $p_a = 0.70$. A power of 0.80 corresponds to 0.84, and the 5% significance level for a one-tailed test corresponds to a critical value of 1.645.

Substituting these values into Equation 8.20, we calculate the sample size n:

$$n = \frac{\left(Z_{1-\alpha}\sqrt{p_o(1-p_o)} + Z_{1-\beta}\sqrt{p_a(1-p_a)}\right)^2}{(p_o - p_a)^2}$$

$$= \frac{\left(1.645\sqrt{0.90(1-0.90)} + 0.84\sqrt{0.70(1-0.70)}\right)^2}{(0.90-0.70)^2}$$

Calculating these yields:

$$n = \frac{(0.8784)^2}{(0.20)^2} = 19.29 \approx 20$$

Since we must round up to the nearest whole number, we conclude that 20 samples are needed.

Next, we calculate the decision rule d^* using Equation 8.21:

$$d^* = n.p_o - Z_{1-\alpha}\sqrt{n \cdot p_o(1-p_o)} = 20 \times 0.90 - 1.645\sqrt{20 \times 0.90(1-0.90)} = 15.79 \approx 15$$

Rounding down to the nearest whole number gives us 15.

If 15 or fewer healthcare workers are non-compliant in the sample of 20, the lot is accepted, and it can be concluded that hand hygiene compliance likely meets the target of at least 70%. If more than 15 are non-compliant, the lot is rejected, indicating that compliance may be below the desired standard.

Note: Table 8.8 can also provide approximate values, but slight differences may occur because Table 8.8 uses exact binomial calculations.

> **Example 8.21:** A new vaccine trial is underway to evaluate its effectiveness in preventing a specific disease. The researchers aim to confirm that the vaccine is successful in preventing the disease in at least 90% of the population. Initial findings suggest that it may be effective in only 80% of cases. Consequently, the researchers must calculate the required sample size to test the vaccine's efficacy and determine the maximum number of vaccine failures that can occur in the sample while still achieving the efficacy goal at a 5% significance level with 90% power.

Solution: Similar to Example 8.10, where $p_0 = 0.90$, $p_a = 0.80$. A power of 0.90 corresponds to a critical value of 1.28, and a 5% significance level for a one-tailed test corresponds to 1.645. Substituting these values into Equations 8.20 and 8.21 allows us to calculate the sample size n and the decision rule d^*:

$$n = \frac{\left(Z_{1-\alpha}\sqrt{p_o(1-p_o)} + Z_{1-\beta}\sqrt{p_a(1-p_a)}\right)^2}{(p_o - p_a)^2}$$

$$= \frac{\left(1.645\sqrt{0.90(1-0.90)} + 1.28\sqrt{0.80(1-0.80)}\right)^2}{(0.90-0.80)^2}$$

Calculating these yields:

$$n = \frac{(1.0055)^2}{(0.10)^2} = 101.1 \approx 102$$

Next, we calculate the decision rule d^* using Equation 8.21:

$$d^* = n. - Z_{1-\alpha}\sqrt{n \cdot p_o(1-p_o)}p_o = 102 \times 0.90 - 1.645\sqrt{102 \times 0.90(1-0.90)} = 86.7 \approx 86$$

Rounding down to the nearest whole number 86 ensures that the threshold is conservative, as required in LQAS.

Therefore, if no more than 86 vaccine failures are observed in the sample of 102 participants, the lot is accepted, and the vaccine is considered to meet the minimum efficacy threshold; in this case, we reject the null hypothesis that the vaccine's efficacy is below the acceptable level. Conversely, if more than 86 failures are observed, the lot is rejected, and we fail to reject the null hypothesis, indicating insufficient evidence that the vaccine achieves the desired efficacy.

Example 8.22: In a large refugee camp, a child health programme aims to achieve a minimum coverage of 70% among all children. However, there are concerns that the current outreach is reaching only 40% of the child population. To evaluate the programme's effectiveness, it is necessary to determine the required sample size and the maximum number of children who can remain unserved while still being considered acceptable. This assessment seeks to test the programme's performance target using a significance level of 5% and a statistical power of 90%.

Solution: The null hypothesis is defined as $H_0 : p_0 = 0.70$, while the alternative hypothesis is $H_0 : p_a = 0.40$. For a one-tailed test at a 5% significance level, the corresponding z-value is 1.645. A power of 90% corresponds to a z-value of 1.28. The required sample size n is calculated using Equation 8.20:

$$n = \frac{\left(Z_{1-\alpha}\sqrt{p_o(1-p_o)} + Z_{1-\beta}\sqrt{p_a(1-p_a)}\right)^2}{(p_o - p_a)^2}$$

Substituting the values:

$$n = \frac{\left(1.645\sqrt{0.70(1-0.70)} + 1.28\sqrt{0.40(1-0.40)}\right)^2}{(0.70-0.40)^2}$$

Calculating this yields:

$$n = \frac{(1.381)^2}{(0.30)^2} = 21.18 \approx 22$$

Next, we calculate the decision rule d^* using Equation 8.21:

$$d^* = n. - Z_{1-\frac{\alpha}{2}}\sqrt{n \cdot p_o(1-p_o)}p_o$$

Substituting the values:

$$d^* = 22 \times 0.70 - 1.645\sqrt{22 \times 0.70(1-0.70)} = 11.86 \approx 11$$

After rounding down, the threshold value is 11.

Therefore, if 11 or fewer children in the sample of 22 are found not to have been reached by the programme, the lot is accepted, and we fail to reject the null hypothesis, indicating that the programme may still meet the 70% coverage threshold. Conversely, if more than 11 children are unserved, the null hypothesis is rejected, indicating that the programme is falling short of its target.

Additionally, the required sample sizes for lot quality assurance sampling (LQAS) across population sizes ranging from 200 to 25,000, as well as for infinite populations, at a 95% confidence level and 80% power, are provided in Table 8.7.

TABLE 8.10

Sample Size and Decision Rule Calculations for Lot Quality Assurance Sampling (LQAS) at a 5% Significance Level and 80% Power of the Test, Based on a One-Sided Alternative Hypothesis, as Extracted from Lemeshow et al. (1988, p. 210, Table 14e)

	p_0																	
	0.5		0.55		0.6		0.65		0.7		0.75		0.8		0.85		0.9	
p_a	d*	n	d*	n	d*	n	d*	n	d*	n	d*	n	d*	n	d*	n	d*	n
0.05	0	5	0	5	–	–	–	–	–	–	–	–	–	–	–	–	–	–
0.1	1	8	1	6	1	5	–	–	–	–	–	–	–	–	–	–	–	–
0.15	2	11	2	8	2	7	1	5	–	–	–	–	–	–	–	–	–	–
0.2	4	15	3	11	2	9	2	7	1	5	–	–	–	–	–	–	–	–
0.25	7	23	5	16	4	12	3	9	2	7	2	5	–	–	–	–	–	–
0.3	13	37	9	24	6	16	5	12	4	9	2	6	2	5	–	–	–	–
0.35	26	67	15	38	10	24	7	16	5	11	3	8	3	6	–	–	–	–
0.4	66	153	30	68	17	38	11	23	8	16	5	11	4	8	2	5	–	–
0.45	288	617	74	154	33	67	19	37	11	22	8	15	5	10	4	7	3	5
0.5	–	–	317	615	80	151	35	65	20	35	12	21	8	13	5	9	4	6
0.55	–	–	–	–	340	600	84	145	37	62	19	32	12	19	8	12	4	7
0.6	–	–	–	–	–	–	353	573	86	136	37	57	19	29	11	16	7	10
0.65	–	–	–	–	–	–	–	–	356	534	85	125	35	50	18	25	9	13
0.7	–	–	–	–	–	–	–	–	–	–	346	483	80	109	32	43	15	20
0.75	–	–	–	–	–	–	–	–	–	–	–	–	321	419	71	91	26	33
0.8	–	–	–	–	–	–	–	–	–	–	–	–	–	–	279	342	58	69
0.85	–	–	219	253	–	–	–	–	–	–	–	–	–	–	–	–		

References

Bonita, R., Beaglehole, R., & Kjellström, T. (2006). *Basic epidemiology*. World Health Organization.

Boslaugh, S. (2007). *Encyclopedia of epidemiology*. Sage Publications.

Daniel, W. W., & Cross, C. L. (2018). *Biostatistics: A foundation for analysis in the health sciences*. John Wiley & Sons.

Indrayan, A., & Holt, M. P. (2016). *Concise encyclopedia of biostatistics for medical professionals*. Chapman and Hall-and CRC Press.

Lemeshow, S., Hosmer Jr, D. W., & Klar, J. (1988). Sample size requirements for studies estimating odds ratios or relative risks. *Statistics in Medicine, 7*(7), 759–764.

Lwanga, S. K., Lemeshow, S., & Organization, W. H. (1991). *Sample size determination in health studies: A practical manual/SK Lwanga and S. Lemeshow*. World Health Organization.

Rosner, B. A. (2006). *Fundamentals of biostatistics* (Vol. 6). Thomson-Brooks.

Rothman, K. J., Greenland, S., & Lash, T. L. (2008). *Modern epidemiology* (Vol. 3). Wolters Kluwer Health and Lippincott Williams & Wilkins Philadelphia.

9

Sample Size for ANOVA Family in Intervention Studies

9.1 Introduction

Analysis of Variance (ANOVA) is a broad family of statistical techniques used to examine differences between the means of *three or more groups*. It extends the t-test, which is limited to comparing the means of two groups. The development of ANOVA dates back to the early 20th century and the pioneering work of *Sir Ronald A. Fisher*, who introduced this method to analyse agricultural experiments – particularly the effects of different fertilisers on crop yields – at the Rothamsted Experimental Station.

In ANOVA, the variables that classify participants into different groups are known as *factors*. The simplest form, *one-way ANOVA*, involves a single factor. When more than one factor is included, the design is referred to as multi-way or factorial ANOVA.

The term *analysis of variance* arises from the partitioning of the total observed variance into distinct components. This decomposition allows researchers to determine the proportion of variance attributable to differences between groups (systematic variation produced by the factors under investigation) and the proportion attributable to differences within groups (random or unsystematic variation among individuals in each group). In this framework, between-group variance reflects systematic effects, whereas within-group variance represents random error or natural variability.

ANOVA has evolved to accommodate increasingly complex experimental designs and data structures. Major extensions include:

- Two-Way ANOVA: Involves two factors, allowing the investigation of interactions between the two factors alongside their individual effects.
- ANCOVA (Analysis of Covariance): Adjusts group means for the influence of other continuous variables, known as covariates, which are not part of the main experimental manipulation.

DOI: 10.1201/9781003749783-9

- Repeated Measures ANOVA: Used when the same participants are measured under different conditions or at various time points, facilitating the analysis of within-subject effects while controlling for individual differences.
- Mixed-Effects Models: Incorporate both fixed effects (factors manipulated or controlled by the experimenter) and random effects (factors sampled from a larger population and not under the experimenter's control).
- Multivariate ANOVA (MANOVA): An extension of ANOVA that involves multiple dependent variables, allowing researchers to assess the effects of one or more independent variables on multiple outcomes simultaneously.

Although the conceptual foundation of ANOVA is straightforward – comparing between-group variance to within-group variance – the underlying mathematics can become complex, especially in the presence of multiple factors, covariates, or repeated measurements. Despite this complexity, ANOVA remains a fundamental tool in statistical analysis across fields such as psychology, medicine, public health, economics, engineering, and the biological sciences.

Determining the sample size for different types of Analysis of Variance (ANOVA) and related methods, such as Analysis of Covariance (ANCOVA) and Multivariate Analysis of Variance (MANOVA), can be challenging and often requires specialised statistical software or dedicated sample size calculators. Nevertheless, this chapter provides streamlined explanations and general formulas to guide sample size estimation for each method.

It is important to note that the formulas presented in this chapter assume equal sample sizes across groups (balanced designs). When sample sizes differ across groups (unbalanced designs), the computations change substantially. In such cases, statistical software programs such as G*Power, SAS, or R offer more accurate and convenient solutions for determining the required sample size.

9.2 Sample Size for Testing the Difference Between Two Variances

When analysing two samples of measurements, each randomly drawn from a normal population, a common question arises: Are the variances of the two populations equal? Let S_1^2 represent an estimate of σ_1^2 from the first sample, and S_2^2 an estimate of σ_2^2 from the second sample. In this context, we can formulate a two-tailed hypothesis with the null and alternative hypotheses stated as:

$$\begin{cases} H_0 : \sigma_1^2 = \sigma_2^2 \\ H_A : \sigma_1^2 \neq \sigma_2^2 \end{cases}$$

To conduct this hypothesis test, we need to determine the minimum sample sizes required to achieve specified test characteristics in our study. The ratio of the two variances follows an F-distribution, expressed as:

$$F = \frac{\sigma_1^2}{\sigma_2^2}$$

Thus, the two-sample variance-ratio test can be formulated as:

$$F = \frac{S_1^2}{S_2^2} \ or \ F = \frac{S_2^2}{S_1^2},$$

whichever is larger. In this formulation, the larger variance is placed in the numerator and the smaller in the denominator. We then assess whether the calculated ratio of sample variances (i.e., F) deviates significantly from 1.0, allowing us to reject H_0 at a given significance level α.

The number of participants required in each sample to test at the α level of significance with a power of 1−β can be determined using the following equation (Zar, 2010, p. 158):

$$n = \left[\frac{Z_{1-\frac{\alpha}{2}} + Z_{1-\beta}}{Ln\left(\frac{S_1^2}{S_2^2}\right)} \right]^2 + 2 \tag{9.1}$$

For researchers who prefer to use "common logarithms" (base 10) instead of "natural logarithms" (base e), the equation can be expressed equivalently as:

$$n = \left[\frac{Z_{1-\frac{\alpha}{2}} + Z_{1-\beta}}{2.30259 \times log\left(\frac{S_1^2}{S_2^2}\right)} \right]^2 + 2 \tag{9.2}$$

These formulas assume that the samples have equal sizes in both groups, which is generally preferred (Zar, 2010, p. 158).

Example 9.1 (Sample Size Calculation for Comparing Variances): Suppose a researcher aims to compare the variances of two different treatments for a specific medical condition. The researcher wants to determine how many samples are needed in each group to test the equality of the two variances with a significance level (α) of 0.05 (5%) and a power ($1-\beta$) of 0.80 (80%). The expected variances are $\sigma_1^2 = 21$ *and* $\sigma_2^2 = 28$. How many samples are needed in each group to conduct this test?

Solution: The corresponding values from the standard normal distribution for a 5% significance level and 80% power are: $Z_{1-\frac{\alpha}{2}} = 1.96$ *and* $Z_{1-\beta} = 0.84$.

Using the larger variance in the numerator, we calculate the F-ratio as follows:

$$F = \frac{S_2^2}{S_1^2} = \frac{28}{21} = 1.333.$$

To determine the required sample size for each group, we apply the following formula:

$$n = \left[\frac{Z_{1-\frac{\alpha}{2}} + Z_{1-\beta}}{Ln\left(\frac{S_1^2}{S_2^2}\right)} \right]^2 + 2$$

Substituting the known values:

$$n = \left[\frac{1.96 + 0.84}{Ln(1.3333)} \right]^2 + 2$$

Calculating the natural logarithm:

$$ln(1.333) \approx 0.2877$$

Substituting this value into the equation:

$$n = \left[\frac{2.80}{0.2877} \right]^2 + 2 = 96.71 \approx 97$$

Rounding up, the required sample size for each group is approximately 97 participants.

9.3 Sample Size Determination for One-Way ANOVA

Calculating the sample size for a one-way ANOVA involves determining the number of observations required to detect a significant difference among group means, given a specified level of power and significance. Several factors influence this process, including the expected effect size, the number of groups, the significance level (commonly set at 0.05 for alpha), and the desired power (typically targeted at 0.80 or 0.90).

TIP

There are several procedures available for estimating the required sample size, each providing slightly different results. We will present three methods that we consider more straightforward than the others.

9.3.1 General Explanation of Sample Size Calculation for One-Way ANOVA

The effect size in ANOVA is often expressed as eta-squared (η^2), which represents the proportion of the total variance attributed to the effect. A larger effect size indicates a greater difference between group means, facilitating the detection of a significant effect with a smaller sample size. The number of groups also impacts the required sample size; as the number of groups increases, a larger sample size is needed to detect significant differences among them.

An estimate of the variability within each group (σ^2) is necessary. This anticipated common variance can be estimated by the mean square error (MSE) from a previous study. The formula for estimating within-group variance is:

$$\sigma^2 = \frac{SSE}{k(n-1)}$$

where SSE is the sum of squares for error, k is the number of groups, and n is the sample size per group.

The sample size per group (n) can be estimated using the formula presented by Chow (Chow et al., 2017, p. 61). This generalised equation for sample size determination serves as an alternative to the specific formula for one-way ANOVA:

$$n = \frac{\lambda}{\Delta} \tag{9.3}$$

In this equation, n represents the required sample size for each group, and λ can be calculated from the chi-squared distribution with k–1 degrees of freedom. The term $\chi^2_{k-1}(.|\lambda)$ denotes the cumulative distribution function of the noncentral chi-squared (χ^2) distribution with k–1 degrees of freedom and noncentrality parameter λ.

TABLE 9.1

The Value of $\chi^2_{k-1}(\chi^2_{\alpha,k-1}|\lambda)=\beta$ from Chow et al. (2017, p. 62)

$1-\beta=0.90$		$1-\beta=0.80$		
$\alpha=0.05$	$\alpha=0.01$	$\alpha=0.05$	$\alpha=0.01$	k
10.51	14.88	7.85	11.68	2
12.66	17.43	9.64	13.89	3
14.18	19.25	10.91	15.46	4
15.41	20.74	11.94	16.75	5
16.47	22.03	12.83	17.87	6
17.42	23.19	13.63	18.88	7
18.29	24.24	14.36	19.79	8
19.09	25.22	15.03	20.64	9
19.83	26.13	15.65	21.43	10
20.54	26.99	16.25	22.18	11
21.20	27.80	16.81	22.89	12
21.84	28.58	17.34	23.57	13
22.44	29.32	17.85	24.22	14
23.03	30.04	18.34	24.84	15
23.59	30.73	18.82	25.44	16
24.13	31.39	19.27	26.02	17
24.65	32.04	19.71	26.58	18
25.16	32.66	20.14	27.12	19
25.66	33.27	20.56	27.65	20

To achieve a power of $1-\beta$, the sample size needed can be determined by solving the following equation (Chow et al., 2017, p. 61):

$$\chi^2_{k-1}(\chi^2_{\alpha,k-1}|\lambda)=\beta$$

This sample size equation for one-way ANOVA typically involves multiple parameters, including λ (the noncentrality parameter), Δ (the effect size), the number of groups (k), the within-group variance (σ^2), the desired significance level (α), and the desired power ($1-\beta$).

Given the complexity of these calculations, it is advisable to use sample size calculators. Table 9.1 from Chow can be referenced to obtain the parameter λ for significance levels of 0.01 and 0.05, as well as power levels of 0.80 and 0.90. The value of Δ can be calculated using the following equations (Chow et al., 2017, p. 61):

$$\bar{\mu}=\frac{1}{k}\sum_{j=1}^{k}\mu_{j.} \quad and \quad \Delta=\frac{1}{\sigma^2}\sum_{i=1}^{k}\left(\mu_i-\bar{\mu}\right)^2 \tag{9.4}$$

Example 9.2: Consider a four-arm (k = 4) parallel-group, randomised clinical trial designed to compare the efficacy of four different treatments. The study will be conducted with a significance level of $\alpha = 0.05$ and a power of 80%. Assuming the within-group standard deviation is $\sigma = 3.5$, and the true mean responses for the four treatment groups are 8.25, 11.75, 12.00, and 13.00, what is the required sample size for each arm of the study?

Solution: To determine the sample size for each group, we first calculate the grand mean (μ), the sum of squares due to the effect (SS(E)), and the variance within groups (σ^2).

The grand mean is calculated as:

$$\bar{\mu} = \frac{8.25 + 11.75 + 12.00 + 13.00}{4} = 11.25$$

Next, we compute Δ, which represents the standardised effect size:

$$\Delta = \frac{1}{\sigma^2}\sum_{i=1}^{k}(\mu_i - \bar{\mu})^2$$

Substituting the values:

$$\Delta = \frac{(8.25-11.25)^2 + (11.75-11.25)^2 + (12.00-11.25)^2 + (13.00-11.25)^2}{12.00}$$

$$= \frac{9 + 0.25 + 0.5625 + 3.0625}{12.25} = \frac{12.875}{12.25} = 1.05$$

From Table 9.1, for a four-group design ($k = 4$), with $\alpha = 0.05$ and power $(1-\beta) = 0.80$, the corresponding parameter value is $\lambda = 10.91$. Thus, the sample size per treatment group can be calculated as:

$$n = \frac{\lambda}{\Delta} = \frac{10.91}{1.05} = 10.39 \approx 11$$

Rounding up to ensure adequate power, we require **11** participants per group.

Example 9.3: A researcher aims to conduct a randomised trial with three parallel groups ($k = 3$) to compare the outcomes of velopharyngeal insufficiency (hyper nasality) in speech across three different treatment programmes. Group A will receive speech therapy, Group B will receive CPAP therapy, and Group C will receive oral motor exercise-based therapies. The objective is to determine the required sample size for each group. The trial will be conducted at a significance level of $\alpha = 0.05$, with a statistical power of 0.80. Although no information is available from similar studies, a pilot study provides the following data for each group:

Group A	$n_A = 3$	$\bar{x}_A = 18$	$Sd_A = 7.2$
Group B	$n_B = 5$	$\bar{x}_B = 14$	$Sd_B = 6.0$
Group C	$n_C = 4$	$\bar{x}_C = 17$	$Sd_C = 6.3$

Solution: To determine the necessary sample size for each group, we will calculate the grand mean, the sum of squares for error (SS(E)), and the variance (σ^2) within the groups. Since the number of subjects in each group is unequal, we will compute the weighted grand mean.

$$\bar{\mu} = \frac{(3\times 18)+(5\times 14)+(4\times 17)}{3+5+4} = 16.0$$

Next, we compute the variance (σ^2) within the groups.

$$\sigma^2 = \frac{SSE}{n-k} = \frac{\Sigma(n_i - 1).Sd_i^2}{n-k}$$

Substituting the values:

$$\sigma^2 = \frac{(3-1)\times 7.2^2 + (5-1)\times 6.0^2 + (4-1)\times 6.3^2}{12-3} = \frac{366.75}{(12-3)} = 40.75$$

Next, we calculate the standardised effect size Δ:

$$\Delta = \frac{1}{\sigma^2}\sum_{i=1}^{k}(\mu_i - \bar{\mu})^2 = \frac{(18-16)^2 + (14-16)^2 + (17-16)^2}{40.75} = 0.221$$

From Table 9.1, the corresponding value for λ with $k = 3$, $\alpha = 0.05$, and $1 - \beta = 0.80$ is $\lambda = 9.64$.

Thus, the sample size per group can be calculated as:

$$n = \frac{\lambda}{\Delta} = \frac{9.64}{0.221} = 43.65 \approx 44$$

Rounding up to ensure adequate power, 44 participants are required per group. Therefore, a total of 44 × 3 = 132 participants should be included in the study.

9.3.2 Alternative Methods for Determining Sample Size in ANOVA

An alternative formula for determining sample size in analysis of variance (ANOVA) is presented by Indrayan and Holt (2016, p. 556), with additional insights from Chow et al. (2017, p. 59) and Indrayan et al. (2024, p. 469). These authors define the minimum medically important effect as the difference between group means that researchers aim to detect, along with general principles for sample size determination.

When analysing three or more groups, ANOVA is used to compare means, whereas chi-square tests are used to compare proportions. Both approaches involve complex formulas for calculating sample sizes. A commonly accepted and simpler method involves calculating the number of pairwise comparisons for K groups, represented by the formula:

$$\tau = \frac{K(K-1)}{2}$$

To adjust the sample size formulas for two groups, replace $z_{1-\frac{\alpha}{2}}$ with $z_{1-\frac{\alpha}{2\tau}}$, where τ represents the number of pairwise comparisons. For example, with four groups, there are six pairwise comparisons: A vs. B, A vs. C, A vs. D, B vs. C, B vs. D, and C vs. D.

All other parameters remain consistent with those used for two-group comparisons; however, a pooled estimate of the variance σ^2 is applied (because ANOVA assumes equal variances among the groups being compared) for both means and proportions. This method is applicable only when the number of subjects in each group is equal. If the effect size δ is consistent across all comparison pairs, a single calculation is sufficient. Conversely, if δ varies among different pairs, the sample size must be calculated for each pairwise difference using the specified δ. The required sample size will then be the largest n per group, or alternatively, the sample size can be determined based on the pairwise comparison with the smallest effect size δ.

The formulas for sample size determination are as follows:

$$n_{ij} = \frac{\left(z_{1-\frac{\alpha}{2\tau}} + z_{1-\beta}\right)^2 \cdot \sigma^2}{\delta^2 = \left(\mu_i - \mu_j\right)^2} \tag{9.5}$$

and

$$n = max\left[n_{ij}, for\, all\, interested\, comparison\right] \tag{9.6}$$

In these equations, the z-value is derived from the Gaussian distribution corresponding to the specified significance level α, while $(1-\beta)$ represents the predetermined power needed to detect a difference between the means (δ).

The σ^2 is the anticipated common variance, which may be estimated by the mean square error (MSE) from previous studies.

This method is applicable under the following conditions:

- The effects are fixed and not random.
- The null hypothesis states that the means in all groups are equal, whereas the alternative hypothesis suggests that at least one mean differs.
- All assumptions of ANOVA are satisfied, including independence of values, homoscedasticity, and adherence to the Gaussian distribution.
- Each subject in each group is either randomly selected or randomly assigned to the groups.

Example 9.4: Determine the required sample size for Example 9.3 using the simplified Equation 9.5.

Solution: To determine the required sample size for each group in the study, we will apply the simplified method outlined in Equation 9.5, using the data from the pilot study and considering pairwise comparisons. In the first step, we define the parameters as follows: Significance level (α)= 0.05, desired power of the test ($1-\beta=0.80$), number of groups (k) = 3, and the number of comparisons:

$$\tau=\frac{K(K-1)}{2}=\frac{3(3-1)}{2}=3.$$

Next, we calculate the pooled variance ($\sigma^2 = MSE$). This is determined using the pilot study data:

$$\sigma^2=\frac{SSE}{n-k}=\frac{(n_A-1).S_A^2+(n_B-1).S_B^2+(n_C-1).S_C^2}{n_A+n_B+n_C-k}$$

Substituting the values:

$$\sigma^2=\frac{(3-1)\times7.2^2+(5-1)\times6.0^2+(4-1)\times6.3^2}{3+5+4-3}=\frac{366.75}{9}=40.75$$

We then calculate the effect size for each comparison:

Group A vs. group B	$\delta^2=(\mu_A-\mu_B)^2=(18-14)^2=16$
Group A vs. group C	$\delta^2=(\mu_A-\mu_C)^2=(18-17)^2=1$
Group B vs. group C	$\delta^2=(\mu_B-\mu_C)^2=(17-14)^2=9$

Next, we find the corresponding values from the standard normal distribution for a power of 0.80 and a significance level of $\alpha = 0.05$:

$$z_{1-\beta} = 0.84$$

$$z_{1-\frac{\alpha}{2\tau}} = z_{1-\frac{0.05}{2\times 3}} = z_{0.99167} = 2.635$$

$$\left(z_{1-\frac{\alpha}{2\tau}} + z_{1-\beta}\right)^2 = (2.635 + 0.84)^2 = 12.075$$

Finally, we substitute the values into Equation 9.5 to calculate the sample sizes for each comparison:

For Group A vs. Group B:

$$n_{AB} = \frac{\left(z_{1-\frac{\alpha}{2\tau}} + z_{1-\beta}\right)^2 \cdot \sigma^2}{\delta^2 = (\mu_A - \mu_B)^2} = \frac{(2.635 + 0.84)^2 \times 40.75}{(18-14)^2} = \frac{492.08}{16} = 31$$

For Group A vs. Group C:

$$n_{AC} = \frac{\left(z_{1-\frac{\alpha}{2\tau}} + z_{1-\beta}\right)^2 \cdot \sigma^2}{\delta^2 = (\mu_A - \mu_B)^2} = \frac{(2.635 + 0.84)^2 \times 40.75}{(18-17)^2} = \frac{492.08}{1} = 492$$

For Group B vs. Group C:

$$n_{BC} = \frac{\left(z_{1-\frac{\alpha}{2\tau}} + z_{1-\beta}\right)^2 \cdot \sigma^2}{\delta^2 = (\mu_A - \mu_B)^2} = \frac{(2.635 + 0.84)^2 \times 40.75}{(17-14)^2} = \frac{492.08}{9} = 55$$

The largest sample size among all pairwise comparisons is 492 per group corresponding to the smallest effect size $\delta^2 = 1$ for Group A vs. Group C. Alternatively, researchers may identify the smallest effect size first and calculate the sample size based solely on that comparison, without needing to calculate the other pairwise comparisons.

Remark: While this simplified method is easy to understand and implement, providing a practical approach, the sample size determined may differ from previous calculations. This discrepancy arises because the method is most appropriate when the assumptions of equal variances and normality are met, assuming equal sample sizes in each group. If these assumptions are violated, alternative methods should be used for sample size determination. Researchers should consider the specific context of their study and consult with a statistician to identify the most suitable method for calculating sample size.

9.3.3 Sample Size Based on the Smallest Detectable Difference

When determining the appropriate sample size for an ANOVA, researchers often consider specific values for the variance components. One such component, $\Sigma\alpha_i^2$, represents the variability among different treatment effects. However, estimating this value can be quite challenging. In the context of fixed effects, $\Sigma\alpha_i^2$ may not provide meaningful information. Instead, it is more practical to focus on the smallest detectable difference between any two treatment effects, denoted as Δ.

Consider a pair of treatments for which the difference in their effects, $|\alpha_i - \alpha_j|$, is at least Δ (for any $i \neq j$). The smallest noncentrality parameter, $\lambda_{\min}$, occurs when only two treatment effects differ by Δ or more, while all other treatment effects are zero ($\alpha_i = 0$ for all $i \neq j$ *and* $i \neq k$). This scenario simplifies the analysis such that the largest treatment effect, $\alpha_{\max}$, and the smallest treatment effect, $\alpha_{\min}$, differ by:

$$\Delta_{\max} = \alpha_{\max} - \alpha_{\min}.$$

For any set of treatment effects $\alpha_i\,(i = 1, 2, \ldots, a)$ that satisfies this condition, the smallest λ is achieved when the remaining treatment effects are equal to the average of $\alpha_{\max}$ and $\alpha_{\min}$ such that:

$$\alpha_i = \frac{\alpha_{\max} + \alpha_{\min}}{2}.$$

Since the sum of all treatment effects (α_i) is zero ($\Sigma\alpha_i = 0$), this implies that:

$$\alpha_{\max} = \frac{\Delta}{2} \text{ and } \alpha_{\max} = -\frac{\Delta}{2},$$

with all other α_i being zero.

If we determine the power of the test $1-\beta$ for $\lambda_{\min}$, the power will be at least as large for all sets of α_i that meet this condition. The formula for $\lambda_{\min}$ is given by:

$$\lambda_{\min} = \frac{n \times 2 \times \frac{\Delta^2}{4}}{2\sigma_e^2} = \frac{n \times \Delta^2}{4 \times \sigma_e^2} \tag{9.7}$$

To find the necessary sample size n for a given Δ, we need to know σ_e, which represents the standard error associated with the treatment effects. Because σ_e is often not precisely known, we use the ratio $C = \frac{\Delta}{\sigma_e}$ instead of Δ itself.

This ratio expresses how large the difference Δ is relative to the variability in the measurements.

Using the formula for the power of the test with

$$\lambda = \frac{n \times \Delta^2}{4 \times \sigma_e^2},$$

we can determine the smallest n such that the actual power $(1-\beta)$ is at least as large as the specified power $1-\beta_0$, ensuring that the actual power meets or exceeds the desired level. When there are only two treatments, this problem becomes equivalent to a two-sample, two-sided Student's t-test. Additionally, research by Nelson (1983) has shown that the sample sizes calculated for fixed effects are generally comparable to those obtained using the analysis of means (ANOM) method. This indicates that the approach described here is robust and widely applicable across different experimental designs (Sahai & Ageel, 2012).

We provide Table 9.2, cited from Sahai and Ageel (2012), which illustrates the minimum sample size per treatment group required in a one-way fixed effects ANOVA design for parameters of $\alpha = 0.10, 0.05, 0.01$; $1-\beta = 0.80$ and 0.90; various $C = \frac{\Delta}{\sigma_e}$ ranging from 1.0 to 2.0 in increments of 0.25, and then 2.5 and 3.0; as well as different numbers of groups ranging from 2 to 11. Here, Δ represents the magnitude of the difference between any pair of treatment groups that is considered meaningful to detect with a probability of at least $1-\beta$.

> **Example 9.5**: Determine the required sample size for Example 9.3 using the Smallest Detectable Differences.

Solution: In this example, we determine the required sample size based on the information provided in Example 9.3. The available data indicates that there are three treatment arms (k = 3), a significance level of $\alpha = 0.05$, and a type II error rate of $\beta = 0.20$. The pilot study provides the following statistics for the three arms: $S_A = 7.2,\ S_B = 6.0,\ S_C = 6.3$, with means $\bar{x}_A = 18,\ \bar{x}_B = 14,\ \bar{x}_C = 17$, and sample sizes $n_A = 3,\ n_B = 5\ and\ n_C = 4$.

First, we calculate the maximum difference $(\Delta_{\max})$ between any two treatment effects:

$$\Delta_{\max} = \alpha_{\max} - \alpha_{\min} = 18 - 14 = 4$$

Next, we calculate the pooled standard deviation (σ) using the formula:

$$\sigma^2 = \frac{SSE}{n-k} = \frac{\Sigma(n_i - 1).Sd_i^2}{n-k} = \frac{366.75}{(12-3)} = 40.75,$$

TABLE 9.2

Minimum Sample Size per Treatment Group Needed for a Given Value of k, α, $1-\beta$, and Effect Size (C) in Terms of Sigma Units

		$1-\beta = 0.80$							$1-\beta = 0.90$						
		C							C						
k	α	1.00	1.25	1.50	1.75	2.00	2.50	3.00	1.00	1.25	1.50	1.75	2.00	2.50	3.00
	0.10	14	9	7	5	4	3	3	18	12	9	7	6	4	3
	0.05	17	12	9	7	6	4	4	23	15	11	8	7	5	4
2	0.01	26	17	13	10	8	6	5	32	21	15	12	10	7	6
	0.10	17	11	8	6	5	4	3	22	15	11	8	7	5	4
	0.05	21	14	10	8	6	5	4	27	18	13	10	8	6	5
3	0.01	30	20	14	11	9	7	5	37	24	18	13	11	8	6
	0.10	19	13	9	7	6	4	3	25	16	12	9	7	5	4
	0.05	23	15	11	9	7	5	4	30	20	14	11	9	6	5
4	0.01	33	22	16	12	10	7	5	40	27	19	15	12	8	6
	0.10	21	14	10	8	6	4	4	27	18	13	10	8	5	4
	0.05	25	17	12	9	7	5	4	32	21	15	12	9	6	5
5	0.01	35	23	17	13	10	7	6	43	28	20	15	12	9	7
	0.10	22	15	11	8	7	5	4	29	19	14	10	8	6	4
	0.05	27	18	13	10	8	6	4	34	23	16	12	10	7	5
6	0.01	38	25	18	13	11	8	6	46	30	21	16	13	9	7

(Continued)

TABLE 9.2 (CONTINUED)

Minimum Sample Size per Treatment Group Needed for a Given Value of k, α, $1-\beta$, and Effect Size (C) in Terms of Sigma Units

		$1-\beta=0.80$							$1-\beta=0.90$						
		C							C						
	0.10	24	16	11	9	7	5	4	31	20	14	11	9	6	5
	0.05	29	19	14	10	8	6	5	36	24	17	13	10	7	3
7	0.01	39	26	18	14	11	8	6	48	31	22	17	13	9	7
	0.10	25	16	12	9	7	5	4	32	21	15	11	9	6	5
	0.05	30	20	14	11	9	6	5	38	25	18	13	11	7	6
8	0.01	41	27	19	15	12	8	6	50	33	23	17	14	9	7
	0.10	26	17	12	9	7	5	4	33	22	16	12	9	6	5
	0.05	31	21	15	11	9	6	5	40	26	18	14	11	8	6
9	0.01	43	28	20	15	12	8	6	52	34	24	18	14	10	7
	0.10	27	18	13	10	8	5	4	35	23	16	12	10	7	5
	0.05	33	21	15	12	9	6	5	41	27	19	14	11	8	6
10	0.01	44	29	21	16	12	8	6	54	35	25	19	15	10	7
	0.10	28	18	13	10	8	6	4	36	23	17	13	10	7	5
	0.05	34	22	16	12	9	7	5	42	28	20	15	12	8	6
11	0.01	46	30	21	16	13	9	7	55	36	26	19	15	10	8

which yields:

$$\sigma = \sqrt{40.75} = 6.384$$

We then compute the ratio C:

$$C = \frac{\Delta}{\sigma_e} = \frac{4}{6.384} = 0.627$$

Referring to Table 9.2, the nearest value of C to 0.627 is 1 (since the table does not provide exact matches, we select the closest value). For C = 1, $\alpha = 0.05$, and a power of $1 - \beta = 0.80$, the required sample size per treatment group is 21.

We also refer to Table 9.3 from Chow on page 445, which presents the sample sizes required for three-arm, four-arm, and five-arm studies with α adjustments for multiple comparisons. This information can be particularly useful for researchers. For instance, a total sample size of 45 subjects (15 subjects per treatment group) is necessary to maintain 80% power for detecting a decrease in illness score by Δ = 1.5 during the active treatment period among treatment groups when σ^* (where σ^{*2} is the sum of the variance components) is 1.25.

9.3.4 Determining Sample Size Using Maximum Effect Size (δ)

Another strategy that simplifies sample size determination is to define the effect size in terms of the number of standard deviations between the largest and smallest anticipated population means. This measure of effect size is designated as $\delta_{\max}$ (Maxwell, S. E., p. 145).

$$\delta_{\max} = \frac{\mu_{\max} - \mu_{\min}}{\sigma_{\varepsilon}} \tag{9.8}$$

where σ_{ε} represents the population within-cell standard deviation. Maxwell et al. noted that the results obtained from this simplified method are similar to those found in tables published by Bratcher et al. (1970) (Maxwell et al., 2017, p. 145). However, this simplification comes at a cost: the expected values of all other means, except for the two most extreme means, do not influence the value of $\delta_{\max}$. In fact, the tables are computed under the assumption that all other means, apart from the two extremes, are equal to the grand mean μ.

Table 9.4, cited from Maxwell et al. (2017, p. 146), allows researchers to easily determine the sample size required for detecting an effect based on various values of $\delta_{\max}$. This table provides a direct reference for the sample sizes needed to detect effects corresponding to different values of $\delta_{\max}$.

The assumptions do not hold; the actual power may be slightly greater than the value indicated by the table.

TABLE 9.3

Sample Size Calculation with α Adjustment for Multiple Comparisons from Chow et al. (2017, p. 445)

		Sample Size per Arm					
		Three Arms		Four Arms		Five Arms	
Power	σ^*	$\Delta = 1.0$	$\Delta = 1.5$	$\Delta = 1.0$	$\Delta = 1.5$	$\Delta = 1.0$	$\Delta = 1.5$
80%	0.75	12	6	14	7	15	7
	0.80	14	6	16	7	17	8
	0.85	16	7	18	8	20	9
	0.90	17	8	20	9	22	10
	0.95	19	9	22	10	25	11
	1.00	21	10	25	11	27	12
	1.05	24	11	27	12	30	14
	1.10	26	12	30	14	33	15
	1.15	28	13	33	15	36	16
	1.20	31	14	35	16	39	17
	1.25	33	15	38	17	42	19
90%	0.75	16	7	18	8	19	9
	0.80	18	8	20	9	22	10
	0.85	20	9	23	10	25	11
	0.90	22	10	25	12	28	13
	0.95	25	11	28	13	31	14
	1.00	28	13	31	14	34	15
	1.05	30	14	34	16	37	17
	1.10	33	15	38	17	41	18
	1.15	36	16	41	19	45	20
	1.20	39	18	45	20	49	22
	1.25	43	19	49	22	53	24

TABLE 9.4

Minimum Sample Size Per Group Needed to Achieve Specified Power with $\alpha = 0.05$ (Maxwell et al., 2017, p. 146)

		δ_{max}							
1-β	Number of Levels	0.20	0.25	0.50	0.75	0.80	1.00	1.25	1.50
1-β = 0.80	2	394	253	64	29	26	17	12	9
	3	483	310	79	36	32	21	14	10
	4	547	350	89	40	36	23	15	11
	5	598	383	97	44	39	25	17	12
1-β = 0.95	2	651	417	105	48	42	27	18	13
	3	774	496	125	56	50	32	21	15
	4	860	551	139	63	55	36	23	17
	5	930	596	150	67	59	39	25	18

Example 9.6 (Reaction-Time Study): In this reaction-time study, you will be examining three groups. Preliminary research and data from the literature indicate that the expected means for these groups are 400 ms, 450 ms, and 500 ms, with a within-group standard deviation of 100 ms. What is the required sample size for each group in your study?

Solution: By substituting the values $\mu_{\text{max}} = 500\text{ ms}$, $\mu_{\text{min}} = 400\text{ ms}$, and $\sigma_{\varepsilon} = 100\text{ ms}$ into the formula, we find:

$$\delta_{\text{max}} = \frac{\mu_{\text{max}} - \mu_{\text{min}}}{\sigma_{\varepsilon}} = \frac{500 - 400}{100} = 1.0$$

Referring to the column labelled 1.00 for a power of 0.80 and a significance level of 0.05, within the row for three levels, we find that n = 21 samples are required for each group. Therefore, the total sample size for the entire study is 3 × 21 = 63.

9.3.5 Determining Sample Size by Iterative Trial and Error

Zar, on page 211, proposed a method for determining sample size in one-way ANOVA using an iterative trial-and-error approach. To employ this method, the user must specify the desired power, significance level, an estimated population variance common to all groups, and k as the number of independent groups being compared in the ANOVA design. The noncentrality parameter, Φ, is then calculated using the following equation:

$$\phi = \sqrt{\frac{n \times \delta^2}{2k \times s^2}} \tag{9.9}$$

where

- Φ is the noncentrality parameter,
- *n* represents the predetermined sample size,
- *δ* is the minimum detectable effect,
- *k* denotes the number of groups, and
- s^2 indicates the estimated variance.

The calculated noncentrality parameter, Φ, is then compared with the figures in Zar's book (Zar, 2010, Appendix B, pp. 859–866). If the preselected sample size satisfies the noncentrality parameter Φ as indicated by the provided figures, the assumed sample size is considered the required sample size. If not, *n* is repeatedly modified until the desired noncentrality parameter Φ is achieved.

Example 9.7: A researcher aims to examine the effect of four dietary regimens on blood HDL levels. He considers a minimum clinically significant effect of 3.5 mg/dL and plans to conduct a study with a power of 80% and a significance level of 5%. Based on past studies involving similar populations, the estimated variance is $s^2 = 9.38$. The question is: how many samples will he need?

Solution: The available information for this study is as follows:

$s^2 = 9.38$	$\delta = 3.5$	$k = 4$	$v = k - 1 = 4 - 1 = 3$

We begin by guessing that $n = 15$ samples are required. The degrees of freedom for the second group (v_2) can be calculated as:

$$v_2 = 4(15 - 1) = 56.$$

Next, we plug these values into Equation 9.9 to calculate the *noncentrality parameter* of Φ:

$$\phi = \sqrt{\frac{n \times \delta^2}{2k \times s^2}} = \sqrt{\frac{15 \times 3.5^2}{2 \times 4 \times 9.38}} = 1.56$$

We then refer to Zar's Figure B.1 to determine whether the predetermined $n = 15$ is sufficient for the desired power or requires adjustment. The horizontal axis of the figure shows the value for Φ. For $v_1 = 3 \, and \, v_2 = 56$, Φ is approximately 0.73. This value is lower than the desired power of 0.80, prompting us to try a larger sample size, say $n = 20$.

$$\phi = \sqrt{\frac{n \times \delta^2}{2k \times s^2}} = \sqrt{\frac{20 \times 3.5^2}{2 \times 4 \times 9.38}} = 1.81$$

Using this Φ value, we recalculate v_2:

$$v_2 = 4(20 - 1) = 76$$

From Zar's Figure B.l, this Φ corresponds to a power of approximately 0.84. Since this power exceeds our target, we will recalculate using $n = 18$:

$$\phi = \sqrt{\frac{n \times \delta^2}{2k \times s^2}} = \sqrt{\frac{18 \times 3.5^2}{2 \times 4 \times 9.38}} = 1.71$$

For $v_2 = 4(18 - 1) = 68$, this Φ indicates a power slightly above 0.80. Therefore, we estimate that using a sample size of at least 18 per group will yield an ANOVA with a power of approximately 80% for the described experiment.

9.4 Sample Size Determination for Two-Way ANOVA

The concepts and procedures for estimating power, sample size, and minimum detectable difference in single-factor ANOVA can be extended to fixed-effects factors in two-factor analyses of variance, also known as multi-way ANOVA (Zar, 2010, p. 275). To determine the sample size for a two-way ANOVA, a simplified approach involves using the standard one-way ANOVA sample size calculation formula, adjusted for the number of "cells" in the design. This method entails allocating an equal sample size to each cell to ensure sufficient power to detect potential interaction effects between the factors.

In a model with two factors, A (with **a** levels) and B (with **b** levels), the analysis results in **a × b** combined cells. To estimate the effect size for all **a × b** cells within the model, the following two methods are applicable:

1. **Simplified Method for Sample Size Determination:** This method is based on the smallest detectable difference (Chow et al., 2017, p. 59; Indrayan & Holt, 2016, p. 556; Indrayan et al., 2024, p. 469). First, determine the sample size required for the cell exhibiting the smallest detectable difference (i.e., the smallest effect size) through comparisons between two groups (see Equation 9.5). This sample size can then be generalised to all other cells for a conservative estimate. This approach ensures equal sample size allocation across all cells.
2. **Generalisation of One-Way ANOVA Equations:** In statistical analysis, either factor A or factor B can be evaluated independently (one at a time), allowing for a focused assessment of each factor's impact. Let k' denote the number of levels for the factor under examination: $k' = a$ for factor A and $k' = b$ for factor B. Correspondingly, let n' represent the number of observations at each level, defined as $n' = b \times n$ for factor A and $n' = a \times n$ for factor B.

Additionally, let $\mathbf{s^2}$ represent the within-cells mean square (MS). The transition from one-way ANOVA to two-way ANOVA is illustrated in Zar (2010, p. 275).

The effect size can be calculated using the following formula:

$$\phi = \sqrt{\frac{n' \times \delta^2}{2k' \times s^2}} \tag{9.10}$$

This comprehensive framework ensures that sample size calculations for both methods in two-way ANOVA are accurate and conservative. It guarantees sufficient statistical power to detect interaction effects while preserving the simplicity of the one-way ANOVA calculation.

Example 9.8: Suppose a researcher wants to study the effect of two different fertilisers (Fertiliser A and Fertiliser B) and two different watering regimes (Regular and High) on plant growth. The researcher aims to detect the smallest effect size (smallest detectable difference) in plant height. How many subjects do we need in each cell of a two-way ANOVA design? The parameters are: smallest detectable difference (effect size, δ) = 5 cm, within-group standard deviation (s) = 10 cm, significance level (α) = 0.05, power of the test ($1-\beta$) = 0.80, number of levels for Fertiliser (a) = 2, and number of levels for Watering (b) = 2.

Solution: To calculate the sample size for a single cell in a one-way ANOVA, we use Equation 9.5:

$$n_{ij} = \frac{\left(z_{1-\frac{\alpha}{2\tau}} + z_{1-\beta}\right)^2 \times \sigma^2}{\delta^2}$$

The corresponding values from a standard normal distribution for a significance level of 0.05 and a test power of 0.80 are 1.96 and 0.84.

Plugging the provided values into the equation above:

$$n_{ij} = \frac{(1.96+0.84)^2 \times 10^2}{5^2} = \frac{784}{25} = 31.36$$

Rounding up, we find that $n = 32$ subjects per cell.

Since there are $2 \times 2 = 4$ cells, this sample size can be applied to all cells, resulting in the total sample size required:

$$n = a \times b \times n = 2 \times 2 \times 32 = 128$$

Therefore, the researcher needs a total sample size of 128 plants, with 32 plants per treatment combination.

Example 9.9: In Example 9.8, the researcher wishes to examine the effect of four dietary regimens on blood HDL levels across three age groups. The question is: how many subjects should participate in this two-way ANOVA study?

Solution: To determine the required sample size for this two-way ANOVA study, we start with the following information:

$$S^2 = 9.38, \quad \delta = 3.5, \quad k = 4, \quad v = k-1 = 4-1$$

$$b = 3(\text{levels of age group})$$

Assuming an initial estimate of 10 subjects per cell ($n = 10$), we calculate the total number of observations for the factor under consideration:

$$n' = b \times n = 3 \times 10 = 30$$

Next, we calculate the degrees of freedom for errors:

$$v_2 = a \times b(n-1) = 4 \times 3 \times (10-1) = 108.$$

Now, we substitute these values into Equation 9.10 to calculate the noncentrality parameter ϕ:

$$\phi = \sqrt{\frac{n' \times \delta^2}{2k' \times s^2}} = \sqrt{\frac{30 \times 3.5^2}{2 \times 4 \times 9{,}38}} = 2.21$$

Next, we consult Zar's Figure B.1 to determine whether the predetermined $n = 10$ is sufficient or needs adjustment. For $v_1 = 3$ and $v_2 = 108$, Φ is approximately 0.95. Since this is higher than the desired power of 0.80, we try a smaller sample size, say $n = 5$:

$$n' = b \times n = 3 \times 5 = 15$$

Calculating the new degrees of freedom for errors gives us:

$$v_2 = a \times b(n-1) = 4 \times 3 \times (5-1) = 48.$$

Now, we substitute the new data into Equation 9.10 to find the new noncentrality parameter Φ:

$$\phi = \sqrt{\frac{n' \times \delta^2}{2k' \times s^2}} = \sqrt{\frac{15 \times 3.5^2}{2 \times 4 \times 9{,}38}} = 1.56$$

According to Zar's Figure B.1, this Φ value, for $v_2 = 48$, corresponds to a power of approximately 0.84. Since this power is still higher than the specified 0.80, we try an even smaller sample size, $n = 4$:

$$n' = b \times n = 3 \times 4 = 12$$

Calculating the new degrees of freedom for errors:

$$v_2 = a \times b(n-1) = 4 \times 3 \times (4-1) = 36.$$

We substitute the new data into Equation 9.10 to find the new noncentrality parameter ϕ:

$$\phi = \sqrt{\frac{n' \times \delta^2}{2k' \times s^2}} = \sqrt{\frac{12 \times 3.5^2}{2 \times 4 \times 9{,}38}} = 1.40$$

For $v_2 = 36$, this Φ value from Zar's Figure B.1 indicates a power of approximately 0.80.

Thus, we estimate that using a sample size of at least four subjects per age group will yield a two-way ANOVA with approximately 80% power for the described experiment.

9.5 Sample Size Determination for Conducting ANCOVA

A straightforward method for determining the sample size required for randomised clinical trials that plan to use analysis of covariance (ANCOVA) is presented by Borm et al. (2007). This method consists of a two-step process (Borm et al., 2007).

First, the sample size is calculated as if a simple *t*-test were to be performed on the follow-up scores (Y_1). This initial calculation assumes that the standard deviation (SD) of the dependent variable (Y_1) is known, as well as the correlation between the baseline (Y_0) and follow-up scores (Y_1). The conditional variance of Y_1 given Y_0 $\mathrm{Var}(Y_1 \mid Y_0)$ is then utilised to derive a *"design factor"*.

The design factor represents the ratio of the number of subjects required for ANCOVA to the number required for a t-test. It adjusts the sample size to account for the covariance inherent in the ANCOVA design. The formula for the initial sample size calculation for the t-test is as follows:

$$n = \frac{2\left(Z_{1-\frac{\alpha}{2}} \times Z_{1-\beta}\right)^2 \times \sigma^2}{\left(\mu_1 - \mu_2\right)^2} \tag{9.11}$$

where μ_1 *and* μ_2 are the mean outcomes for the two groups, σ is the standard deviation of the response variable, $Z_{1-\frac{\alpha}{2}}$ is the critical value from the standard normal distribution corresponding to the desired significance level, and $Z_{1-\beta}$ is the critical value corresponding to the desired power.

TIP

The standard deviation (Sd) used in the ANCOVA calculation refers to the dependent or outcome variable Y_1.

To determine the required sample size for ANCOVA n_{ANCOVA}, the number of subjects calculated for the *t*-test is multiplied by the design factor, which is $(1-\rho^2)$, where ρ is the correlation between Y_0 and Y_1. Additionally, one extra subject per group is added to account for the difference in variance explained by ANCOVA compared to the *t*-test. The proposed formula is:

$$n_{ANCOVA} = 2n\left(1-\rho^2\right)+2 \tag{9.12}$$

For small sample sizes, Borm and colleagues (2007) recommend a slight modification to the formula to enhance accuracy:

$$n_{ANCOVA} = 2(n+1)\left(1-\rho^2\right)+2 \tag{9.13}$$

Furthermore, they advise including additional subjects in the calculated sample size to compensate for potential missing data or non-evaluable observations, thereby ensuring that the study maintains its intended power (Borm et al., 2007).

> **Example 9.10:** Consider a hypothetical clinical trial aimed at comparing the effectiveness of two treatments (A and B) for reducing blood pressure. The primary outcome (Y_1) is the systolic blood pressure measured after treatment, while the baseline systolic blood pressure (Y_0) is also recorded. Assuming a standard deviation (σ) of Y_1 of 10 mmHg and an expected difference in means ($\mu_1 - \mu_2$) of 5 mmHg, we need to determine the required sample size for each group at a significance level of 0.05 and a power of 0.80. Previous literature indicates a correlation between Y_0 and Y_1 (ρ) of 0.50.

Solution: First, we calculate the sample size required for a *t*-test (n) using the following formula, with $Z_{1-\frac{0.05}{2}} = 1.96$ *and* $Z_{1-0.20} = 0.84$:

$$n = \frac{2\left(Z_{1-\frac{\alpha}{2}} \times Z_{1-\beta}\right)^2 \times \sigma^2}{\left(\mu_1-\mu_2\right)^2} = \frac{2(1.96\times 0.84)^2\times 10^2}{(5)^2} = \frac{1568}{25} = 62.72 \approx 63$$

Next, we calculate the sample size for ANCOVA (n_{ANCOVA}) using the correlation ($\rho = 0.5$):

$$n_{ANCOVA} = 2n\left(1-\rho^2\right)+2 = 2\times 63\times\left(1-0.5^2\right)+2 = 96.5 \approx 97$$

Thus, the required sample size for ANCOVA in this clinical trial is **97** subjects per group.

Example 9.11: Consider a hypothetical medical study designed to compare the effectiveness of three different treatments (Treatment A, Treatment B, and placebo) in lowering cholesterol levels among patients. The primary outcome is the change in LDL cholesterol levels from baseline to the end of the study period, with a specific focus on post-intervention LDL levels (Y_1). The correlation between baseline LDL (Y_0) and post-intervention LDL (Y_1) is 0.65. To conduct this study effectively using an ANCOVA model at a significance level of 0.05 and a power of 0.80, we need to determine the required sample size for each group. The expected difference in means ($\mu_1 - \mu_2$) is 10 mg/dL, and the standard deviation (σ) is 20 mg/dL. How many samples are needed in each group?

TIP

A higher correlation between repeated measures generally reduces the required sample size because the design becomes more efficient at detecting within-subject changes.

Solution: First, we calculate the sample size required for a *t*-test (n) using the following formula. We will use $Z_{1-\frac{0.05}{2}} = 1.96$ and $Z_{1-0.20} = 0.84$ along with the expected difference in means ($\mu_1 - \mu_2$) = 10 mg/dL, as follows:

$$n = \frac{2\left(Z_{1-\frac{\alpha}{2}} \times Z_{1-\beta}\right)^2 \times \sigma^2}{\left(\mu_1 - \mu_2\right)^2} = \frac{2(1.96 \times 0.84)^2 \times 20^2}{(10)^2} = \frac{1568}{25} = 62.72 \approx 63$$

Next, we calculate the sample size for ANCOVA (n_{ANCOVA}) using the design factor of $(1 - 0.65^2)$:

$$n_{ANCOVA} = 2n\left(1 - \rho^2\right) + 2 = 2 \times 63 \times \left(1 - 0.65^2\right) + 2 = 74.77 \approx 75$$

Therefore, the required sample size for ANCOVA in this clinical trial is **75** subjects per group.

9.6 Sample Size Determination for Repeated Measures ANOVA

In clinical research, it is common to conduct parallel-group clinical trials that involve multiple assessments. This design entails measuring the dependent variable (outcome) repeatedly over time, such as at baseline (before intervention), immediately after interventions, and at one or more follow-up points. This approach facilitates the evaluation of clinical efficacy and safety throughout the study. The data collected from these assessments are typically analysed using repeated measures ANOVA.

The primary advantage of a repeated measures design is its ability to control for variability among subjects, as each subject serves as their own control. In essence, repeated measures ANOVA is a statistical test used to determine whether there are significant differences between the means of three or more conditions when the same participants are involved in each condition. Calculating the sample size is a critical step in planning clinical trials and other types of research to ensure that the study has sufficient participants to detect a statistically significant effect, if one exists.

Here, we provide formulas for calculating sample size in a design with multiple assessments using the repeated measures ANOVA method. The sample size for repeated measures ANOVA can be calculated using estimates of both the within-subject standard deviation (σ_w) and the effect size (Δ), similar to parallel group studies (Chow et al., 2017, p. 443; Julious, 2023, p. 75). The formula for total sample size is

$$n = \frac{2 \times \sigma_w^2 \times \left(Z_{1-\frac{\alpha}{2}} + Z_{1-\beta} \right)^2}{\Delta^2} \tag{9.14}$$

where

- n is the total sample size,
- Δ is the effect size, defined as the difference between the means you wish to detect, standardised by the within-subject standard deviation.

$$\text{Effect Size } (\Delta) = \frac{\text{Difference Between Means}}{\text{Within} - \text{Subject Standard Deviation}}$$

- σ_w is the within-subject (intra-subject) standard deviation, measuring the variability of the repeated measurements within the same subject. It is calculated as $\sigma_w^2 = \sigma^2(1-\rho)$, where σ^2 is the total variance and ρ is the correlation between repeated measures. Alternatively, it can be derived from the residual line of an ANOVA model and quantifies the expected variation among repeated measurements on the same individual (Julious, 2023, p. 75).
- $Z_{1-\frac{\alpha}{2}}$ *and* $Z_{1-\beta}$ are the critical values from the standard normal distribution for the desired significance level (α) and power ($1 - \beta$), respectively.

To utilise this formula, both σ_w and Δ can be estimated based on previous research or pilot studies. It is essential to note that the correlation between repeated measures (ρ) is also a crucial parameter that influences the sample size calculation in repeated measures designs. A higher correlation between repeated measures typically results in a smaller required sample size, as the design is more efficient at detecting changes within subjects.

> **Example 9.12:** Consider a hypothetical clinical trial aimed at determining the impact of a new treatment on blood pressure over time. Our objective is to detect a difference of 15 mmHg in systolic blood pressure between baseline measurements and follow-up assessments, using a significance level of 5% and a power of 80%. We need to determine the required number of participants for the study using repeated measures ANOVA.

Solution: The provided information indicates that a 5% significance level corresponds to a critical value of 1.96 for a two-tailed test, while a power of 0.80 corresponds to a critical value of 0.84. The detectable difference is 15 mmHg, and previous studies suggest that the within-subject standard deviation (σ_w) is at most 6 mmHg. Therefore, the effect size can be calculated as follows:

$$\Delta = \frac{15}{6} = 2.5\ mmHg$$

We also estimate the correlation between repeated measures to be $\rho = 0.5$, indicating a moderate correlation. This assumption is based on the premise that individual blood pressure measurements remain relatively consistent over time.

By substituting these values into Equation 9.9, we can calculate the required sample size:

$$n = \frac{2 \times \sigma_w^2 \times \left(Z_{1-\frac{\alpha}{2}} + Z_{1-\beta}\right)^2}{\Delta^2} = \frac{2 \times 36 \times (1.96 + 0.84)^2}{2.5^2}$$

Calculating these yields:

$$n = \frac{2 \times 36 \times 7.84}{6.25} = 90.32 \approx 91$$

Rounding up to the nearest whole number, we conclude that approximately 91 participants are needed in total to detect the desired effect size with the specified power and significance level. This calculation is based on the assumed within-subject standard deviation of 6 mmHg.

References

Borm, G. F., Fransen, J., & Lemmens, W. A. J. (2007). A simple sample size formula for analysis of covariance in randomized clinical trials. *Journal of Clinical Epidemiology, 60*(12), 1234–1238.

Bratcher, T. L., Moran, M. A., & Zimmer, W. J. (1970). Tables of sample sizes in the analysis of variance. *Journal of Quality Technology, 2*, 156–164.

Chow, S.-C., Shao, J., Wang, H., & Lokhnygina, Y. (2017). *Sample size calculations in clinical research.* Chapman and Hall and CRC Press.

Indrayan, A., & Holt, M. P. (2016). *Concise encyclopedia of biostatistics for medical professionals.* Chapman and Hall and CRC Press.

Indrayan, A., Mishra, A., & Bhaskarapillai, B. (2024). Simplified sample size formulas for detecting a medically important effect. *Indian Journal of Community Medicine, 49*(3), 464–471.

Julious, S. A. (2023). *Sample sizes for clinical trials.* Chapman and Hall and CRC Press.

Maxwell, S. E., Delaney, H. D., & Kelley, K. (2017). *Designing experiments and analyzing data: A model comparison perspective.* Routledge.

Nelson, P. R. (1983). A comparison of sample sizes for the analysis of means and the analysis of variance. *Journal of Quality Technology, 15*(1), 33–39.

Sahai, H., & Ageel, M. I. (2012). *The analysis of variance: Fixed, random and mixed models.* Springer Science & Business Media.

Zar, J. H. (2010). *Biostatistical analysis.* Pearson Education India.

10

Sample Size for Correlation and Regression Analysis

10.1 Introduction

In experimental research, scientists frequently encounter multiple random variables and seek to identify associations between two quantitative measurements. These measurements may include weight, height, age, blood pressure, waist circumference, hip circumference, or other relevant variables, depending on the study's focus. Statistical analyses are used to explore the relationships among these variables within a defined study population. An association implies that as one measurement increases, the other tends to either increase or decrease correspondingly.

Correlation is a statistical measure that quantifies the strength and direction (positive or negative) of a linear relationship between two quantitative variables. This measure is applicable when the variables are paired, such as when they are obtained from the same subjects at a specific time point (e.g., the correlation between systolic and diastolic blood pressure readings in a group of participants). The correlation coefficient, denoted by ρ (rho), provides a numerical representation of the association between the variables. A correlation coefficient of $\rho = 0$ indicates no linear relationship, while $\rho = +1$ or $\rho = -1$ signifies a perfect positive or perfect negative linear relationship, respectively. It is important to note that the correlation coefficient measures *only the strength of linear relationships* between two variables and does not capture non-linear associations.

TIP

Correlation quantifies the strength and direction of the association between variables, whereas regression is used to predict the value of one variable based on another (or multiple other variables). Notably, the mathematical equations underlying correlation and simple (bivariate) regression are closely related.

DOI: 10.1201/9781003749783-10

Regression analysis is used when the objective is to predict the value of one variable based on the known values of another. This statistical technique estimates the mathematical relationship between variables, aiming to determine how an independent variable (predictor) can account for variation in a dependent variable (response).

This chapter will cover various aspects of regression and correlation analyses, including:

- Determining the appropriate sample size for estimating correlation coefficients,
- Comparing different correlation coefficients,
- Conducting hypothesis tests for correlation coefficients across populations,
- Estimating regression models,
- Comparing regression coefficients, and
- Performing hypothesis tests for regression coefficients in both simple and multiple regression contexts.

10.2 Sample Size for Estimating a Correlation Coefficient

To estimate the correlation coefficient (r), two methods are commonly used. The first method is derived from the standard error of the correlation coefficient, $Se(r)$, which depends on both the correlation itself and the sample size:

$$Se(r) = \sqrt{\frac{1-r^2}{n-2}} \tag{10.1}$$

This equation shows that the standard error of the distribution is determined by the magnitude of the correlation and the sample size, thereby eliminating the need to estimate the standard error separately. By algebraically manipulating $Se(r)$, the necessary sample size for estimating the correlation coefficient with a significance level α and a power of $1-\beta$ can be derived (Norman & Streiner, 2008, p. 316):

$$n = \left(\frac{z_{1-\frac{\alpha}{2}} + z_{1-\beta}\sqrt{1-r^2}}{r} \right)^2 + 2 \tag{10.2}$$

It is important to note that when the goal is to estimate a correlation coefficient rather than to test it, the concept of power $(1-\beta)$ remains relevant. This pertains to the precision of the estimation and the probability of detecting the true effect size if it exists. Therefore, the power is included in the calculations, though the sample size formula may not directly utilise $z_{1-\beta}$ in the same manner as a hypothesis test.

The second approach, proposed by Fisher, involves a transformation designed to better approximate a normal distribution. This transformation is necessary because the sample correlation coefficient r exhibits a skewed distribution for non-zero ρ, which cannot be accurately approximated by a normal distribution. Fisher's transformation corrects this skewness and provides an approximately normal distribution with a variance of $1/\sqrt{n-3}$.

$$U_\rho = \frac{1}{2} ln\left(\frac{1+\rho_0}{1-\rho_0}\right) \tag{10.3}$$

The required sample size to detect a correlation of at least ρ with a two-sided significance level α and a specified power of $1-\beta$ can be calculated using Equation 10.4 (Indrayan & Holt, 2016, p. 577; Rosner, 2006, p. 499):

$$n = \left(\frac{z_{1-\frac{\alpha}{2}} + z_{1-\beta}}{U_\rho}\right)^2 + 3 \tag{10.4}$$

In this equation, U_ρ represents the Fisher z-transformation of the minimum correlation ρ to be detected. The notation U_ρ is used instead of z to avoid confusion with the standard normal probabilities $z_{1-\frac{\alpha}{2}}$ and $z_{1-\beta}$. The Fisher z-transformation closely approximates r for small values of r but deviates increasingly for larger values.

TIP

When using the Fisher z-transformation to determine sample size for expected negative correlation coefficients, the absolute value of $r(\rho_0)$ should be used, ignoring its sign. This is because the Fisher transformation normalises the distribution of the correlation coefficient, emphasising the magnitude of ρ_0 rather than its direction.

$$U_\rho = \frac{1}{2} ln\left(\frac{1-|\rho_0|}{1+|\rho_0|}\right)$$

Table 10.1 provides the Fisher z-transformed values for r ranging from 0.02 to 0.96.

TABLE 10.1

Fisher's z-Transformation of Correlation Coefficient, adopted from Rosner (2006, p. 887)

r	U_ρ	r	U_ρ	r	U_ρ
0.02	0.020	**0.34**	0.354	**0.66**	0.793
0.04	0.040	**0.36**	0.377	**0.68**	0.829
0.06	0.060	**0.38**	0.400	**0.70**	0.867
0.08	0.080	**0.40**	0.424	**0.72**	0.908
0.10	0.100	**0.42**	0.448	**0.74**	0.950
0.12	0.121	**0.44**	0.472	**0.76**	0.996
0.14	0.141	**0.46**	0.497	**0.78**	1.045
0.16	0.161	**0.48**	0.523	**0.80**	1.099
0.18	0.182	**0.50**	0.549	**0.82**	1.157
0.20	0.203	**0.52**	0.576	**0.84**	1.221
0.22	0.224	**0.54**	0.604	**0.86**	1.293
0.24	0.245	**0.56**	0.633	**0.88**	1.376
0.26	0.266	**0.58**	0.662	**0.90**	1.472
0.28	0.288	**0.60**	0.693	**0.92**	1.589
0.30	0.310	**0.62**	0.725	**0.94**	1.738
0.32	0.332	**0.64**	0.758	**0.96**	1.946

We present the sample size calculations in Table 10.2, which include various correlation coefficients ranging from 0.05 to 0.90. These calculations are based on Equation 10.2 rather than Fisher's z transformation, as Equation 10.2 provides a slightly more conservative estimate, ensuring adequate precision.

> **Example 10.1:** The goal of a study is to estimate the correlation coefficient between two attributes in a population. The researcher aims to detect a correlation coefficient at a 5% significance level with 80% power of the test. The hypothesised correlation coefficient is approximately −0.60. How many participants are needed in the sample?

Solution: Since $|r| = |-0.60| = 0.60$, a 5% significance level corresponds to $z =$ 1.96 for a two-tailed test, and 80% power corresponds to $z = 0.84$. Substituting these values into Equations 10.2, 10.3, and 10.4 gives the required sample size.

$$n = \left(\frac{z_{1-\frac{\alpha}{2}} + z_{1-\beta}\sqrt{1-r^2}}{r} \right)^2 + 2 = \left(\frac{1.96 + 0.84\sqrt{1-0.6^2}}{0.60} \right)^2 + 2 = 21.25 \approx 22$$

TABLE 10.2

Required Sample Sizes for Estimating Population Correlation Coefficients Using Equation 10.2 for r Values Ranging from 0.05 to 0.90, Considering Significance Levels of 0.01, 0.05, and 0.10, with Test Powers of 0.80 and 0.90

$\alpha = 0.10$		$\alpha = 0.05$		$\alpha = 0.01$		
$1\text{-}\beta$		$1\text{-}\beta$		$1\text{-}\beta$		
0.90	0.80	0.90	0.80	0.90	0.80	r
3421	2471	4197	3136	5942	4665	0.05
854	618	1048	784	1484	1166	0.10
379	275	465	349	658	518	0.15
213	155	261	196	369	291	0.20
136	99	166	126	235	186	0.25
94	69	115	87	162	129	0.30
69	51	84	64	119	95	0.35
52	39	64	49	90	72	0.40
41	31	50	39	71	57	0.45
33	25	40	31	57	46	0.50
27	21	33	26	46	38	0.55
22	17	27	22	38	32	0.60
19	15	23	18	32	27	0.70
16	13	19	16	27	23	0.75
14	11	17	14	23	20	0.80
12	10	14	12	20	17	0.85
10	9	12	10	17	15	0.90

Using the Fisher z-transformation (Equations 10.3 and 10.4):

$$U_\rho = \frac{1}{2} ln\left(\frac{1+|\rho_0|}{1-|\rho_0|}\right) = 0.5ln\left(\frac{1.60}{0.40}\right) = 0.693$$

This value (0.693) also appears in Table 9-1 for $r = 0.60$.

Now, calculating the sample size using the Fisher z-transformation:

$$n = \left(\frac{z_{1-\alpha} + z_{1-\beta}}{U_\rho}\right)^2 + 3 = \left(\frac{1.96 + 0.84}{0.693}\right)^2 + 3 = 19.31 \approx 20$$

The sample size should be rounded up to the nearest whole number.

A sample size of approximately 22 (from Equation 10.2) to 20 (from Fisher's z-transformation) is required to estimate a correlation coefficient of 0.60 with 95% confidence and 80% power.

Equation 10.2 yields a slightly more conservative estimate, as expected.

Thus, the researcher should plan to enrol 20–22 paired observations.

10.3 Sample Size Determination for Correlations with Specified Confidence Interval

A 95% confidence interval (CI) for a correlation coefficient indicates that there is a 95% probability that the interval contains the true population correlation coefficient (ρ). The confidence interval is defined by the lower and upper limits, calculated as follows:

$$\text{Lower Limit (LL): } LL = r - Z_{1-\frac{\alpha}{2}} \times \sigma_r$$

and

$$\text{Upper Limit (UL): } UL = r - Z_{1-\frac{\alpha}{2}} \times \sigma_r$$

Here, σ_r is the standard error of the correlation coefficient (r), given by:

$$\sigma_r = \frac{1-r^2}{\sqrt{n-1}}$$

When a researcher aims to estimate the required sample size based on a desired confidence interval width, the half-width of the confidence interval (w) is defined as Equation 10.5:

$$w = Z_{1-\frac{\alpha}{2}} \times \frac{1-r^2}{\sqrt{n-1-6r^2}} \tag{10.5}$$

The term $6r^2$ represents a small-sample correction. The sample size needed to estimate a correlation coefficient with a pre-specified confidence interval width can be calculated using the following formula (Moinester & Gottfried, 2014, p. 127):

$$n = \frac{Z^2_{\frac{1-\alpha}{2}}\left(1-r^2\right)^2}{w^2} + 1 + 6r^2 \tag{10.6}$$

This method is particularly useful for researchers who want to ensure their correlation estimates are sufficiently precise for meaningful inferences.

TIP

When researchers cannot accurately predict the correlation coefficient and have a range of plausible values, they should use the smallest coefficient in sample size formulas. This conservative approach yields a larger sample size, providing a margin of error and increasing the likelihood of detecting the true effect size if it exists.

Table 10.3 provides a quick reference for determining the required sample size for 95% confidence levels and pre-specified confidence interval widths. This table serves as a valuable tool for researchers who prefer not to perform the calculations themselves or who need a rapid reference for study planning.

TABLE 10.3

Sample Size Requirements for Desired 95% Confidence Interval Half-Widths for Different Pearson Correlation Values (| *r* |), cited from Moinester and Gottfried (2014, p. 126)

	w								
|r|	**0.05**	**0.10**	**0.15**	**0.20**	**0.25**	**0.30**	**0.35**	**0.40**	**0.45**
0.05	1530	383	171	97	62	43	32	25	20
0.10	1507	378	168	95	61	43	32	25	20
0.15	1469	368	164	93	60	42	31	24	19
0.20	1418	355	159	90	58	41	30	23	19
0.25	1352	339	151	86	55	39	29	22	18
0.30	1274	320	143	81	53	37	28	21	17
0.35	1185	298	133	76	49	35	26	20	16
0.40	1086	273	123	70	46	32	24	19	15
0.45	980	247	111	64	42	30	22	18	14
0.50	867	219	99	57	37	27	20	16	13
0.55	751	190	86	50	33	24	18	15	12
0.60	633	161	74	43	29	21	16	13	11
0.65	517	132	61	36	25	18	14	12	–
0.70	404	105	49	30	20	15	12	–	–
0.75	299	79	38	23	17	13	–	–	–
0.80	205	56	28	18	13	–	–	–	–
0.85	125	36	19	13	–	–	–	–	–
0.90	62	20	12	–	–	–	–	–	–
0.95	22	–	–	–	–	–	–	–	–

10.4 Sample Size Determination to Compare a Correlation Coefficient with a Known Value

In statistical analyses, when comparing the correlation coefficient of a population with a predetermined value, a hypothesis test is conducted. This test is formulated with the null hypothesis $H_0 : \rho = \rho_0$ and the alternative hypothesis $H_A : \rho \neq \rho_0$. The required sample size for this test is influenced by the difference between the true population correlation coefficient and value specified under the null hypothesis, as well as the desired significance level (α) and the power of the test (1–β).

To calculate the appropriate sample size for testing a correlation coefficient against a non-zero value ($H_0 : \rho = \rho_0$, where $\rho_0 \neq 0$), we can use an equation reported in Zar's text (Zar, 2010, p. 388). For a two-tailed test, the power is determined using the following expression:

$$Z_{1-\beta} = \frac{\left|z - z_0\right| - Z_{1-\alpha/2}}{\sqrt{n-3}}$$

This formula parallels that used when estimating the sample size for a correlation coefficient based on Fisher's *z*-transformation, applied here to both z and z_0. The required sample size (n) is then calculated using the following equation, referred to as Equation 10.7 for simplicity:

$$n = \left(\frac{Z_{1-\beta} + z_{1-\frac{\alpha}{2}}}{\left|U - U_0\right|} \right)^2 + 3 \tag{10.7}$$

In this equation, U *and* U_0 represent the Fisher transformations of ρ *and* ρ_0, respectively.

> **Example 10.2:** We aim to test the hypothesis that the true correlation coefficient is $\rho_0 = 0.30$ with a significance level of 0.05 and a power of 0.80. What is the required sample size for this test?

Solution: First, we need to calculate U *and* U_0, the Fisher transformations of ρ and ρ_0. These values can also be obtained from Table 10.1, which provides Fisher *z*-values of 0.5493 and 0.3095, respectively. Given a significance level of $\alpha = 0.05$ and a desired power of $1–\beta = 0.80$, the corresponding *z*-scores are 1.96 and 0.84.

Substitute these values into the sample size equation to determine the required sample size for this study:

$$n = \left(\frac{Z_{1-\beta} + z_{1-\frac{\alpha}{2}}}{\left|U - U_0\right|} \right)^2 + 3$$

We obtain

$$n = \left(\frac{0.84 + 1.96}{|0.5493 - 0.3095|} \right)^2 + 3 = 139.34 \approx 140$$

Thus, the required sample size is approximately 140 participants.

If a correlation coefficient has not been anticipated in advance, calculating the Fisher *z*-transformation may be challenging. In such cases, the sample size can instead be determined by applying the Fisher transformation to the smallest detectable correlation coefficient that the researcher wishes to distinguish from ρ_0.

10.5 Sample Size for Comparing Two Correlation Coefficients

When testing the hypothesis $H_0 : \rho_0 = \rho_1 \quad vs \quad H_A : \rho_0 \neq \rho_1$, such as when comparing correlation coefficients from two populations, two common approaches are used. The first method is based on the *t*-distribution, and the second uses the Fisher *z* transformation. The sample sizes obtained from these two methods are usually similar, with only minor differences.

The following equation, provided by Indrayan and by Zar, is based on the Fisher *z* transformation and is used to estimate the required sample size when comparing two correlations (Indrayan & Holt, 2016, p. 557; Zar, 2010, p. 392):

$$n = \left(\frac{z_{1-\alpha} + z_{1-\beta}}{U_0 - U_1} \right)^2 + 3 \qquad (10.8)$$

In this equation, U_0 and U_1 represent the Fisher *z* transformations of the expected correlations ρ_0 and ρ_1 in the two populations. The term $|U_0 - U_1|$ reflects the minimum detectable difference between the two correlations. In practice, all parameters are replaced with their corresponding estimated values.

> **Example 10.3:** A researcher aims to compare the correlation coefficients between age and systolic blood pressure in female and male populations. Previous studies report correlation coefficients of 0.55 for women and 0.65 for men. We want to determine the required sample size at a 5% significance level and 80% power.

Solution: Given the information: $r_0 = 0.55$ and $r_1 = 0.65$, significance level of 5% (for a two-sided test) corresponds to a *z*-score of 1.96, and an 80% power corresponds to a z-score of 0.84. Using Equation 10.8, we can calculate the necessary sample size.

First, we calculate the Fisher transformations $U_{\rho 0}$ and $U_{\rho 1}$:

$$U_{\rho 0} = \frac{1}{2} ln\left(\frac{1+\rho_0}{1-\rho_0}\right) = \frac{1}{2} ln\left(\frac{1.55}{0.45}\right) = 0.6184$$

$$U_{\rho 1} = \frac{1}{2} ln\left(\frac{1+\rho_0}{1-\rho_0}\right) = \frac{1}{2} ln\left(\frac{1.65}{0.35}\right) = 0.7753$$

Substitute these values into the sample size equation:

$$n = \left(\frac{z_{1-\alpha} + z_{1-\beta}}{U_0 - U_1}\right)^2 + 3$$

This results in

$$n = \left(\frac{1.96 + 0.84}{0.7753 - 0.6184}\right)^2 + 3 = 321.47 \approx 322$$

A total sample size of approximately 322 participants is required for this study.

10.6 Sample Size for Estimating Regression Coefficient

Regression and correlation are two statistical methods used to analyse the relationship between variables X and Y. *Correlation* measures the strength and direction of the linear relationship between two variables, whereas *regression* is used to predict the value of one variable based on the value of another. In simple linear regression, the objective is to find the best-fitting straight line that describes the relationship between X and Y. This line is obtained by minimising the sum of the squared distances between the observed data points and the fitted line, which passes through the means of X and Y.

In certain research studies, evidence suggests a linear association between observed y and x values, although this relationship may not necessarily pass through the origin. In such situations, the additional information provided by the auxiliary variable x can be incorporated through a regression estimator of the mean μ_y. To apply this estimator, however, the population mean μ_x must be known, similar to ratio estimation of μ_y.

TIP

To determine the appropriate sample size for comparing a regression coefficient to a specific value, or for conducting hypothesis tests involving regression coefficients between two populations, researchers should first calculate the corresponding correlation coefficient. This approach is also applicable when estimating sample size for comparing correlation coefficients or performing hypothesis tests on correlations across populations.

The line representing the basic relationship between y and x values is known as the **regression line of y on x**. When fitting a straight line through a set of paired observations (x_i, y_i), the resulting equation takes the form:

$$y_i = a + b.x_i$$

where a is the intercept and b is the regression coefficient. The regression coefficient b is defined as the product of the correlation coefficient (ρ or r) and the ratio of the standard deviations of y and x, as shown below (Tabachnick et al., 2013, p. 57):

$$b = \rho \frac{\sigma_y}{\sigma_x} = r \frac{S_y}{S_x} \Leftrightarrow r = b \frac{S_x}{S_y} \tag{10.9}$$

The sample size required for testing the null hypothesis $H_0 : \beta = 0$ (where β is the regression coefficient) is the same as the sample size required for testing the null hypothesis $H_0 : \rho = 0$ (where ρ is the correlation coefficient), provided that both X and Y are standardised. This equivalence arises because if the true regression coefficient is zero $(\beta = 0)$, then the true correlation coefficient would also be zero $(\rho = 0)$, according to Equation 10.9. Therefore, the sample size for estimating a regression coefficient β can be calculated using either Equations 10.10 or 10.11 (Hsieh et al., 1998, p. 1625; Kleinbaum et al., 2013, p. 888).

$$n = \left(\frac{z_{1-\frac{\alpha}{2}} + z_{1-\beta}\sqrt{1-r^2}}{r = b\frac{S_x}{S_y}} \right)^2 + 2 \tag{10.10}$$

$$n = \left(\frac{z_{1-\frac{\alpha}{2}} + z_{1-\beta}}{U_\rho} \right)^2 + 3 \tag{10.11}$$

where U_ρ is defined in Equation 10.3.

Example 10.4: A pharmaceutical researcher aims to investigate the impact of a drug at varying concentrations (denoted as x) on a specific factor present in the blood serum (denoted as y) of patients with type II diabetes. The study will consider a change statistically significant at a 95% confidence level if the average shift in this factor is at least 0.2 mg per unit increase in drug concentration. Based on the researcher's experience, the standard deviation of drug concentration is approximately 5 units, while the standard deviation of the factor is 2 units. The objective is to determine the required sample size of patients for this study.

Solution: The statement that the factor changes by an average of 0.2 mg for each unit increase in drug concentration indicates that the slope of the regression line (regression coefficient) is $b = 0.2$. Additionally, we have $\sigma_Y = 2$ and $\sigma_X = 5$. The correlation coefficient can be calculated using Equation 10.9:

$$r = b \times \frac{\sigma_X}{\sigma_Y} = 0.2 \times \frac{5}{2} = 0.5$$

The sample size can then be determined using Equation 10.10 for a power of 0.80 ($z_{1-\beta} = 0.84$) and a significance level of 0.05 ($z_{1-\alpha/2} = 1.96$):

$$n = \left[\frac{z_{1-\frac{\alpha}{2}} + z_\beta \sqrt{1-r^2}}{r}\right]^2 + 2 = \left[\frac{1.96 + 0.84\sqrt{1-0.5^2}}{0.5}\right]^2 + 2 = 30.88 \cong 31$$

Using the Fisher z-transformation (Equation 10.11) provides a slightly refined estimate:

$$U_{\rho 0} = \frac{1}{2} ln\left(\frac{1+\rho_0}{1-\rho_0}\right) = \frac{1}{2} ln\left(\frac{1.50}{0.50}\right) = 0.549$$

$$n = \left(\frac{z_{1-\frac{\alpha}{2}} + z_{1-\beta}}{U_\rho}\right)^2 + 3 = \left(\frac{1.96 + 0.84}{0.549}\right)^2 + 3 = 29.01 \cong 30$$

Therefore, the required sample size for this study is approximately 30 patients. Using the correlation-based formula provides a slightly more conservative estimate of 31 patients, while the Fisher z-transformation yields 30 patients. Both approaches are appropriate for planning the study.

Example 10.5: Researchers intend to examine the association between APGAR scores recorded immediately after birth and infant blood pressure measured five hours post-delivery. The study will employ a significance level of 0.05 and a type II error rate of 0.15 to detect a correlation of at least $r = 0.25$. The objective is to determine the appropriate sample size of infants to include in the study.

Solution: Given that $r = 0.25$, the significance level $\alpha = 0.05$ corresponds to $z_{1-\alpha/2} = 1.96$, and the desired power $1-\beta = 0.85$ corresponds to $z_{1-\beta} = 1.04$. Substituting these values into Equation 10.10 provides an initial estimate of the required sample size:

$$n = \left[\frac{z_{1-\frac{\alpha}{2}} + z_{\beta}\sqrt{1-r^2}}{r}\right]^2 + 2 = \left[\frac{1.96 + 1.04\sqrt{1-0.25^2}}{0.25}\right]^2 + 2 = 142.85 \cong 143$$

Using the Fisher z-transformation (Equation 10.11) for a slightly refined estimate:

$$U_{\rho 0} = \frac{1}{2} ln\left(\frac{1+\rho_0}{1-\rho_0}\right) = \frac{1}{2} ln\left(\frac{1.25}{0.25}\right) = 0.2554$$

$$n = \left(\frac{z_{1-\frac{\alpha}{2}} + z_{1-\beta}}{U_{\rho}}\right)^2 + 3 = \left(\frac{1.96 + 1.04}{0.2554}\right)^2 + 3 = 140.96 \cong 141$$

The required sample size for this study is approximately 141 infants. Using the correlation-based formula provides a slightly more conservative estimate of 143 infants.

10.7 Sample Size for Comparing Two Slopes of Linear Regression

Researchers must determine the appropriate sample size when comparing a population's regression coefficient to a specified value. This involves testing the null hypothesis $H_0 : \beta = \beta_0$ against the alternative hypothesis $H_A : \beta \neq \beta_0$. Additionally, when conducting hypothesis testing on regression coefficients between two populations, the null hypothesis $H_0 : \beta_1 = \beta_2$ is tested against the alternative hypothesis $H_A : \beta_1 \neq \beta_2$.

The formulae used in these cases are similar to those for determining sample size when comparing correlation coefficients. This includes testing $H_0 : \rho = \rho_0$ versus $H_A : \rho_1 \neq \rho_2$, or when assessing correlation coefficients between two populations, $H_0 : \rho_1 = \rho_2$ versus $H_A : \rho_1 \neq \rho_2$.

To test the null hypothesis $H_0 : \beta_1 = \beta_2$ against $H_0 : \beta_1 \neq \beta_2$, the minimum sample size required can be determined using the following equation (Darling & Treatment, 2020, p. 820):

$$n = \sigma_R^2 \times \left(\frac{z_{1-\frac{\alpha}{2}} + z_{1-\beta}}{b_1 - b_2} \right)^2 \tag{10.12}$$

where b_1 and b_2 are the slopes of the first and second regression lines, respectively, and σ_R^2 is the variance of the regression errors for both groups, calculated as:

$$\sigma_R^2 = \sigma_p^2 \left(\frac{1}{k \times \sigma_1^2} + \frac{1}{\sigma_2^2} \right)$$

Here, σ_p^2 represents the pooled variance.

> **Example 10.6:** We aim to compare the relationship between pulse rate and body weight in adult patients without cancer (Group 1) and those with cancer (Group 2). The objective is to determine the required sample size for both groups.

Solution: Assume the standard deviations for pulse rate are $\sigma_1 = 11$ beats per minute in Group 1 and $\sigma_2 = 10$ beats per minute in Group 2. The groups will be allocated in a ratio of $k = 2:1$ (i.e., $r = 2$). A rough estimate of the regression slopes is $b_1 = 0.04$ kg/beat per minute for Group 1 and $b_2 = 0.06$ kg/beat per minute for Group 2.

Assuming a pooled standard deviation of $\sigma_p = 0.54$, we first calculate the variance of the regression errors:

$$\sigma_R^2 = \sigma_p^2 \left(\frac{1}{k \times \sigma_1^2} + \frac{1}{\sigma_2^2} \right) = 0.54^2 \left(\frac{1}{2 \times 11^2} + \frac{1}{10^2} \right) = 0.004121$$

Next, we calculate the sample size for patients with cancer (Group 2):

$$n_{Cancer} = \sigma_R^2 \times \left(\frac{z_{1-\frac{\alpha}{2}} + z_{1-\beta}}{b_1 - b_2} \right)^2 = 0.004121 \times \left(\frac{1.96 + 0.84}{0.06 - 0.04} \right)^2 = 80.77 \approx 81$$

For Group 1 (non-cancer), the sample size is proportional to the group ratio:

$$n_{\text{non-Cancer}} = k \times n_{\text{Cancer}} = 2 \times 81 = 162$$

Conclusion: The total sample size required for the study is:

$$n_{\text{total}} = 162 + 81 = 243 \text{ patients}$$

10.8 Sample Size Determination for Multiple Linear Regression

In multiple linear regression models, the Variance Inflation Factor (VIF) can be calculated for p covariates, allowing researchers to adjust sample size when a regression model includes multiple predictors. In simple linear regression model, the correlation coefficient ρ and the regression parameter β_1 are related by the equation

$$\rho = \beta_1 \frac{\sigma_X}{\sigma_Y}.$$

Therefore, $\rho = 0$ if and only if $\beta_1 = 0$. When both X and Y are standardised, testing the hypotheses $\rho = 0$ and $\beta_1 = 0$ becomes equivalent, and the required sample sizes are the same (Hsieh et al., 1998, p. 1625). Below, we describe four commonly used methods for determining sample size in multiple linear regression.

10.8.1 A Simple Approach

In multiple regression models where one independent variable is of primary interest and the remaining predictors serve mainly to control for confounding, the sample size can be approximated using formulas for simple linear regression. If n_s represents the sample size required for a simple linear regression of Y on X_1, then the sample size n for a multiple regression – where the dependent variable Y is regressed on several independent variables $X_1, X_2, \ldots, X_k$ – can be estimated using the following equation (Hsieh et al., 1998, p. 1625; Kleinbaum et al., 2013, p. 888):

$$n = \frac{n_s}{1 - \rho^2_{X_1(X_2,\cdots,X_k)}} = n_s \times VIF \tag{10.13}$$

The VIF for the variable X_1 is calculated as the reciprocal of the term $1 - \rho^2_{X_1(X_2,\cdots,X_k)}$, expressed as:

$$VIF = \frac{1}{1 - \rho^2_{X_1(X_2,\cdots,X_k)}}.$$

This formula provides a simplified approximation and may not fully capture the complexity of sample size determination in multiple regression. Here, n_s represents the sample size required for simple linear regression, and $\rho^2_{X_1(X_2,\cdots,X_k)}$ denotes the expected population squared multiple correlation between the main independent variable of interest, X_1, and the remaining predictors $X_2, \ldots, X_k$. This value indicates the proportion of variance in X_1 that is explained by the other independent variables.

The denominator term $1-\rho^2_{X_1(X_2,\ldots,X_k)}$ represents the variance inflation factor (VIF), which adjusts for multicollinearity among the predictors. If no multicollinearity is present, $\rho^2_{X_1(X_2,\ldots,X_k)}=0$, resulting in a required sample size equal to n_s. However, as multicollinearity increases and $\rho^2_{X_1(X_2,\ldots,X_k)}$ approaches 1, the required sample size increases substantially.

TIP

For multiple regression analyses (both logistic and ordinary), the sample sizes should be multiplied by the Variance Inflation Factor ($VIF=\dfrac{1}{(1-\eta 2)}$), where η represents the coefficient of determination. This can also be expressed using the multiple correlation coefficient R or its equivalent in linear regression. The same VIF is applicable to both logistic and linear regression models. As with all sample size calculations, the parameter values should be substituted with anticipated values derived from prior studies (Indrayan & Holt, 2016, p.558).

The Variance Inflation Factor (VIF) serves as an indicator of the degree of multicollinearity among predictors in multiple regression. It is computed for each independent variable, and a high VIF indicates that the variable is strongly correlated with the other predictors. The underlying principle is that the sample size required for simple linear regression should be multiplied by the VIF associated with the primary independent variable. Hsieh et al. (1998) demonstrated that this approximation is reasonably accurate for both normally and non-normally distributed independent variables.

> **Example 10.7:** Suppose you are studying the relationship between daily caloric intake (Y) and several independent variables, including age (X_1), physical activity level (X_2), and daily consumption of fruits and vegetables (X_3). Initial data indicate that the squared multiple correlation coefficient between age (X_1) and the other independent variables (X_2 and X_3) is $\rho^2_{X_1(X_2,\cdots X_k)}=0.50$, and the Pearson correlation between daily caloric intake (Y) and age (X_1) is $r=0.30$. To estimate the regression coefficients with a significance level of 0.05 and a statistical power of 0.85, how many samples are needed for the study?

Solution: Given a Pearson correlation coefficient of r = 0.30 between daily caloric intake (Y) and age (X_1), along with a power of 0.85 and a significance level of 0.05, the corresponding critical values are $z_{1-\beta}=1.04$ and $z_{1-\frac{\alpha}{2}}=1.96$.

The number of independent variables in this study is $k = 3$: age, physical activity level, and daily consumption of fruits and vegetables.

First, we need to determine Fisher's z-transformation of ρ using the following equation:

$$U_\rho = \frac{1}{2} ln\left(\frac{1+\rho_0}{1-\rho_0}\right) = \frac{1}{2} ln\left(\frac{1+0.30}{1-0.30}\right) = 0.3095$$

Next, we calculate the sample size n_s for simple linear regression:

$$n_s = \left(\frac{z_{1-\frac{\alpha}{2}} + z_{1-\beta}}{U_\rho}\right)^2 + 3 = \left(\frac{1.96+1.04}{0.3095}\right)^2 + 3 = 96.96 \approx 97$$

Now, to account for the squared multiple correlation coefficient $\rho^2_{X_1(X_2,\cdots,X_k)} = 0.50$, the total sample size n for multiple regression is calculated as follows:

$$n = \frac{n_s}{1-\rho^2_{X_1(X_2,\cdots,X_k)}} = \frac{97}{1-0.5} = 194$$

Thus, a total of 194 samples are required for this study.

10.8.2 The PEAR Method

Determining the sample size for multiple linear regression with k independent variables requires consideration of several factors beyond those used in simpler approaches. The PEAR method, which stands for "Precision Efficacy Analysis for Regression", was proposed by Brooks and Barcikowski (2012). This method provides a systematic strategy for estimating sample size in multiple linear regression and helps researchers determine the number of observations required to achieve adequate statistical power, particularly when dealing with multiple predictors (Brooks & Barcikowski, 2012, p.7). The formula for the PEAR method is as follows:

$$n = \left(\frac{2-2\rho^2+\varepsilon}{\varepsilon}\right)(K+1) \tag{10.14}$$

where

- k is the number of predictors (independent variables) in the regression model. As the number of predictors increases, a larger sample size is generally required to maintain the same level of statistical power.

- ρ^2 is the *a priori* effect size, representing the proportion of variance in the dependent variable explained by the set of predictors.
- ε (epsilon) is the *a priori* shrinkage tolerance, which allows researchers to determine how closely the sample-based estimate of ρ^2 should approximate the population value – either in absolute terms (e.g., $\varepsilon = 0.10$) or relative terms (e.g., $\varepsilon = 0.25\rho^2$). When using a proportional definition of shrinkage tolerance, the formula simplifies because ρ^2 appears in both the numerator and denominator and thus cancels out.

The level of precision efficacy in the resulting sample size depends on the chosen shrinkage tolerance value.

TIP

The PEAR method for determining sample size in multiple linear regression emphasises the precision and effectiveness of the regression analysis, particularly in estimating the effect size and the number of predictors. Although the method does not explicitly incorporate the significance level (α) or statistical power ($1 - \beta$) into its formula, these parameters are implicitly accounted for in the application of the method.

Estimating the expected value of ρ^2 without preliminary information can be challenging, as ρ^2 is an empirical measure that typically requires data for accurate estimation. However, several strategies may assist in forming a reasonable estimate:

1. **Literature Review:** Reported ρ^2 values from similar studies can provide a useful benchmark.
2. **Expert Opinion:** Field experts may offer informed estimates based on their experience.
3. **Pilot Study:** A small preliminary study can yield an initial estimate of ρ^2.
4. **Theoretical Considerations:** Conceptual models and theory-based expectations regarding relationships among variables can guide the anticipated magnitude of ρ^2. Strong theoretical relationships imply higher expected ρ^2, while weaker relationships imply lower values.

It is important to remember that the estimate of ρ^2 is only an approximation. Researchers should exercise caution when selecting this value to ensure that the study maintains adequate statistical power. In general, it is preferable to slightly overestimating the effect size and obtaining a larger sample than necessary, rather than risking an underpowered study due to underestimation.

> **Example 10.8:** Consider a study similar to Example 10.6 that involves three predictors: age (X_1), physical activity level (X_2), and daily consumption of fruits and vegetables (X_3), with daily caloric intake (Y) as the dependent variable. Initial data indicate that the squared multiple correlation coefficient between age (X_1) and the other independent variables (X_2 and X_3) is $\rho^2_{X_1(X_2,\cdots X_k)} = 0.50$, and the shrinkage tolerance is ε = 0.15. How many samples are needed to estimate the regression coefficients with a significance level of 0.05 and a statistical power of 0.85 using the PEAR method?

Solution: The squared multiple correlation coefficient between age (X_1) and the other independent variables is $\rho^2_{X_1(X_2,\cdots X_k)} = 0.50$. The number of predictors is $k = 3$ (age, physical activity level, and daily consumption of fruits and vegetables). Using a power of 0.85 and a significance level of 0.05, which correspond to critical values of 1.04 and 1.96, the sample size required for multiple regression according to the PEAR method is calculated as follows:

$$n = \left(\frac{2-2\rho^2+\varepsilon}{\varepsilon}\right)(K+1) = \left(\frac{2-2\times 0.50+0.15}{0.15}\right)(3+1) = \frac{1.15}{0.15}\times 4 = 30.66 \approx 31$$

Thus, the required sample size for the study is **31** participants.

> **Example 10.9:** Consider a study investigating the factors that influence clinic pricing. The dependent variable is Y (clinic price), and the model includes four predictors: X_1 (square footage), X_2 (number of examination rooms), X_3 (number of clinicians), and X_4 (history and background of the clinic). Based on previous research and expert opinion, the a priori effect size is estimated as $\rho^2 = \rho^2_{X_1(X_2,\cdots X_k)} = 0.60$. To obtain a relatively precise estimate of the effect size, we select a proportional shrinkage tolerance of $\varepsilon = 0.20\rho^2$. Our objective is to achieve a statistical power of 0.90 at a significance level of 0.05.

Solution: The squared multiple correlation coefficient between square footage (X_1) and the other predictors is $\rho^2 = \rho^2_{X_1(X_2,\cdots X_k)} = 0.60$. With a power of 0.90 and a significance level of 0.05, the corresponding critical values are 1.28 and 1.96. The number of independent variables is k = 4.

The shrinkage tolerance is calculated as:

$$\varepsilon = 0.20\rho^2 = 0.20\times 0.60 = 0.12$$

Using the PEAR method (Eq. 10.14):

$$n = \left(\frac{2-2\rho^2+\varepsilon}{\varepsilon}\right)(K+1) = \left(\frac{2-2\times 0.60+0.12}{0.12}\right)(4+1) = \frac{0.92}{0.12}\times 5 = 38.33 \approx 39$$

Therefore, the study requires a sample size of approximately 39 clinics to achieve a statistical power of 0.90 with a proportional shrinkage tolerance of 0.20 and an estimated effect size of 0.60.

10.8.3 Most Important Predictor Approach

A key consideration in multiple regression analysis, represented by the equation

$$Y = b_0 + b_1.x_1 + b_2.x_2 + b_3.x_3 + \cdots + b_n.x_n,$$

is the identification of the independent variable that is of primary interest to the researcher. The sample size required to estimate the slope of this independent variable, as if it were part of a simple linear regression, can serve as an estimate for the multiple regression model. This is important because the significance of the coefficient for this variable forms the basis for determining the necessary sample size.

If multiple independent variables are of interest, a separate sample size estimate should be calculated for each variable. The largest sample size among these estimates is then used as the criterion for the overall study.

To further justify the importance of the primary independent variable in determining sample size, it is useful to consider the squared multiple correlation coefficient between this variable and the other predictors in the model. This is denoted as $R^2_{X \cdot X_j}$,, where X_j represents the independent variable of interest, and X represents the set of all other independent variables in the model.

This measure indicates the proportion of variance in X_j that can be explained by the remaining predictors and is critical for adjusting the sample size to account for multicollinearity.

> **Example 10.10:** The goal of this study is to examine the relationship between blood pressure (BP, measured in mmHg) as the dependent variable and several independent variables, including Age (in years), Body Mass Index (BMI), and Cholesterol Level (in mg/dL) in patients. The objective is to determine the number of participants needed to estimate the regression coefficients accurately.

Solution: The multiple linear regression model incorporating these three predictor variables can be expressed as:

$$BP = b_0 + b_1.\ Age + b_2.\ BMI + b_3.\ Cholestrol + e$$

In this equation:

- b_0 represents the intercept,
- b_1 is the coefficient for age, representing the expected change in BP for each additional year of age while holding other variables constant,
- b_2 is the regression coefficient for BMI, representing the expected change in BP for each additional unit of BMI while holding other variables constant,
- b_3 is the regression coefficient for Cholesterol, representing the expected change in BP for each additional mg/dL while holding other variables constant, and
- e denotes the residual (error term).

Literature suggests that BMI and Age are more significant predictors of systolic blood pressure (SBP) than Cholesterol. Specifically, the correlation between BMI and SBP is $r = 0.26$ (upper bound $U_p = 0.266$), and the correlation between Age and SBP is $r = 0.24$ (upper bound $U_p = 0.245$).

Using Equation 10.11 for sample size estimation with a significance level $\alpha = 0.05$ and power $1 - \beta = 0.84$, the required sample sizes are:

- For BMI: $n = 114$
- For Age: $n = 134$

Therefore, to ensure adequate precision for all predictors, a total sample size of 134 participants is sufficient for conducting the multiple linear regression analysis.

10.8.4 Rules of Thumb for Determining Sample Size in Multiple Regression Analysis

Several rules of thumb have been proposed for determining the minimum sample size required for multiple regression analysis. Tabachnick and Fidell discuss these under the section titled *"Ratio of Cases to IVs"* (Tabachnick et al., 2013, p.123), while Green provides guidance on the necessary number of cases (Green, 1991, p. 508). Table 10.4 summarises some commonly used rules of thumb:

TABLE 10.4

Rules of Thumb for Determining Sample Size in Multiple Regression Analysis

Rule	Use
$n = 50 + 8k$	For testing multiple correlation/regression.
$n = 104 + k$	For testing individual predictors, assuming a medium-sized relationship between the independent variables (IVs) and the dependent variable (DV), with $\alpha = 0.05$ and $\beta = 0.20$.
$n = 20 + 5k$	When power estimates are not feasible, using reliability as a criterion to determine the minimum sample size.
$n = \frac{8}{f^2} + (k-1)$	When the anticipated effect size is known. More cases are needed to detect a small effect than a large effect, with $\alpha = 0.05$ and $\beta = 0.20$. Values of f^2 are 0.02, 0.15, and 0.35 for small, medium, and large effect sizes, respectively.
$n = 8 + 2kf$	For estimating the minimum sample size based on the number of predictors (k) and the anticipated effect size (f).

In these formulas:

- k represents the number of predictors (independent variables) in the regression model, and
- f is the effect size, defined as $f^2 = \frac{R^2}{1-R^2}$.

These methods are widely recognised and commonly employed approaches for determining sample size in multiple regression analysis. The choice of method depends on the specific requirements of the study, including the number of predictors, desired effect size, and required statistical power.

If the dependent variable is not normally distributed (i.e., skewed) and transformations are not applied, a larger sample size may be necessary. Additionally, if the independent or dependent variables have low reliability, greater measurement error will necessitate a larger sample size.

TIP

If you are interested in both the overall correlation and the individual independent variables (IVs), calculate the sample size N using both methods and choose the larger number of cases.

Example 10.11: Suppose we want to explore how lifestyle factors – such as exercise, diet, and stress levels – impact blood pressure. How many samples are required to conduct a multiple linear regression analysis using the rule-of-thumb formulas provided above?

Solution: We have three predictors ($k = 3$). Assuming a medium effect size ($f^2 = 0.15$), the calculations using the rules of thumb are as follows:

- For testing the overall regression:

$$n = 50 + 8k = 50 + 8 \times 3 = 74$$

- For testing individual predictors:

$$n = 104 + k = 104 + 3 = 107$$

- Considering the effect size of the model:

$$n = \frac{8}{f^2} + (k - 1) = \frac{8}{0.15} + (3 - 1) = 55.33 \approx 56$$

Thus, depending on the approach, the recommended sample size ranges from 55 to 107, with the larger value ensuring sufficient power for testing individual predictors.

Example 10.12: Now, suppose we aim to predict the mortality rate using six different health indicators. How many samples are required to perform a multiple linear regression analysis using the aforementioned rule-of-thumb formulas?

Solution: For a study with six predictors ($k = 6$) and an expected small effect size ($f^2 = 0.02$), the sample size calculations using the rules of thumb are:

- For testing the overall regression:

$$n = 104 + k = 104 + 6 = 110$$

- For testing individual predictors:

$$n = 104 + k = 104 + 6 = 110$$

- Considering the effect size of the model:

$$n = \frac{8}{f^2} + (k - 1) = \frac{8}{0.02} + (6 - 1) = 405$$

Therefore, to account for a small effect size, a sample size of 405 participants is recommended to ensure adequate power for detecting significant effects in the model.

Supplementary Remark: The wide range of sample sizes in each example illustrates the sensitivity of these rules of thumb to both the number of predictors and, particularly, the effect size. Green compared sample sizes determined by power analysis with those obtained using rule-of-thumb methods, demonstrating that the estimates from both approaches are generally quite similar (Green, 1991). These calculations are presented in Table 10.5.

TABLE 10.5

Sample Size Required to Test the Hypothesis that the Population Multiple Correlation Is Equal to Zero, with a Power of 0.80 and Alpha of 0.05

	Sample Sizes Based on Power Analysis			Sample Sizes Based on the Rule-of-Thumb		
	Effect Size			Effect Size		
Number of Predictors	Small	Medium	Large	Small	Medium	Large
1	390	53	24	400	53	23
2	481	66	30	475	63	27
3	547	76	35	545	73	31
4	599	84	39	610	81	35
5	645	91	42	670	89	38
6	686	97	46	725	97	41
7	726	102	48	775	103	44
8	757	108	51	820	109	47
9	788	113	54	860	115	49
10	844	117	56	895	119	51
15	952	138	67	1045	139	60
20	1066	156	77	1195	159	68

10.9 Sample Size Determination for Confidence Intervals of Multiple Regression Coefficient

In regression analysis, the required sample size can be determined based on the expected confidence interval of the regression coefficients of interest. Similar to other confidence intervals, a symmetric confidence interval is defined by upper and lower bounds, with w representing half the width of the interval. Consequently, the total width of the confidence interval is $2w$. The value of w is critical for accurate estimation, as the width of the interval directly affects the precision of the estimated regression coefficient.

TIP

Any increase in $R^2_{x.x_j}$ or decrease in the confidence interval width (w) will result in a reduction in the required sample size for the multiple regression coefficient.

The formula for determining the sample size required to ensure that confidence intervals around a specific population regression coefficient (β_j) have a specified width is as follows (Kelley & Maxwell, 2003, p.309):

$$n = \left(\frac{Z_{1-\frac{\alpha}{2}}}{W} \right)^2 \times \left(\frac{1-R^2}{1-R^2_{x.x_j}} \right) + P + 1 \quad (10.15)$$

where

- P is the number of predictors (independent variables, covariates, or regressors),
- R^2 is the observed multiple correlation coefficient of the full regression model,
- $R^2_{x.x_j}$ is the squared multiple correlation coefficient predicting the jth predictor (X_j) from the remaining $(p-1)$ predictors,
- n is the required sample size, which is the same as presented in Equation 10.15 (Kelley & Maxwell, 2003, p.309).

The calculated sample size n should be rounded up to the nearest whole number. In practice, both R^2 and $R^2_{x.x_j}$ must be estimated prior to data collection, and w should be set as small as feasible (typically less than 0.50) to ensure greater precision of the regression coefficient estimates.

> **Example 10.13:** To study the relationship between gender and daily salt intake on average systolic blood pressure (SBP), how many participants should be selected to ensure a 95% confidence interval with an expected width of 0.30 (i.e., $w = 0.15$)? Assume the multiple correlation coefficient of the regression model is at least 0.20, and based on the literature, the correlation between gender and daily salt intake is 0.40.

Solution: Given $Z_{1-\alpha/2} = 1.96$, $P = 2$, $R^2 = 0.20$, $w = 0.15$, and $R^2_{x.x_j} = 0.40 \times 0.40 = 0.16$, the required sample size can be calculated as follows:

$$n = \left(\frac{1.96}{0.15} \right)^2 \cdot \left(\frac{1-0.20}{1-0.16} \right) + 2 + 1 = 165.60 \approx 166$$

If the confidence interval width is decreased to $w = 0.10$, the new sample size becomes:

$$n = \left(\frac{1.96}{0.10} \right)^2 \cdot \left(\frac{1-0.20}{1-0.16} \right) + 2 + 1 = 368.86 \approx 369$$

In studies with multiple predictors, $R^2_{x.x_j}$ can vary between 0 and 1. It is recommended to use the highest anticipated value of $R^2_{x.x_j}$ to ensure a sufficiently large and reliable sample size. For example, if $R^2_{x.x_j} = 0.80 \times 0.80 = 0.64$ instead of $0.40 \times 0.40 = 0.16$, the required sample size would be:

$$n = \left(\frac{1.96}{0.15}\right)^2 \cdot \left(\frac{1-0.20}{1-0.64}\right) + 2 + 1 = 382.42 \approx 383$$

10.10 Sample Size Estimation for Simple Logistic Regression

Regression analysis is a versatile tool in statistical research, with the choice of regression type depending on the research objectives and the nature of the variables involved. Linear regression, a widely used method, is applied to continuous outcomes under the assumption of a linear relationship between the outcome variable and the independent variables.

However, linear regression is not appropriate for all types of outcomes, particularly when dealing with binary events such as mortality. In such cases, logistic regression is the preferred method. Logistic regression can accommodate one or more independent variables, and models with multiple predictors provide deeper insights by quantifying the unique contribution of each variable while controlling for the others.

In logistic regression, the setup for independent variables (X) and their corresponding coefficients (β) is analogous to linear regression, as illustrated by the following equation:

$$p(Y) = \frac{e^{\beta_0 + \beta_1 x_1 + \beta_2 x_2 + \ldots + \beta_k x_k}}{1 + e^{\beta_0 + \beta_1 x_1 + \beta_2 x_2 + \ldots + \beta_k x_k}}$$

This equation estimates the probability of an event occurring in one category of a binary outcome compared to the other, expressed on the logit scale. The logit transformation is defined as:

$$\text{logit}(p) = \log\left(\frac{p}{1-p}\right) = \beta_0 + \beta_1 x_1 + \beta_2 x_2 + \cdots + \beta_k x_k$$

The strength of logistic regression lies in its ability to model binary outcomes while retaining characteristics analogous to linear regression on the logit scale. Logistic regression provides valuable insights into the relationships between independent variables and binary outcomes, allowing for estimation of odds ratios and interpretation of the effect size of predictors.

10.11 Continuous Covariate

Hsieh, Bloch, and Larsen simplified the process of calculating sample size for logistic regression by relating it to the more familiar formulas for comparing two means or two proportions. They recognised that the sample size required for logistic regression could be estimated using concepts analogous to those used in comparing two groups – a common and well-understood scenario in statistics. Their method conceptualises the logistic regression model as a comparison between two groups: those with and without the outcome of interest (Hsieh et al., 1998).

By adopting this approach, they expressed the sample size formula for logistic regression in terms of the effect size (logistic regression coefficient or corresponding odds ratio), the proportion of subjects with the outcome, and the desired significance level and statistical power. This method allows researchers to calculate the required sample size for logistic regression analyses in a straightforward and intuitive manner (Hsieh et al., 1998, p. 1624).

Equation 10.16 shows their simplified formula for determining the sample size needed to detect a logistic regression coefficient β_0:

$$n = \frac{\left(Z_{1-\frac{\alpha}{2}} + Z_{1-\beta}\right)^2}{p(1-p) \times \beta_0^2} \tag{10.6}$$

where

- n is the required total sample size,
- β_0 is logistic regression coefficient to be detected (corresponding to the minimum effect size or odds ratio of interest), and
- p is anticipated probability of the outcome at the mean value of the covariate X.

This formula provides a practical and intuitive approach to estimate the total sample size needed for logistic regression when assessing the effect of a continuous covariate, ensuring that the study achieves the desired significance level and statistical power.

> **Example 10.14:** A medical researcher aims to investigate the relationship between a continuous biomarker (e.g., blood glucose level) and the risk of developing a specific disease (e.g., diabetes). The researcher plans to use logistic regression to model the binary outcome (disease status: yes/no) as a function of the continuous biomarker. The question is: How many participants are needed for this study?

Solution: To determine the required sample size, we will use Equation 10.16 derived from (Hsieh et al., 1998), which is suitable for simple logistic regression with a single continuous predictor. We set the confidence level at 95% ($\alpha = 0.05$), giving $Z_{1-\frac{\alpha}{2}} = 1.96$. We desire a power of 80% ($\beta = 0.20$), giving $Z_{1-\beta} = 0.84$.

We estimate the disease prevalence in the population to be 30%, so $p = 0.3$. We aim to detect an odds ratio of 2, which corresponds to a logistic coefficient of $\beta_0 = ln(2) = 0.6931$.

Substituting these values into the sample size formula, Equation 10.16:

$$n = \frac{\left(Z_{1-\frac{\alpha}{2}} + Z_{1-\beta}\right)^2}{p(1-p) \times \beta_0^2} = \frac{(1.96 + 0.84)^2}{0.30(1-0.30) \times 0.6931^2}$$

Calculating this gives

$$n = \frac{2.8^2}{0.10088} = 77.71 \approx 78$$

Rounding up, the required sample size for this study is 78 participants. This calculation assumes a simple logistic regression model with a single continuous predictor, a two-sided test, and equal allocation of subjects when applicable. For models with multiple predictors, additional adjustments to the sample size may be necessary to maintain adequate power.

10.12 Binary Covariate

When the covariate is a binary variable, represented by $X = 1$ or $X = 0$, corresponding to categories such as "Yes" or "No", the log-odds coefficient $b_1 = 0$ indicates that the two event rates are equal. In this context, logistic regression with a binary predictor is mathematically equivalent to comparing two independent proportions. Hsieh et al. (1998) derived a sample size formula for this situation by treating the logistic model as a comparison between two groups defined by the binary covariate. This approach enables researchers to determine the number of subjects required to detect a meaningful difference in event rates between the two groups.

The total sample size required to compare two independent event rates is given by the following equation (Hsieh et al., 1998, p. 1630):

$$n = \frac{p(1-p)}{B(1-B)} \times \frac{\left(Z_{1-\frac{\alpha}{2}} + Z_{1-\beta}\right)^2}{(p_1 - p_2)^2} \tag{10.17}$$

where

- B is the proportion of the population with $X = 1$,
- p_1 is the event rate when $X = 0$,
- p_2 is the event rate when $X = 1$, and
- p is the overall event rate, typically calculated as $p = B.p_2 + (1-B).p_1$.

> **Example 10.15:** In an underdeveloped country, the incidence of low-birth-weight births is 15% (B = 0.15). It is also known that up to 60% of mothers of low-birth-weight babies have anaemia ($p_1 = 0.60$). The health administration has implemented an iron supplementation programme for pregnant women, aiming to reduce the anaemia rate to 40% or less ($p_2 = 0.40$).

How many subjects are required to detect this decline with a power of 0.90 and a significance level of 0.025 (one-sided, since the supplementation programme is not expected to increase anaemia rates)?

Solution: We first calculate the overall (average) prevalence of anaemia:

$$p = \frac{p_1 + p_2}{2} = \frac{0.60 + 0.40}{2} = 0.50.$$

Next, we apply Equation 10.17:

$$n = \frac{p(1-p)}{B(1-B)} \times \frac{\left(Z_{1-\frac{\alpha}{2}} + Z_{1-\beta}\right)^2}{(p_1 - p2)^2}$$

Substituting these values:

$$n = \frac{0.50(1-0.50)}{0.15(1-0.15)} \times \frac{(1.96 + 1.28)^2}{(0.60 - 0.40)^2} = 515$$

A field trial with a sample size of 515 pregnant women would provide sufficient statistical power to demonstrate that the supplementation programme can reduce anaemia levels to 40% or lower in this population.

Remark: The sample size required for detecting an odds ratio r remains unchanged if the odds ratio is reversed to $\frac{1}{r}$. For example, the sample size needed to detect an odds ratio of *2.5* is the same as that required to detect an odds ratio of *0.4* (Hsieh, 1989, p. 796; Hsieh et al., 1998, p. 1627).

When multiple covariates are included in the model, *multiple logistic regression* can be used to estimate the effect of a covariate on the outcome while adjusting for the influence of other covariates. In such cases, the required sample size is larger than that for a single covariate. To calculate the necessary sample size, first determine the sample size for one covariate using Table 10.6. Then, divide this value by the factor $1-\rho^2$, where ρ is the multiple correlation coefficient between the covariate of interest and the remaining covariates in the model. This adjustment accounts for shared variance among predictors.

Table 10.6 provides the required sample size for logistic regression with a single covariate (risk factor) at a significance level of $\alpha = 0.05$ and power $1-\beta = 0.80$. To use the table, two inputs are needed:

- the probability P of the event at the mean value of the covariate, and
- the odds ratio r (where $r = \exp(b_1)$), corresponding to a one–standard deviation increase from the mean of the covariate.

10.13 Sample Size Estimation for Multiple Logistic Regression

When conducting multiple logistic regression with several predictors, the primary objective is often to evaluate the effect of a specific factor while controlling for the influence of others. The corresponding hypotheses are:

$$\begin{cases} H_0: \text{The effect of the first factor}\,(\beta_1)\,\text{is zero.} \\ H_A: \text{The effect of the first factor}\,(\beta)\,\text{is not zero.} \end{cases}$$

Here, β_1 represents the regression coefficient corresponding to the first factor.

Research has shown that for normally distributed predictors X, the variance of β_1 in a multiple logistic regression model can be estimated by adjusting the variance from a single-predictor model using a factor that reflects the degree of multicollinearity among predictors. This same adjustment can be applied to estimate the required sample size for a multiple-predictor model based on the sample size needed for a univariate logistic regression model.

TABLE 10.6

Sample Size Required for Univariate Logistic Regression with an Overall Event Proportion of *P* and an Odds Ratio r Evaluated at One Standard Deviation Above the Mean of the Covariate, with $\alpha = 0.05$ and $1 - \beta = 0.80$, adopted from Hsieh (1989, p. 797)

	Odds Ratio (*r*)															
P	0.6	0.7	0.8	0.9	1.1	1.2	1.3	1.4	1.5	1.6	1.7	1.8	1.9	2.0	2.5	3.0
0.01	2334	4872	12580	56741	69359	18889	9076	5485	3751	2771	2158	1746	1453	1237	690	480
0.02	1199	2492	642 1	28935	35367	9637	4635	2804	1921	1422	1110	900	751	642	367	267
0.03	821	1699	4368	19666	24037	6554	3155	1911	1311	972	760	618	517	444	260	196
0.04	632	1302	3342	15031	18371	5012	2414	1464	1006	747	585	477	401	344	206	160
0.05	518	1064	2726	12251	14912	4086	1970	1196	823	612	481	392	330	285	174	139
0.06	443	905	2315	10397	12706	3470	1674	1018	701	522	411	336	284	245	152	125
0.07	389	792	2022	9073	11087	3029	1463	890	614	458	361	296	250	217	137	115
0.08	348	707	1802	8080	9873	2699	1304	794	548	410	323	266	225	196	125	107
0.09	317	641	1631	7307	8929	2442	1181	720	497	372	294	242	206	179	116	101
0.10	291	588	1494	6689	8174	2236	1082	660	457	342	27 1	223	190	166	109	96
0.12	254	509	1289	5762	7041	1928	934	571	396	297	236	195	167	146	98	89
0.14	227	452	1142	5100	623 1	1708	828	507	352	265	21 1	175	150	132	91	84
0.16	206	410	1032	4604	5624	1542	749	459	320	241	192	160	137	121	85	80
0.18	191	377	947	4218	5152	1414	687	422	294	222	178	148	128	113	80	77
0.20	178	350	878	3909	4774	1311	638	392	274	207	166	139	120	106	77	75
0.25	155	303	755	3352	4095	1126	549	339	237	180	145	122	106	94	70	71
0.30	140	271	673	2982	3641	1003	490	303	213	162	131	111	96	86	66	68
0.35	129	248	614	2717	3318	915	448	277	195	149	121	103	90	81	63	66
0.40	121	231	570	2518	3075	848	416	258	182	140	114	96	85	76	61	64
0.45	115	218	536	2364	2886	797	391	243	172	132	108	92	81	73	59	63
0.50	110	207	509	2240	2735	756	372	231	164	126	103	88	78	70	57	62

Note: To obtain sample sizes for multiple logistic regression, divide the sample size obtained from the table by the factor of $1 - p^2$, where p^2 is the multiple correlation coefficient relating the covariate of interest to the remaining covariates in the model.

TIP

When multiple covariates are included in the logistic model, multiple logistic regression estimates the relationship between a covariate of interest and the disease outcome while adjusting for the effects of the other covariates. The sample size required to detect such a relationship is larger than that needed when only a single covariate is considered. To calculate the required sample size, first determine the sample size for the single covariate using Table 10.6. Then, divide this value by the factor $1-\rho^2$ to obtain the required sample size for the multiple logistic regression model, where ρ^2 is the multiple correlation coefficient relating the covariate of interest to the remaining covariates.

Specifically, the required sample size for a logistic regression model with multiple predictors (n_p) can be obtained from the sample size needed for a single-predictor model (n_1) using the following formula (Hsieh et al., 1998, p. 1625):

$$n_p = \frac{n_1}{1-\rho^2_{1.2.3\cdots p}} \tag{10.18}$$

where $\rho^2_{1.2,3,\ldots,p}$ is the multiple correlation coefficient measuring the linear relationship between the first predictor and all remaining predictors.

This formula adjusts the sample size upward according to the degree of multicollinearity and is applicable to both continuous and binary predictors. Thus, the variance inflation factor (VIF), defined as $\dfrac{1}{1-\rho^2_{1.2,3,\ldots,p}}$, provides a practical tool for determining sample size requirements in multiple logistic regression models (Hsieh et al., 1998, p. 1625).

Example 10.16: Consider a study aimed at determining whether a new drug (X_1) reduces the risk of heart disease, while also accounting for other factors such as age (X_2), gender (X_3), and blood pressure (X_4). The researchers aim to ensure a sufficient number of participants to accurately assess the drug's effect.

Solution: If the sample size required for a study that considers only the drug as a factor is $n_1 = 100$, and the multicollinearity among the predictors is characterised by $\rho^2_{1.2.3\cdots p} = 0.50$, then the sample size needed for the study incorporating all predictors (n_p) can be calculated using Equation 10.18:

$$n_p = \frac{n_1}{1-\rho^2_{1.2.3\cdots p}} = \frac{100}{(1-0.50)} = 200$$

Thus, the researchers would need approximately 200 participants to adequately account for the additional predictors in their multiple logistic regression analysis.

References

Brooks, G. P., & Barcikowski, R. S. (2012). The PEAR method for sample sizes in multiple linear regression. *Multiple Linear Regression Viewpoints, 38*(2), 1–16.

Darling, H. J. (2020). Basics of statistics–4: Sample size calculation (ii): A narrative review. *Cancer Research, Statistics, and Treatment, 3*(4), 817–828.

Green, S. B. (1991). How many subjects does it take to do a regression analysis. *Multivariate Behavioral Research, 26*(3), 499–510.

Hsieh, F. Y. (1989). Sample size tables for logistic regression. *Statistics in Medicine, 8*(7), 795–802.

Hsieh, F. Y., Bloch, D. A., & Larsen, M. D. (1998). A simple method of sample size calculation for linear and logistic regression. *Statistics in Medicine, 17*(14), 1623–1634.

Indrayan, A., & Holt, M. P. (2016). *Concise encyclopedia of biostatistics for medical professionals*. Chapman and Hall and CRC Press.

Kelley, K., & Maxwell, S. E. J. (2003). Sample size for multiple regression: Obtaining regression coefficients that are accurate, not simply significant. *Psychological Methods, 8*(3), 305.

Kleinbaum, D. G., Kupper, L. L., & Muller, K. E. (2013). *Applied regression analysis and other multivariable methods* (2nd ed.). PWS-Kent.

Moinester, M., & Gottfried, R. (2014). Sample size estimation for correlations with pre-specified confidence interval. *The Quantitative Methods for Psychology, 10*(2), 124–130.

Norman, G. R., & Streiner, D. L. (2008). *Biostatistics: The bare essentials*. PMPH USA (BC Decker).

Rosner, B. A. (2006). *Fundamentals of biostatistics* (Vol. 6). Thomson-Brooks.

Tabachnick, B. G., Fidell, L. S., & Ullman, J. B. (2013). *Using multivariate statistics* (Vol. 6). Pearson.

Zar, J. H. (2010). *Biostatistical analysis*. Pearson Education India.

11

Sample Size Estimation for Survival Studies

11.1 Introduction

Survival analysis encompasses a range of statistical methods used to examine data in which the primary outcome is the time until an event occurs, such as the duration until a patient recovers or experiences a relapse. In some instances, the event may not be observed within the study period, resulting in incomplete or "censored" data. It is assumed that censored individuals have the same survival prospects as those who continue to be followed, rendering the censoring process non-informative.

Survival data are typically characterised and modelled using two fundamental functions: the survivor function and the hazard function. The survivor function represents the probability that an individual will survive beyond a specified time from the start of the study. This function is commonly estimated using the Kaplan–Meier method, while the log-rank test is employed to compare survival curves across different groups, such as treatment cohorts.

The hazard function quantifies the instantaneous risk of an event occurring at a given time, conditional on the individual having survived up to that moment. This function is particularly valuable for comparing treatments or prognostic groups and can be adjusted for patient-related factors that may influence survival time. Failure to account for these factors may lead to biased or misleading conclusions.

In this chapter, we will focus on determining the appropriate sample size for various survival analyses, including the hazard ratio, survival function, Cox proportional hazards regression, log-rank test, and Kaplan–Meier estimation.

11.2 The Required Total Number of Deaths (Events)

To determine the required sample size for a study, it is essential to calculate the number of individuals needed to achieve a specified probability of

DOI: 10.1201/9781003749783-11

declaring θ significantly different from zero when the true log-hazard ratio, θ_R, is unknown. The value of θ_R serves as the reference point for θ, indicating the magnitude of the treatment difference we aim to detect through significance testing. Typically, θ_R is chosen based on the desired increase in median survival time or the probability of survival beyond a specific time frame.

The necessary number of deaths is calculated to ensure a $1-\beta$ probability of declaring the observed log-hazard ratio significantly different from zero, assuming $\theta = \theta_R$, with a specified significance level of α. The value $1-\beta$ represents the power of the test, which is the probability of correctly rejecting the null hypothesis when it is false. Both α and β are generally small, with common values of $\alpha = 0.05$ and $\beta = 0.10$ or 0.20. The specific values selected will vary depending on the context of the study. The required total number of deaths, denoted by *d*, can be calculated using the following equation (Collett, 2023, p. 408):

$$d = \frac{4}{\theta_R^2} \times \left(z_{1-\frac{\alpha}{2}} + z_{1-\beta} \right)^2 \tag{11.1}$$

where θ_R is the reference value of θ, and $z_{1-\frac{\alpha}{2}}$ and $z_{1-\beta}$ are values derived from the standard normal distribution corresponding to the upper tail probabilities of $\frac{\alpha}{2}$ and β, respectively.

Freedman has proposed an alternative formula for determining the necessary number of deaths, which replaces $\frac{4}{\theta_R^2}$ with the following expression:

$$\left(\frac{1+\theta_R}{1-\theta_R} \right)^2 \times \left(z_{1-\frac{\alpha}{2}} + z_{1-\beta} \right)^2 \tag{11.2}$$

The calculated sample size using the above equations is intended for the entire study, typically with half of the participants allocated to each treatment group.

However, when θ_R is small, the two expressions tend to yield similar results, as the left-hand sides of Equations 11.1 and 11.2 become approximately equal:

$$\left(\frac{1+\theta_R}{1-\theta_R} \right)^2 \approx \frac{4}{\theta_R^2}$$

The derivation of the result in Equation 11.1 assumes an equal number of individuals will be assigned to each treatment group. If this assumption does not hold, a modification is necessary. Specifically, if the proportions of individuals allocated to Groups I and II are p_1 *and* p_2, respectively (where $p_1 + p_2 = 1$), then the required total number of deaths can be calculated using Equation 11.3 as follows:

$$d = \frac{\left(z_{1-\frac{\alpha}{2}} + z_{1-\beta}\right)^2}{p_1 \times p_2 \times \theta_R^2} \tag{11.3}$$

TIP

It should be noted that any imbalance between the two treatment groups will increase the total number of deaths required. In addition, because the calculation is only an approximation, the estimated number of deaths may be lower than what is actually needed. Therefore, it is recommended that the calculated value be rounded upward to ensure adequate precision.

Example 11.1: Balanced Groups (Equal Allocation): In this example, we design a clinical trial to compare a new treatment (Group I) with a standard treatment (Group II) for a specific disease. Our goal is to detect a hazard ratio of 0.7 ($\theta_R = -0.357$, since the hazard ratio is on the exponential scale) with a power of 90% ($\beta = 0.10$) at a significance level of 0.05 ($\alpha = 0.05$). We need to determine the required sample size for the study.

Solution: To derive $\theta_R = -0.357$ from a hazard ratio of 0.7, we first need to understand the concept of hazard ratios. The hazard ratio represents the ratio of hazard rates between two groups, indicating the rate at which an event occurs. A hazard ratio of 0.7 signifies a 30% reduction in risk with the new treatment. Values below 1 indicate a lower risk in the treatment group.

The log-hazard ratio (θ_R) is the natural logarithm of the hazard ratio, providing a more symmetric distribution, particularly for hazard ratios close to zero. This logarithmic transformation is essential for statistical tests that assume normally distributed differences in log-hazard ratios. For a hazard ratio of 0.7, the log-hazard ratio is calculated as:

$$\theta_R = \ln(0.7) = -0.357$$

indicating a reduced risk associated with the new treatment. This value is crucial for calculating the required number of events (deaths) in hypothesis testing and sample size determination.

By substituting $\theta_R = -0.357$, $z_{1-\frac{\alpha}{2}} = 1.96$, and $z_{1-\beta} = 1.28$ into Equation 11.1, we find that the total number of deaths required is 330:

$$d = \frac{4}{\theta_R^2} \times \left(z_{1-\frac{\alpha}{2}} + z_{1-\beta} \right)^2 = \frac{4}{0.357^2} \times (1.96 + 1.28)^2 = 329.47 \approx 330$$

Thus, we would need approximately 330 deaths in total, with 165 deaths in each group, to achieve the desired statistical power.

Example 11.2: Unbalanced Groups (Unequal Allocation): In this scenario, we modify the allocation from Example 11.1 due to ethical or practical considerations, assigning 60% of patients to the new treatment (Group I) and 40% to the standard treatment (Group II). We will use Equation 11.3 with the same parameters as before.

Solution: By substituting $\theta_R = -0.357$, $z_{1-\frac{\alpha}{2}} = 1.96$, $z_{1-\beta} = 1.28$, $p_1 = 0.60$, and $p_2 = 0.40$ into Equation 11.3, we calculate the required total number of deaths as 344:

$$d = \frac{\left(z_{1-\frac{\alpha}{2}} + z_{1-\beta} \right)^2}{p_1 p_2 \times \theta_R^2} = \frac{(1.96 + 1.28)^2}{0.60 \times 0.40 \times 0.357^2} = 343.20 \approx 344$$

Therefore, we would need approximately 344 deaths in total, with 206 deaths in Group I (344 × 0.60) and 138 deaths in Group II (344 × 0.40), to achieve the desired power.

11.3 Determining the Number of Participants Needed for a Survival Study

To calculate the required number of participants for a survival study, we must account for the probability of death during the study period. Patients are typically enrolled over a specified duration known as the accrual period, denoted as "*a*". Following this, there is a follow-up period, referred to as "*f*". Consequently, the total duration of the study is represented as "*a* + *f*". It is crucial to note that if "*f*" is short or even zero, a larger sample size will be necessary to observe the desired number of deaths.

Once we have estimated the probability of a patient dying during the study, we can calculate the total number of participants needed using Equation 11.4:

$$n = \frac{d}{p(\text{death})} \qquad 11.4)$$

Here, "*d*" represents the required number of deaths, which can be determined using Equation 11.1. This number is often based on the desired statistical power and effect size of the study. The probability of death can be calculated using Equation 11.5:

$$\mathrm{P}(death) = 1 - \left[\frac{\bar{S}(f) + 4\bar{S}(0.5a + f) + \bar{S}(a + f)}{6} \right] \tag{11.5}$$

where

$$\bar{S}(t) = \frac{S_S(t) + S_N(t)}{2} \tag{11.6}$$

In this context, $S_S(t)$ and $S_N(t)$ are the estimated survivor functions for individuals receiving standard and new treatments, respectively, at time t.

For a simplified approach, if we assume that survival times follow an exponential distribution, with mean survival times under the standard and new treatments being λ_S^{-1} and λ_N^{-1}, respectively, the average survivor function, $\bar{S}(t)$, is given by

$$\bar{S}(t) = \frac{e^{-\lambda St} + e^{-\lambda Nt}}{2} \tag{11.7}$$

The above equations outline how to calculate the necessary number of participants for a trial with an accrual period of *"a"* and a follow-up period of *"f"*. The specific durations of the accrual and follow-up periods will depend on the recruitment rate.

Assuming a recruitment rate of *"m"* patients per month and a requirement for *"d"* deaths, if *"n"* patients are to be enrolled over *"a"* months, we need to recruit $\frac{n}{a}$ patients each month. In practice, we often have information regarding the expected accrual rate, m. The total number of patients recruited over an accrual period of length *"a"* is then $m \times a$, and the expected number of deaths in the study is (Collett, 2023, p. 413):

$$m \times a \times P(death).$$

To identify values for *"a"* and *"f"* that approximate the required number of deaths, we can numerically test different combinations. This process can be automated using a computer algorithm and optimisation methods to minimise the difference between *"d"* and $\left[m \times a \times P(death)\right]$. Alternatively, we could determine the value of *"f"* that achieves the desired outcome for various values of *"a"*. A two-way table illustrating the required number of participants for different combinations of *"a"* and *"f"* would be beneficial for study planning.

$$d - \left[m \times a \times P(death)\right]$$

Example 11.3: In a study investigating chronic active hepatitis, researchers determined that observing 140 deaths was necessary to ensure the study had sufficient power to detect a significant hazard ratio of 0.57 at the 5% significance level. The study design includes recruiting patients over an 18-month period, followed by an additional 24 months of follow-up. Our objective is to calculate the total number of participants required for this study.

Solution: The overall duration of the study will be:

$$a + f = 18 + 24 = 42 \text{ months.}$$

To ascertain the total number of participants needed, we will utilise Equation 11.4, which requires calculating the probability of death using Equation 11.5. Before proceeding, we must determine the average survival probabilities at various time points using Equation 11.6:

$$\bar{S}(f) = \bar{S}(24\ months),$$
$$\bar{S}(0.5a + f) = \bar{S}(0.5 \times 18 + 24) = \bar{S}(33\ months)$$
$$\bar{S}(a + f) = \bar{S}(18 + 24) = \bar{S}(42\ months)$$

The following survival probabilities are derived from the estimated survivor functions or their graphical representation (Figure 11.1), based on the collected data for both the new and standard treatments:

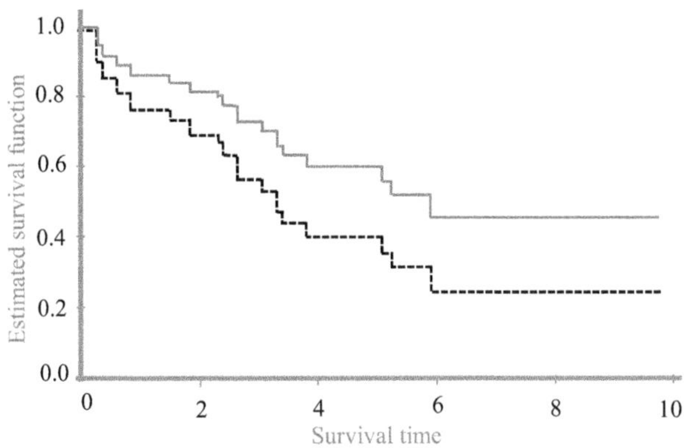

FIGURE 11.1
Estimated survivor functions for individuals receiving standard treatment (green) and those undergoing the new treatment (red). Adapted from Collett, 2023, p. 412.

$$S_S(24\ months) = 0.70 \qquad S_N(24\ months) = 0.82$$
$$S_S(33\ months) = 0.53 \qquad S_N(33\ months) = 0.73$$
$$S_S(42\ months) = 0.45 \qquad S_N(42\ months) = 0.63$$

Using Equation 11.6, we calculate the average survival probabilities as follows:

$$\bar{S}(24)=\frac{S_S(24)+S_N(24)}{2}=\frac{0.70+0.82}{2}=0.76$$

$$\bar{S}(33)=\frac{S_S(33)+S_N(33)}{2}=\frac{0.53+0.73}{2}=0.63$$

$$\bar{S}(42)=\frac{S_S(42)+S_N(42)}{2}=\frac{0.45+0.63}{2}=0.54$$

Next, we calculate the probability of death over the 42-month study period using Equation 11.5:

$$\mathrm{P}(death)=1-\left[\frac{\bar{S}(f)+4\bar{S}(0.5a+f)+\bar{S}(a+f)}{6}\right]$$

$$=1-\left[\frac{\bar{S}(24)+4\bar{S}(0.5\times 18+24)+\bar{S}(18+24)}{6}\right]$$

Substituting the values, we obtain:

$$\mathrm{P}(death)=1-\left[\frac{\bar{S}(24)+4\bar{S}(33)+\bar{S}(42)}{6}\right]=1-\left[\frac{0.76+4\times 0.63+0.54}{6}\right]$$

$$=1-0.6367=0.3633$$

Finally, we apply the required number of deaths and the calculated probability of death in Equation 11.4 to determine the number of patients needed:

$$n=\frac{d}{p(death)}=\frac{140}{0.3633}=385.35\approx 386$$

Thus, a total of **386** participants are required for the study.

11.4 An Approximate Procedure

This section outlines a simplified method for determining the necessary number of patients in a survival study aimed at comparing two treatments. The method assumes that the average probability of a patient surviving beyond time τ is the mean of the survivor functions for the standard treatment $S_S(t)$ and the new treatment $S_N(t)$ at time τ, represented as:

$$\frac{S_S(t)+S_N(t)}{2}$$

The probability of death from the start of the study to time τ can be approximated by

$$1-\frac{S_S(t)+S_N(t)}{2}$$

Using Equation 11.4, the required number of patients n can be calculated as:

$$n=\frac{2d}{2-S_S(t)-S_N(t)} \tag{11.8}$$

where "d" represents the required number of deaths.

A reasonable choice for τ in this calculation is the average length of the follow-up period for patients in the study, calculated as:

$$\tau = f+\left(\frac{a}{2}\right)$$

where f is the follow-up period and a is the accrual period.

This method is considered approximate because it does not account for patient follow-up times that extend beyond τ, which may lead to an overestimation of the required sample size (Collett, 2023, p. 417).

> **Example 11.4:** Utilising the Approximate Method to Determine the Required Number of Patients for a Study on Chronic Active Hepatitis (Example 11.3).

Solution: As in Example 11.3, suppose patients are recruited over 18 months, followed by an additional 24-month follow-up. The average length of the follow-up period for a patient would then be:

$$\tau = f+\left(\frac{a}{2}\right)=24+\frac{18}{2}=33 \text{ months.}$$

From the survivor functions, we have $S_N(33)=0.73$ and $S_S(33)=0.57$ for the standard treatment. The average survival probability at 33 months is given by

$$\bar{S}(33)=\frac{S_N(33)+S_S(33)}{2}=\frac{0.73+0.57}{2}=0.65$$

The approximate probability of death from 0 to 33 months is therefore:

$$P(death) = 1 - \bar{S}(33) = 1 - 0.65 = 0.35$$

The denominator of Equation 11.8 can also be calculated as:

$$2 - S_S(t) - S_N(t) = 2 - 0.57 - 0.73 = 0.70$$

The number of patients required, according to Equation 11.8, to observe 140 deaths is

$$n = \frac{2d}{2 - S_S(t) - S_N(t)} = \frac{2 \times 140}{2 - 0.57 - 0.73} = \frac{280}{0.70} = 400.$$

In this illustration, the sample size produced by the approximate method is the same as that obtained using the more complex procedure in Example 11.3; however, this may not always be the case.

11.5 Determining Sample Size for the Log-Rank Test

The log-rank test, developed by Peto et al. in 1977, is a widely used non-parametric method for comparing survival distributions among different patient groups. It does not assume a specific distribution of survival times, making it particularly useful for analysing survival curves across various treatment arms or prognostic groups.

The log-rank test calculates the expected number of events in each group at each event time, assuming no difference between the groups. These expected numbers are then summed to obtain the total expected number of events for each group, denoted as E_i for the i_{th} group. The observed number of events, O_i , for group i, is compared to the expected number using the following test statistic (Clark et al., 2003, p. 235):

$$\chi^2 = \sum_{i=1}^{g} \frac{(O_i - E_i)^2}{E_i} \tag{11.9}$$

This calculated value is compared to a χ^2 distribution with (g–1) degrees of freedom, where g is the number of groups. The resulting p-value indicates the statistical significance of the differences between the survival curves.

TIP

A non-parametric log-rank test compares survival distributions across patient groups without assuming a specific survival-time distribution, making it useful for evaluating differences among treatment arms or prognostic categories. Assuming no group differences, the test calculates the expected number of events at each event time for each group, sums these expected events, E_i, and compares them with the observed events O_i to compute the test statistic.

The formula for calculating the sample size for the log-rank test, as proposed by Freedman in 1982, is based on the expected number of events under the null hypothesis and the difference in survival proportions between the groups. This formula incorporates the hazard ratio, the type I error rate (α), the power ($1-\beta$), and the survival proportions in each group. The sample size formula for each group can be represented as:

$$n = \frac{\left[\frac{\theta+1}{\theta-1}\right]^2 \times \left(z_{1-\frac{\alpha}{2}} + z_{1-\beta}\right)^2}{2 - S_1 - S_2} \tag{11.10}$$

Here, θ is the hazard ratio assumed to be constant over time, defined as:

$$\theta = \frac{\log(S_1)}{log(S_2)}$$

The critical values $z_{1-\frac{\alpha}{2}}$ and $z_{1-\beta}$ correspond to the two-sided significance level (α) and the power of the test ($1-\beta$), respectively. S_1 and S_2 are the survival proportions in groups 1 and 2 at a specific time point (Freedman, 1982, p. 124; Ryan, 2013, p. 311).

> **Example 11.5:** Suppose we are designing a clinical trial to compare two treatments for a specific disease. We expect the survival proportion at a certain time point to be 0.6 in group 1 ($S_1 = 0.60$) and 0.4 in group 2 ($S_2 = 0.40$). We aim to determine how many samples are needed to detect a hazard ratio between the two groups with a power of 90% ($\beta = 0.10$) at a significance level of 5% ($\alpha = 0.05$).

Solution: The hazard ratio θ can be calculated as follows:

$$\theta = \frac{\log(S_1)}{\log(S_2)} = \frac{\log(0.60)}{\log(0.40)} = \frac{-0.2218}{-0.3979} = 0.5574$$

The critical values for a two-sided test with α = 0.05 and a power of $1-\beta$ = 90% are 1.96 and 1.28, respectively. We can now substitute these values into the formula:

$$n = \frac{\left[\frac{\theta+1}{\theta-1}\right]^2 \times \left(z_{1-\frac{\alpha}{2}} + z_{1-\beta}\right)^2}{2 - S_1 - S_2}$$

$$n = \frac{\left[\frac{0.5574+1}{0.5574-1}\right]^2 \times (1.96+1.28)^2}{2-0.6-0.4} = \left(\frac{11.40}{1}\right)^2 = 129.98 \approx 130$$

Thus, we would need approximately 130 subjects in each group to achieve the desired power with the specified hazard ratio and survival proportions.

11.6 Determining Sample Size for Hazard Ratio (HR)

The hazard ratio (HR) is a statistical measure used in survival analysis to compare the likelihood of an event occurring in two different groups. It quantifies the relative risk of an event, such as death or disease progression, over time. The HR is calculated by dividing the hazard rate of one group by that of another, typically an experimental group versus a control group. An HR of 1 indicates no difference in risk between the groups. An HR greater than 1 signifies a higher risk in the first group, while an HR less than 1 suggests a lower risk.

The hazard ratio can be estimated using the following formula (Clark et al., 2003, p. 236):

$$HR = \frac{O_1 / E_1}{O_2 / E_2} \tag{11.11}$$

where O_i / E_i represents the observed-to-expected event ratio in group i. If the HR is constant over time, it can also be expressed as:

$$HR = \frac{\log \pi_A}{\log \pi_B} \tag{11.12}$$

From this, we can derive π_B (response rate in group B) in terms of π_A (response rate in group A) or vice versa:

$$\log \pi_A = HR \times \log \pi_B \Leftrightarrow \pi_A = e^{HR \times \log \pi_B} \tag{11.13}$$

In practice, the Cox proportional hazards regression model is commonly employed to estimate the HR. This model accommodates multiple variables, adjusting for potential confounders to provide a more accurate assessment of the effect of an intervention or exposure on the risk of an event. The Cox model assumes that the HR remains constant over time, which is a critical assumption for its validity.

The hazard ratio serves as a concise metric to convey the strength of the association between an exposure and an outcome. It is widely reported in clinical trials and observational studies to communicate the impact of treatments or risk factors on survival or disease progression.

TIP

The hazard ratio (HR) is a measure used in survival analysis to compare the likelihood of an event between two groups over time. The HR is calculated by dividing the hazard rate of one group (typically the experimental group) by that of another (typically the control group). An HR of 1 indicates no difference in risk, an HR greater than 1 indicates higher risk in the first group, and an HR less than 1 indicates lower risk.

To estimate the sample size needed to determine the hazard ratio in each group, we must consider the survival rates at the end of the study: π_A and π_B for treatment groups A and B. Therefore, the sample size n_A in each group (assuming $n_A = n_B$) can be calculated using the following equation (Julious, 2023, p. 357):

$$n_A = \frac{2E}{2 - \pi_B - \pi_A} \tag{11.14}$$

where E represents the number of events, π_A and π_B are the anticipated response rates of treatment groups A and B.

$$E = \frac{\left(z_{1-\frac{\alpha}{2}} + z_{1-\beta}\right)^2 (HR+1)^2}{2(HR-1)^2} \tag{11.15}$$

In most trials, some patients will be lost during the follow-up period, classified as censored in the analysis, which will affect the required sample size per group. If we anticipate that a proportion "w" of patients will be lost to follow-up, we need to adjust the total sample size per group in Equation 11.14, as shown in Equation 11.16 (Julious, 2023, p. 358):

$$n_{Aw} = \frac{n_A}{1-w} \tag{11.16}$$

For quick estimates at 90% power and a two-sided significance level of 5%, we can use the following formula (Julious, 2023, p. 333):

$$E = \frac{5.25(HR+1)^2}{(HR-1)^2} \tag{11.17}$$

For calculations at 80% power, the following formula can be applied:

$$E = \frac{4(HR+1)^2}{(HR-1)^2} \tag{11.18}$$

Example 11.6: A 2-year study is being conducted to investigate a new treatment compared to a control group, with the primary endpoint being progression-free survival. The target effect size of interest is a Hazard Ratio (HR) of 1.2 compared to the control treatment, which corresponds to an HR of 0.83 in favour of the investigative treatment. For a two-tailed significance level of 5% and 90% power, we need to determine the required sample size in each arm of the study.

Solution: Based on the provided information, with HR = 1.2 and $\pi_A = 0.80$, the sample size (in terms of the number of events), assuming only hazards, is calculated as follows using Equation 11.17:

$$E = \frac{5.25(HR+1)^2}{(HR-1)^2} = \frac{5.25(1.2+1)^2}{(1.2-1)^2} = 635.25 \approx 636$$

Next, we calculate:

$$\log \pi_A = \log(0.80) - 0.0969.$$

Using the HR, we find:

$$\log \pi_B = \frac{\log \pi_A}{HR} = \frac{-0.0969}{1.2} = -0.08076.$$

Taking the antilogarithm, we calculate π_B:

$$\pi_B = \text{antilog}(-0.08076) = e^{-0.08076} = 0.83$$

This indicates that approximately 83% of patients are expected to survive on the investigative treatment.

TABLE 11.1

Number of Events for Various Hazard Ratios at a Two-Sided 5% Significance Level with 80% and 90% Power (Assuming Hazards Only)

	Number of Events	
Hazard Ratio	**80% Power**	**90% Power**
0.6	63	85
0.7	127	169
0.8	318	426
0.9	1417	1897
1.1	1731	2317
1.2	475	636
1.3	231	309
1.4	142	190
1.5	99	132
1.6	74	99
1.7	59	79
1.8	49	65
1.9	41	55
2.0	36	48

Using this data, we can calculate the anticipated total sample size per arm to ensure detection of the desired hazard ratio using Equation 11.14:

$$n_A = \frac{2E}{2-\pi_B-\pi_A} = \frac{2\times 636}{2-0.83-0.80} = 3438$$

If we anticipate losing 10% of patients to follow-up, we must adjust the total sample size as calculated using Equation 11.16 (Julious, 2023, p. 358):

$$n_{Aw} = \frac{n_A}{1-w} = \frac{3438}{1-0.10} = 3820$$

For the convenience of readers, we have provided the number of events required for different Hazard Ratios at a two-sided 5% significance level and 80% and 90% power (assuming hazards only) in Table 11.1.

11.7 Determining Sample Size for Cox Proportional Hazards Regression

The Cox proportional hazards (Cox PH) model, introduced by Cox in 1972, is the most commonly used multivariate approach for analysing survival time data in medical research. This survival analysis regression model describes the relationship between the incidence of an event, as expressed by the hazard function, and a set of covariates.

TIP

The Cox proportional hazards (Cox PH) model is a multivariate regression model used to analyse survival-time data in medical research. It examines the relationship between the occurrence of an event, represented by the hazard function, and a set of covariates.

In brief, the hazard represents the instantaneous probability of an event occurring at a given time, or the likelihood that an individual under observation will experience the event during a period centred around that specific time. Mathematically, the Cox model can be expressed as:

$$h(t) = h_0(t) \times \exp\{b_1 x_1 + b_2 x_2 + \cdots + b_p x_p\} \quad or \quad \log \frac{h(t)}{h_0(t)} = b_1 x_1 + b_2 x_2 + \cdots + b_p x_p \tag{11.19}$$

In this formulation, the hazard function $h(t)$ depends on a set of p covariates $(x_1, x_2, \cdots, x_p)$, with their effects quantified by the corresponding coefficients $(b_1, b_2, \cdots, b_p)$. The term $h_0(t)$ represents the baseline hazard, which is the hazard value when all covariates x_i are equal to zero (since $\exp(0) = 1$). The variable t in $h(t)$ indicates that the hazard may vary over time.

A notable feature of the Cox model is that the baseline hazard function is estimated non-parametrically. Unlike many other statistical models, the Cox model does not assume that survival times follow a specific statistical distribution (Bradburn et al., 2003, Part II, p. 432).

To calculate the sample size and the number of events required when comparing two groups in a univariate model, the group indicator X_1 is binary, and $b_1 = \log \Delta$ represents the log hazard ratio between the two groups. When there is only one binary covariate X_1, the score test is equivalent to the Mantel-Haenszel test and the log-rank test, provided there are no ties in survival times.

It is well established that the power of the log-rank test is influenced by the sample size solely through the number of deaths, which simplifies the sample size formula. For comparing two groups, we utilise the following equation from F.Y. Hsieh derived by Schoenfeld (Hsieh & Lavori, 2000, p. 2):

$$D = \frac{\left(Z_{1-\alpha} + Z_{1-\beta}\right)^2}{P(1-P)(\log \Delta)^2} \tag{11.20}$$

In this equation, P represents the proportion of the sample assigned to the first treatment group, D is the total number of deaths, and $Z_{1-\alpha}$ and $Z_{1-\beta}$ are the standard normal deviates at the desired one-sided significance level α and power β, respectively (Hsieh & Lavori, 2000, p. 2).

> **Example 11.7 (With a Binary Covariate):** In a survival study aimed at investigating the effect of a treatment on subjects' survival times, the covariate of interest is binary. This covariate determines whether a subject is assigned to the experimental group (receiving the treatment) or the control/placebo group (receiving a placebo). Prior to conducting the study, researchers must estimate the sample size required to detect a hazard ratio of 0.5, where

$$\beta_{1a} = ln(0.5) = -0.6931$$

between the experimental and control groups, with 80% power using a two-sided 5% significance level test. Assuming a 1:1 randomisation, each subject has a 50% chance of being assigned to the treatment group ($p = 0.50$).

Solution: The binary covariate for this study follows a Bernoulli distribution, where the probability of a subject receiving treatment is $p = 0.5$. The standard deviation of the covariate is calculated as:

$$\sqrt{p(1-p)} = \sqrt{0.5(1-0.5)} = 0.5$$

These study parameters align with the default values of Power Cox. To calculate the required sample size for the study, we use Equation 11.20:

$$D = \frac{(Z_{1-\alpha} + Z_{1-\beta})^2}{P(1-P)(\log\Delta)^2}$$

Substituting the values:

$$D = \frac{(1.64 + 0.84)^2}{0.50(1-0.50)(-0.693)^2} = 51.23 \approx 52$$

For a two-tailed test, the number of deaths/events is calculated as:

$$D = \frac{\left(Z_{1-\frac{\alpha}{2}} + Z_{1-\beta}\right)^2}{P(1-P)(\log\Delta)^2}$$

Substituting the values:

$$D = \frac{(1.96 + 0.84)^2}{0.50(1-0.50)(-0.693)^2} = 65.30 \approx 66$$

Note: If a researcher wishes to calculate the sample size based on the effect size, they can use a regression coefficient or a hazard ratio in place of the effect size in the equation above, resulting in the same sample size of 66. If an effect size is not specified, a hazard ratio of 0.5 is assumed (StataCorp, 2023, p. 526).

In a univariate model with continuous (non-binary) covariates, and without making assumptions about the distributions of covariate X_1 and survival time T, the total number of deaths required can be determined using a similar formula to Equation 11.19:

$$D = \frac{\left(Z_{1-\alpha} + Z_{1-\beta}\right)^2}{\sigma^2 \left(\log \Delta\right)^2} \tag{11.21}$$

where σ^2 represents the variance of X_1, and $\log \Delta = b^*$ is the logarithm of the hazard ratio associated with a one-unit change in X_1.

Equation 11.21 is analogous to Equation 11.20, except that $P(1-P)$ in Equation 11.20 is replaced by the more general term σ^2. The required sample size is then calculated as the number of deaths divided by the overall proportion of deaths. In practice, investigators often have a good understanding of the overall death rate.

> **Example 11.8 (With a Continuous Covariate):** Consider a study by Hsieh and Lavori (2000) involving multiple myeloma patients treated with alkylating agents. In this study, 17 out of 65 survival times were censored. The covariate of interest, X_1, represents the natural logarithm of the blood urea nitrogen (BUN) levels measured in patients. Our objective is to determine the necessary sample size for a one-sided test at a 5% significance level to detect a coefficient (log hazard ratio) of 1 for a unit increase in X_1, with a power of 80%. To estimate the sample size, we will input b_1 as an argument, select the standard deviation option (0.3126), and specify the one-sided test option.

Solution: The standard deviation of LOGBUN is 0.3126, and the overall death rate is calculated as:

$$1 - \frac{17}{65} = 0.738$$

The corresponding values from the standard normal distribution for 80% power and a one-sided significance level of 5% are 0.84 and 1.645, respectively. Assuming we want to detect a log hazard ratio of $\log \Delta = 1$, we can calculate the required number of deaths using Equation 11.21:

$$D = \frac{\left(Z_{1-\alpha} + Z_{1-\beta}\right)^2}{\sigma^2 \left(\log \Delta\right)^2}$$

Substituting the values:

$$D = \frac{(1.645 + 0.84)^2}{(0.3126)^2 (1)^2} = 63.19 \approx 64$$

Thus, applying Equation 11.21 with no other covariates, the required number of deaths is 64. Equivalently, the necessary sample size is

$$\frac{64}{0.738} = 86.72 \approx 87$$

Now, assuming that the squared multiple correlation between X_1 and the remaining covariates $\rho^2_{X_1(X_2,\cdots,X_k)}$ is 0.18, suppose we want to adjust the sample size to account for other covariates due to potential confounding effects. The approximate Variance Inflation Factor (VIF) for the model, as discussed in Chapter 10 on multiple regression, is given by

$$VIF = \frac{1}{1 - \rho^2_{X_1(X_2,\cdots,X_k)}} = \frac{1}{1 - 0.18} = 1.219 \approx 1.22$$

The required total sample size for a full model can be approximated by:

$$(87 \times 1.22) = 106.14 \approx 107.$$

Note: Rosner proposed Equation 11.22 for estimating required sample size under the Cox Proportional-Hazards Model (Rosner, 2006, p. 838).

When comparing survival curves between an experimental group (Group E) and a control group (Group C) in a clinical trial, where the ratio of participants in Group E (n_1) to those in Group C (n_2) is represented by k, and the maximum follow-up time is t, we aim to detect a hazard ratio of IRR for Group E compared with Group C. We also wish to conduct a two-sided test with a significance level of α. The number of participants required in each group to achieve a power of $1-\beta$ is given by Rosner (2006, p. 838):

$$n_1 = \frac{m \times k}{K \times p_E + p_C}, \quad n_2 = \frac{m}{K \times p_E + p_C} \tag{11.22}$$

where

$$m = \frac{1}{k}\left(\frac{k \times IRR + 1}{IRR - 1}\right)^2 \times \left(Z_{1-\frac{\alpha}{2}} + Z_{1-\beta}\right)^2$$

and

- $k = {}^{n_1}/_{n_2}$ is allocation ratio,
- IRR is hazard ratio

- p_E *and* p_C cumulative probabilities of event detection, and
- K is adjustment factor for number of events in the experimental group vs. control.

Example 11.9: Let us consider an example from Rosner on page 939 regarding cancer research. Suppose researchers want to enrol 10,000 postmenopausal women who have not had cancer in a clinical trial. Of these, 5,000 women would be randomly assigned to receive estrogen-replacement therapy (ERT), while the other 5,000 would receive a placebo. The study's endpoint is breast cancer incidence, and participants would be followed for an average of 5 years (with a range of 4 to 6 years). The expected incidence rate in the control group is 0.003 per person-year. If it is hypothesised that ERT increases the incidence rate of breast cancer by 25%, we need to determine the required sample size for this study under the Cox Proportional-Hazards Model.

Solution: We have IRR = 1.25, $\alpha = 0.05$, $\beta = 0.20$, and $k = 1$. Thus,

$$m = \frac{1}{k}\left(\frac{k \times IRR + 1}{IRR - 1}\right)^2 \times \left(Z_{1-\frac{\alpha}{2}} + Z_{1-\beta}\right)^2$$

Calculating m:

$$m = \frac{1}{1}\left(\frac{1.25+1}{1.25-1}\right)^2 \times (1.96 + 0.84)^2 = 635.04$$

To determine the sample size estimate for each group, we use the Kaplan-Meier estimator to estimate p_C and p_E as follows:

$$p_C = 1 - (1 - 0.003)^5 = 1 - 0.98509 = 0.01491$$

$$p_E = 1 - (1 - 0.00375)^5 = 1 - 0.98139 = 0.01861$$

Thus, the number of participants needed in each group is

$$n_1 = n_2 = \frac{635.04}{0.01861 + 0.01491} = 18945 \quad \text{participants per group.}$$

11.8 Determining Sample Size for Kaplan-Meier Estimator

The Kaplan-Meier (KM) estimator, introduced by Kaplan and Meier in 1958, is a widely used non-parametric method for estimating survival probabilities in the presence of time-varying incidence rates. This technique adeptly manages both censored and uncensored data, enabling researchers to calculate survival probabilities based on observed survival times (Rosner, 2006, p. 811). Survival duration is defined as the time until an event occurs, often necessitating specialised statistical methods due to skewed distributions and the presence of censored data – instances where complete durations are not recorded due to dropout or other reasons (Indrayan & Holt, 2016, p. 313).

In a study involving k patients experiencing events at distinct times

$$t_1 < t_2 < t_3 < t_4 < t_5 < \cdots < t_k,$$

it is assumed that these events occur independently. The cumulative survival probability is calculated by multiplying the probabilities of surviving each interval. The survival probability at time t_j, denoted as $S(t_j)$, is determined using Equation 11.23 (Clark et al., 2003, Part I, p. 233):

$$S(t_j) = S(t_{j-1})\left(1 - \frac{d_j}{n_j}\right) = \prod\left(1 - \frac{d_j}{n_j}\right) \tag{11.23}$$

where

- $S(t_{j-1})$ is the probability of being alive at t_{j-1} (the previous time point),
- n_j is the number of patients alive just before t_j, and
- d_j is the number of events at t_j.

The initial conditions are $t_0 = 0$ and $S(0) = 1$. The estimated survival probability forms a step function, changing only at the occurrence of each event and remaining constant between these times.

The KM estimator maintains the survival probability $S(t)$ constant between events, resulting in a step function that only changes at event times. This method incorporates each patient's data from the study's start until their event or censoring. If all patients experience an event without any censoring, the estimator reflects the fraction of event-free individuals at time t compared to the total study group. Additionally, confidence intervals for survival probabilities can be calculated.

To calculate the sample size needed for single-arm survival studies using the Kaplan-Meier (KM) estimator, Kengo Nagashima and colleagues have developed a formula. The KM estimator is a statistical method used to estimate the survival function from observed survival times, providing insights into how long patients can expect to survive after receiving a treatment. The formula helps researchers determine the number of participants required to ensure that their findings are statistically significant and reliable.

The required sample size for KM estimator can be obtained using Equation 11.24 (Nagashima et al., 2021, p. 4/22):

$$n_1 = \left[\frac{\tau_1 \left(z_{1-\frac{\alpha}{2}} + z_{1-\beta} \right)}{\epsilon} \right]^2 \tag{11.24}$$

In this formula:

- τ_1 is the variance of the survival times, which reflects the variability in the time until the event occurs.
- $z_{1-\frac{\alpha}{2}}$ and $z_{1-\beta}$ are *z*-scores that correspond to the desired significance level (α) and power (β) of the study.
- ϵ represents the margin of error or the level of precision desired in the survival estimates.

Example 11.10: Let us consider a clinical trial evaluating a new treatment for patients with a specific type of cancer. The researchers want to estimate the survival function using the Kaplan-Meier method and need to determine how many patients they should enrol in the study to achieve reliable results.

Solution: In this example, the Study Duration τ_I is set to *6 months*. This means that patients will be followed for up to 6 months to observe their survival outcomes. The researchers chose a significance level of 0.05 (5%), which corresponds to a *z*-score of 1.96. The desired power of the study is 0.80 (80%), corresponding to a *z*-score of 0.84. The researchers also want a margin of error (precision) of 0.1 (10%) in their survival estimates.

Substituting the provided information into Equation 11.24 gives:

$$n_1 = \left[\frac{\tau_1 \left(z_{1-\frac{\alpha}{2}} + z_{1-\beta} \right)}{\epsilon} \right]^2 = \left[\frac{6(1.96+0.84)}{0.1} \right]^2 = \left[\frac{16.8}{0.1} \right]^2 = 28224$$

Based on the calculations, the researchers would need to follow up approximately 28,224 patients to conduct the study effectively. This large sample size ensures that the study is adequately powered to detect significant differences in survival outcomes, which is crucial for validating the effectiveness of the new treatment.

11.9 Logarithmic Transformation

There is another method to determine sample size that is frequently used in one-sample survival studies. This method is based on the logarithmic transformation of the survival function,

$$g(S(t)) = \log S(t).$$

To estimate the sample size under this transformation, Equation 11.25 is used (Nagashima et al., 2021, p. 5/22):

$$n_0 = \left(\frac{\tau_1 z_{1-\frac{\alpha}{2}} + \tau_0 z_{1-\beta}}{\epsilon} \right)^2 \quad (11.25)$$

where τ_1 and τ_0 are the asymptotic variances of survival times under the alternative and null hypotheses, respectively, for the transformed survival function.

> **Example 11.11:** In a clinical trial aimed at evaluating the effectiveness of a new cancer treatment, researchers need to determine the appropriate sample size to ensure reliable results. To do this, they utilise the Kaplan-Meier (KM) estimator, which is commonly used for analysing time-to-event data. In this scenario, the researchers define $\tau_0 = 1.5$ as the variance of survival times under the null hypothesis (i.e., the current standard treatment) and $\tau_1 = 2.5$ as the variance under the alternative hypothesis (i.e., the new treatment), reflecting their expectations about the variability in survival times for both treatment groups. They aim for a 95% confidence level ($\alpha = 0.05$) and 80% power ($\beta = 0.20$), which are standard thresholds in clinical research. The effect size, ϵ, representing the minimum clinically significant difference they wish to detect, is set at 0.1.

Solution: Using these parameters ($z_{1-\frac{\alpha}{2}} = 1.96$ for 5% significance level, $z_{1-\beta} = 0.84$ for 80% power, $\tau_0 = 1.5$, $\tau_1 = 2.5$ and a precision of ϵ = 0.10), the required sample size is calculated using Equation 11.25:

$$n_0 = \left(\frac{\tau_1 z_{1-\frac{\alpha}{2}} + \tau_0 z_{1-\beta}}{\epsilon} \right)^2 = \left(\frac{2.5 \times 1.96 + 1.5 \times 0.84}{0.10} \right)^2 = \left(\frac{6.16}{0.10} \right)^2 = 3794.56 \cong 3795$$

Thus, the required sample size n_0 is approximately 3,795 participants. This indicates the number of subjects needed to achieve the desired statistical power and confidence level in the survival study based on the KM estimator.

References

Bradburn, M. J., Clark, T. G., Love, S. B., & Altman, D. G. (2003). Survival analysis part II: Multivariate data analysis–an introduction to concepts and methods. *British Journal of Cancer, 89*(3), 431–436.

Clark, T. G., Bradburn, M. J., Love, S. B., & Altman, D. G. (2003). Survival analysis part I: Basic concepts and first analyses. *British Journal of Cancer, 89*(2), 232–238.

Collett, D. (2023). *Modelling survival data in medical research.* Chapman and Hall and CRC Press.

Freedman, L. S. (1982). Tables of the number of patients required in clinical trials using the logrank test. *Statistics in Medicine, 1*(2), 121–129.

Hsieh, F., & Lavori, P. W. (2000). Sample-size calculations for the Cox proportional hazards regression model with nonbinary covariates. *Controlled Clinical Trials, 21*(6), 552–560.

Indrayan, A., & Holt, M. P. (2016). *Concise encyclopedia of biostatistics for medical professionals.* Chapman and Hall and CRC Press.

Julious, S. A. (2023). *Sample sizes for clinical trials.* Chapman and Hall and CRC Press.

Nagashima, K., Noma, H., Sato, Y., & Gosho, M. (2021). Sample size calculations for single-arm survival studies using transformations of the Kaplan–Meier estimator. *Pharmaceutical Statistics, 20*(3), 499–511.

Rosner, B. A. (2006). *Fundamentals of biostatistics* (Vol. 6). Thomson-Brooks.

Ryan, T. P. (2013). *Sample size determination and power.* John Wiley & Sons.

StataCorp LLC. (2023). *Stata 18 power, precision, and sample-size reference manual.* StataCorp LLC.

12

Sample Size Estimation for Reliability Studies

12.1 Introduction

Reliability and validation studies are essential for understanding measurement error in epidemiological research. Accurate information about measurement error is crucial for obtaining valid estimates and making reliable inferences, particularly when using methods such as regression calibration or maximum likelihood estimation. These studies typically involve repeated measurements of error-prone variables, allowing researchers to assess consistency and reliability.

The validity of these approaches relies on a well-defined error model, expressed as:

$$\text{Error Model: } Y = X + \epsilon$$

where Y is the observed measurement, X is the true value, and ϵ represents the measurement error. Understanding this error is vital for correctly interpreting the results of epidemiological studies.

By quantifying measurement error, researchers can adjust their analyses to account for bias, leading to more accurate and reliable conclusions. This adjustment is particularly important in fields where precise measurements are critical for understanding the relationship between exposures and health outcomes. Ultimately, improving measurement reliability enhances the quality of epidemiological research and supports informed public health decision-making (Donna, 2005, p. 4945).

12.2 Reliability Studies

The concept of reliability is fundamentally linked to the repeatability and reproducibility of measurements. For any measurement to be considered

DOI: 10.1201/9781003749783-12

useful, it must demonstrate consistency, producing similar results for an individual upon repeated administration. High reliability indicates that a measure yields comparable results across different occasions, which is essential for establishing the measure's validity, although reliability alone does not guarantee validity.

It is important to recognise that no measurement is entirely free of error; some degree of measurement error is always present. Understanding reliability allows researchers to quantify this margin of error. Generally, tests with high reliability exhibit a smaller margin of error compared to those with low reliability.

TIP

Reliability allows researchers to quantify the margin of error in data collection, as some degree of measurement error is always present. Highly reliable tests indicate a smaller margin of error, whereas tests with low reliability indicate larger margins. In other words, high reliability corresponds to low measurement error, while low reliability increases the likelihood of substantial discrepancies in results.

In essence, high reliability corresponds to low measurement error, while low reliability can lead to significant discrepancies in the results.

This concept can be illustrated using the following equation:

$$O = T \pm E \tag{12.1}$$

where

- O represents the observed value,
- T denotes the true value, and
- E indicates the error, reflecting the discrepancy between the true value and the observed value.

This equation highlights that observed values cluster around the true value, with the magnitude of the error determining the spread of these observed values. A smaller error (E) signifies higher reliability, indicating that the observed values are closely aligned with the true value.

The required sample size for assessing reliability depends on the method used to calculate the reliability coefficient. Different methods have varying sample size requirements due to their distinct statistical properties and assumptions. The primary methods for calculating reliability include:

- Internal Consistency (e.g., Cronbach's Alpha)
- Intraclass Correlation Coefficient (ICC)
- Kuder-Richardson Formula
- Split-Half Method
- Equivalent-Forms Reliability
- Test-Retest Reliability

Each method evaluates reliability from a different perspective, and the choice of method influences both the precision of the reliability estimate and the sample size needed for robust assessment.

12.3 Sample Size Determination for Coefficient Alpha

Coefficient alpha, commonly referred to as Cronbach's alpha, is a widely used measure of reliability that serves as an intraclass correlation coefficient. It assesses the reliability of a scale composed of k items, which often represent different raters or quantitatively scored questions (Bonett, 2002a, p. 335). As a measure of internal consistency, Cronbach's alpha estimates the degree to which items in a questionnaire measure the same underlying construct, with values ranging from 0 to 1. An alpha of 0 indicates that the true score is not captured at all, whereas an alpha of 1.0 indicates that all items perfectly measure the true score without error.

Although originally designed for psychometric instruments, higher alpha values suggest that the items are measuring the same dimension. Conversely, a low alpha value (near zero) indicates that some or all items may not adequately measure the intended construct. Therefore, researchers must consider Cronbach's alpha when evaluating the reliability of their measurement tools to ensure that the items accurately capture the target construct (Bujang et al., 2018, p. 87).

To determine the sample size required for testing a hypothesis regarding a single coefficient alpha with a desired statistical power, or for estimating a single coefficient alpha with a specified precision, the following formula can be used (Bonett, 2002a):

$$n = \frac{2k}{k-1} \times \frac{\left(z_{1-\frac{\alpha}{2}} + z_{\beta}\right)^2}{ln\left(\tilde{\delta}\right)} + 2 \qquad (12.2)$$

where

- $z_{1-\frac{\alpha}{2}}$ and z_β are critical values from the standard normal distribution,
- K denotes the number of items or raters,
- $\tilde{\delta} = \dfrac{1-\rho_0}{1-\rho_1}$
- ρ_0 is Cronbach's alpha under the null hypothesis, and
- ρ_1 is the expected or target value of Cronbach's alpha.

The values of ρ_0 and ρ_1 can range from –1 to 1; however, it is essential that $\rho_1 \neq \rho_0$. As with all sample size calculations, the value of n obtained from Equation 12.2 should be rounded up to the nearest integer to ensure an adequate sample size for reliable estimation of Cronbach's alpha.

TIP

As the number of raters or items increases, the proportion of k/(k-1) decreases, and consequently the sample size required to estimate Cronbach's alpha also decreases.

Example 12.1: The study aims to evaluate the internal consistency of a particular questionnaire, referred to as "A". Questionnaire "A" consists of 15 items, each rated on a five-point Likert scale. The null hypothesis (ρ_0) assumes a Cronbach's alpha of 0.0, while the alternative hypothesis (ρ_1) assumes a Cronbach's alpha of 0.70. Based on a significance level of 0.05 and a desired power of 80%, the goal is to determine the minimum sample size required for this study.

Solution: The parameters for this calculation are

- $\rho_0 = 0.0$ and $\rho_1 = 0.7$,
- Significance level (α) = 0.05 (corresponding to $z_{1-\frac{\alpha}{2}} = 1.96$),
- Power ($1-\beta$) = 0.80 (corresponding to $z_{1-\beta} = 0.84$),
- Number of items (k) = 15.

First, calculate the planning value of $\tilde{\delta}$:

$$\tilde{\delta} = \frac{1-\rho_0}{1-\rho_1} = \frac{1-0}{1-0.7} = \frac{1}{0.3} = 3.333$$

Next, use Equation 12.2 to calculate the required sample size:

$$n = \frac{2k}{k-1} \times \frac{\left(z_{1-\frac{\alpha}{2}} + z_{1-\beta}\right)^2}{ln\left(\tilde{\delta}\right)} + 2$$

Substituting the values:

$$n = \frac{2 \times 15}{15-1} \times \frac{(1.96+0.84)^2}{ln(3.333)} + 2 = \frac{30}{14} \times \frac{7.84}{1.204} + 2 = 15.93 \approx 16$$

Since the sample size must be a whole number, we round up to the nearest integer: $n = 16$

The minimum sample size required to evaluate the internal consistency of questionnaire "A" is 16 participants. If the questionnaire contains a different number of items, researchers should recalculate the sample size using Equation 12.2, adjusting for the specific number of items and the expected Cronbach's alpha.

12.4 Sample Size for Comparing Two Alphas

Bonett provided a formula for calculating the sample size required to test the equality of two coefficient alphas, given a desired power of $1-\beta$ and a significance level of α (Bonett, 2003).

$$\boldsymbol{n} = 2\left(\frac{k_1}{k_1-1} + \frac{k_2}{k_2-1}\right) \times \frac{\left(z_{1-\frac{\alpha}{2}} + z_{\beta}\right)^2}{ln\left(\tilde{\delta}\right)^2} + 2 \qquad (12.3)$$

where

- k_1 and k_2 are the number of items or raters for each alpha,
- $z_{1-\alpha/2}$ and z_{β} are the critical values from the standard normal distribution corresponding to the chosen significance level and desired power, and
- $\tilde{\delta} = \frac{1-\rho_0}{1-\rho_1}$, where ρ_0 and ρ_1 are the Cronbach's alpha coefficients under the null and alternative hypotheses, respectively.

This formula allows researchers to determine the minimum total sample size required to reliably test whether two scales or sets of raters differ in internal consistency.

Example 12.2: A screening test for adolescent attention deficit disorder consists of 25 behavioural descriptions, each rated by a parent on a scale from 0 to 3. Results from a pilot study suggest that the internal consistency reliabilities are approximately 0.70 for male adolescents and 0.85 for female adolescents. The objective is to determine the minimum number of subjects required to compare these two alphas.

Solution: The following parameters are identified:

- $\rho_0 = 0.70$ and $\rho_1 = 0.85$ for null and alternative hypotheses,
- Significance level $\alpha = 0.05$ (corresponding to $z_{1-\frac{\alpha}{2}} = 1.96$),
- Power $(1-\beta) = 0.80$ (corresponding to $z_{1-\beta} = 0.84$),
- Number of items $k_1 = k_2 = 25$.

Next, calculate the planning value of $\tilde{\delta}$:

$$\tilde{\delta} = \frac{1-\rho_0}{1-\rho_1} = \frac{1-0.70}{1-0.85} = \frac{0.30}{0.15} = 2$$

We use Equation 12.3 to calculate the required Sample Size to test $H_0 : \rho_0 = \rho_1$:

$$n = 2\left(\frac{k_1}{k_1-1} + \frac{k_2}{k_2-1}\right)\frac{\left(z_{1-\frac{\alpha}{2}} + z_\beta\right)^2}{ln\left(\tilde{\delta}\right)^2} + 2$$

Substituting the values:

$$n = 2\left(\frac{25}{24} + \frac{25}{24}\right)\frac{(1.96+0.84)^2}{ln(2)^2} + 2 =$$

$$n = 2 \times 2.083 \times \frac{7.84}{0.480} + 2 \approx 68.06 + 2 \approx 2 \approx 70.06$$

Since the sample size must be a whole number, we round up to the nearest integer: $n = 71$

The minimum sample size required to compare the two alphas for the screening test is 71 subjects. It is important to note that the accuracy of this sample size estimate depends on the precision of the planning value of $\tilde{\delta}$.

12.5 Sample Size Calculation for Intraclass Correlation Coefficient

The intraclass correlation coefficient (ICC), denoted as ρ, serves as an extension of Cohen's κ for situations in which raters evaluate items on a continuous scale rather than a binary scale. Importantly, the ICC allows for comparisons involving more than two raters. Mathematically, the ICC is defined as:

$$\rho = \frac{\sigma_B^2}{\sigma_B^2 + \sigma_W^2} \tag{12.4}$$

where σ_B^2 represents the between-rater variance, and σ_W^2 denotes the within-rater variance (Machin et al., 2018, p. 235).

To estimate the required sample size for achieving a specified ICC, Walter et al. provide the following formula (Walter et al., 1998):

$$n = 1 + \frac{2k\left(z_{1-\frac{\alpha}{2}} + z_{1-\beta}\right)^2}{(k-1)(ln\ C_0)^2} \tag{12.5}$$

where

$$C_0 = \frac{1 + k\theta_0}{1 + k\theta_1}$$

- K is the number of raters (must be 2 or more),
- ρ_0 is the value of ICC under the null hypothesis,
- ρ_1 is the value of ICC under the alternative hypothesis,
- α is the pre-specified significance level, typically set at 0.05, and
- $1-\beta$ is the pre-specified power of the test, commonly set at 0.80 or 0.90.

Example 12.3: In a study involving three raters ($k = 3$), the raters aim to measure the reliability of their assessments, with an acceptable reliability (null hypothesis) of $\rho_0 = 0.0$ and an expected reliability (alternative hypothesis) of $\rho_1 = 0.2$. The power is set to a minimum of 80%, and the significance level is $\alpha = 0.05$. How many subjects are required for this study?

Solution: The following parameters are identified:

- Number of items ($k = 3$),
- Null and alternative hypotheses: $\rho_0 = 0.0$ and $\rho_1 = 0.2$,

- Significance level (α) = 0.05 (corresponding to $z_{1-\frac{\alpha}{2}} = 1.96$), and
- Power ($1-\beta$) = 0.80 (corresponding to $z_{1-\beta} = 0.84$),

Calculating the planning θ_0 and θ_1:

$$\tilde{\delta} = \frac{1-\rho_0}{1-\rho_1} = \frac{1-0.00}{1-0.20} = \frac{1}{0.80} = 1.25$$

We use Equation 12.3 to calculate the required Sample Size to reject $\boldsymbol{H_0} : \rho_0 = \rho_1$. First compute θ_0 and θ_1:

$$\theta_0 = \frac{\rho_0}{1-\rho_0} = \frac{0}{1-0} = 0$$

$$\theta_1 = \frac{\rho_1}{1-\rho_1} = \frac{0.2}{1-0.2} = 0.25$$

Plugging these values into C_0:

$$C_0 = \frac{1+k\theta_0}{1+k\theta_1} = \frac{1+3\times 0}{1+3\times 0.25} = \frac{1}{1.75} = 0.5714$$

Substitute C_0 into Equation 12.5 to calculate the sample size:

$$n = 1 + \frac{2k\left(z_{1-\frac{\alpha}{2}} + z_{1-\beta}\right)^2}{(k-1)(\ln C_0)^2}$$

Substituting the known values:

$$n = 1 + \frac{2\times 3(1.96+0.84)^2}{(3-1)(\ln 0.5714)^2} = 1 + \frac{47.04}{0.62645} = 76.09 \approx 77$$

Rounding up, the minimum sample size required for this study to estimate the ICC with the specified parameters is 77 subjects.

It is essential to recognise that the accuracy of these sample size calculations depends on the precision of the planning values for ρ_0 and ρ_1.

To assist the reader, Table 12.1 presents the required sample sizes for the Intraclass Correlation Coefficient (ICC) for hypothesis testing with a one-sided $\alpha = 0.05$ and a power of 0.80 ($1-\beta = 0.80$). The sample sizes are calculated using Equation 12.5 for 2, 3, 4, and 5 observers.

TABLE 12.1

Sample Sizes Required to Observe a Given ICC Using the Hypothesis Testing Approach with One-Sided $\alpha = 0.05$ and Power of 0.80 for Different Numbers of Observers, k, according to Equations 12.5

		Number of Observers, k			
$\rho 0$	$P1$	2	3	4	5
0.1	0.2	591	252	157	115
	0.3	143	65	43	33
	0.4	61	30	20	16
	0.5	32	17	12	10
	0.6	19	11	8	7
	0.7	12	7	6	5
	0.8	8	5	4	4
	0.9	5	4	3	3
0.2	0.3	544	262	178	140
	0.4	128	65	46	37
	0.5	53	29	21	18
	0.6	27	16	12	10
	0.7	15	10	8	7
	0.8	9	6	5	5
	0.9	5	4	3	3
0.3	0.4	476	252	184	151
	0.5	109	61	46	38
	0.6	44	26	20	17
	0.7	21	10	11	9
	0.8	11	6	6	6
	0.9	6	4	4	4
0.4	0.5	393	226	173	147
	0.6	87	52	41	36
	0.7	33	21	17	15
	0.8	15	10	9	8
	0.9	7	5	5	4
0.5	0.6	300	184	147	129
	0.7	63	40	33	29
	0.8	22	15	13	11
	0.9	9	6	6	5
0.6	0.7	205	134	110	99
	0.8	39	27	22	20
	0.9	12	9	7	7
0.7	0.8	117	80	68	62
	0.9	18	13	12	11
0.8	0.9	46	33	29	27

12.6 Sample Size Calculation for ICC with a Confidence Interval

The hypothesis testing approach may not always be suitable for planning a reliability study, as it requires specifying both ρ_0 *and* ρ_1, which can be challenging in practice (Bonett, 2002b; Giraudeau & Mary, 2001). An alternative approach is to focus on the width of the confidence interval (CI) for ρ. In single-sample situations, the results of a reliability study are typically presented as a point estimate of ρ along with its associated CI. Therefore, sample size calculations aim to achieve an interval estimate with sufficient precision.

To determine the sample size needed for an exact CI for ρ with a specified width w, one can use the formula:

$$w = 2z_{1-\alpha/2}\sqrt{\text{var}(r)}$$

Substituting ρ with the "planning value" $\bar{\rho}$, the required sample size to achieve the desired width w of the CI for ρ is given by

$$n = \frac{8 \times z_{1-\frac{\alpha}{2}}^2 (1-\bar{\rho})^2 \{1+(k-1)\bar{\rho}\}^2}{w^2 \times k \times (k-1)} \tag{12.6}$$

This value is then rounded up to the nearest integer. Bonett suggests an approximation that requires one additional sample compared to Equation 12.6 (Shoukri et al., 2004, p. 6).

TIP

The ICC serves as an extension of Cohen's κ, applying to situations in which two or more raters evaluate items on a continuous scale rather than a binary one. Similar to Cronbach's alpha, increasing the number of raters tends to decrease the ICC.

Example 12.4: A reliability study is being conducted to assess the consistency of a new blood pressure measurement device, with the outcome measured on a continuous scale. How many subjects should participate in this study if a confidence interval with a width of $w = 0.1$ is desired, a planning value of $\bar{\rho} = 0.85$, and a significance level of $\alpha = 0.05$ is assumed? Additionally, assume $k = 2$ (two measurements per subject).

Solution: The provided information is: α = 0.05, corresponding to a value of $z_{1-\alpha/2} = 1.96$, k = 2, w = 0.1, and $\bar{\rho}$ = 0.85. Substitute values into the sample size Equation 12.6:

$$n = \frac{8 \times z^2_{1-\frac{\alpha}{2}} (1-\bar{\rho})^2 \{1+(k-1)\bar{\rho}\}^2}{w^2 \times k \times (k-1)}$$

Substituting the values:

$$n = \frac{8 \times \left[1.96(1-0.85)^2\right] \times \{1+(2-1)\times 0.85\}^2}{0.1^2 \times 2 \times (2-1)}$$

Calculating the final sample size:

$$n = \frac{2.4733}{0.02} = 123.665 \approx 124$$

The required sample size is n = 124 subjects. Therefore, to achieve a confidence interval with a width of 0.1 for the reliability estimate of the blood pressure measurement device, a sample size of 124 subjects is required.

To aid the reader, Table 12.2 presents the required sample sizes for estimating the Intraclass Correlation Coefficient (ICC) with a 95% confidence interval (α = 0.05), a pre-specified width, and a power of 0.80 ($1 - \beta = 0.80$). The sample sizes are calculated using Equation 12.6 for 2, 3, and 4 observers.

For example, in a study with 2 raters (k = 2), an ICC of ρ = 0.80, and a desired 95% CI width of W = 0.10, Table 12.2 shows that m = 205 subjects are required. Thus, the total number of observations is: $n = k \times m = 2 \times 205 = 410$.

12.7 Sample Size for ICC in Test-Retest Reliability

Test-retest reliability studies evaluate the consistency between two numerical ratings taken at different times. Although some researchers have used Pearson's correlation coefficients for this purpose, this approach can be misleading, as it does not account for systematic biases (Bartko, 1976). The Intraclass Correlation Coefficient (ICC) is recommended for a more accurate measure of consistency with quantitative variables.

Test-retest reliability is essential in validating questionnaire designs, especially during initial pilot testing. For example, in a validation study of the Children's Depression Inventory, the ICC was used to measure the test-retest reliability of total scores for evaluating depression among children (Tan et al., 2013). This approach helps determine the extent to which the total scores

TABLE 12.2

Sample Sizes Required to Estimate an ICC for a 95% Confidence Interval Width Using Equation 12.6. Each cell gives the number of subjects, m subjects. Hence, the total number of observations for the study is n = k × m subjects

		Planned Width of Two-Sided CI, $W\rho$			
k	ρ	0.05	0.10	0.15	0.20
2	0.60	2,519	631	281	159
	0.65	2,051	514	229	130
	0.70	1604	405	183	105
	0.75	1,182	299	136	79
	0.80	802	205	94	55
	0.85	479	120	58	35
3	0.60	1,588	398	178	101
	0.65	1,329	333	149	84
	0.70	1,064	267	120	68
	0.75	802	202	90	52
	0.80	555	140	63	36
	0.85	338	86	39	23
4	0.60	1,286	323	144	82
	0.65	1,094	275	123	70
	0.70	887	223	100	57
	0.75	678	171	77	44
	0.80	475	120	54	31
	0.85	292	74	34	20

remain consistent across two different time points. Researchers typically aim for a high level of agreement between these scores to ensure that the questionnaire is reliable.

To detect ICC values of 0.5, 0.6, and 0.7, the minimum required sample sizes are 22, 15, and 10, respectively (Table 12.3). These sample sizes are calculated using Equation 12.5.

When planning to determine the level of agreement for a specific score in a questionnaire between responses collected at two time points, researchers might state: "The objective of this study is to determine the level of agreement for the score assessing respondent satisfaction at two different periods (time 1 and time 2) by evaluating its test-retest reliability." Sample size calculations for ICC can be derived using PASS software and the above equation. With a significance level (α) of 0.05 and a power lower than 80%, a minimum sample size of 22 is sufficient to detect an ICC of 0.50 (Table 12.3). The sample size should be adjusted by adding a typical dropout rate.

A small sample size is often adequate for estimating ICC, which is beneficial since test-retest reliability studies are typically conducted during initial pilot phases with a limited number of participants. Additionally, reliability

TABLE 12.3

Sample Size Requirement for ICC (Test-Retest) with Power = 80% and 90%; One-Sided Alpha = 0.05, Two Observations per Subject, and R0 is set at 0. Using Equation 12.5 (Bujang & Baharum, 2017b, p. 7)

ICC	1-β = 0.80	1-β = 0.90
0.2	152	210
0.3	66	91
0.4	36	50
0.5	22	30
0.6	15	20
0.7	10	13
0.7	7	9
0.9	5	6

studies may be costly, as incentives might be required to encourage respondents to participate again during follow-up assessments.

In conclusion, although Pearson's correlation provides some insights, the ICC is a more robust and appropriate measure for evaluating test-retest reliability in quantitative rating studies (Bujang & Baharum, 2017b, p. 3).

Note: We do not provide an example here, as the exercises are solved using Equation 12.5, which is the same method used in the previous section.

12.8 Sample Size Determination to Estimate Kappa Coefficient

The sample size determination formula for estimating the Kappa coefficient is essential in various research contexts, particularly when planning studies to assess inter-rater agreement. Researchers use this formula to calculate the minimum sample size necessary to achieve a desired level of precision for the Kappa estimate, thereby ensuring that the results are both statistically valid and reliable. This formula is especially valuable in pilot studies, where the Kappa coefficient is being estimated for the first time, as it helps maintain a consistent statistical foundation, enhancing the validity of the conclusions drawn. Overall, it plays a crucial role in study design by allowing researchers to set confidence intervals, determine statistical power, and adjust for variability, ultimately leading to more meaningful and generalisable results. The minimum sample size required to estimate Kappa is represented by Equation 12.7 (Machin et al., 2018, p. 324):

$$n = \frac{4(1-\kappa)z^2_{1-\frac{\alpha}{2}}}{w^2}\left[(1-\kappa)(1-2\kappa)+\frac{\kappa(2-\kappa)}{2\pi(1-\pi)}\right] \tag{12.7}$$

where

- κ: Expected Kappa coefficient.
- w: Width of the confidence interval.
- π: Proportion of agreement by chance.
- $z_{1-\frac{\alpha}{2}}$: Z-score corresponding to the desired confidence level (e.g., 1.96 for a 95% confidence interval).

> **Example 12.5:** Consider a scenario in which we aim to assess the level of agreement between two radiologists interpreting chest images for the diagnosis of a specific disease. Each radiologist independently indicates the presence or absence of the disease in the images. Based on previous studies, the researcher anticipates a Kappa coefficient (κ) of 0.70, which reflects substantial agreement beyond chance. To ensure adequate precision in estimating this coefficient, the researcher specifies a confidence interval width (w) of 0.10 at a 95% confidence level. Additionally, the probability that the disease is present in the chest X-ray is $\pi = 0.40$, meaning that 40% of the chest X-rays are expected to show evidence of the disease. This value is required for determining the necessary sample size for reliable estimation. How many samples should be included in the study?

Solution: Given information is: Expected Kappa coefficient, $\kappa = 0.70$; Desired width of the confidence interval, $w = 0.10$; Probability of the disease being evident in the chest X-ray, $\pi = 0.4$; and Z-score for a 95% confidence level, $z_{1-\frac{\alpha}{2}} = 1.96$. Using these values in Equation 12.7 gives the necessary sample size for kappa estimation:

$$n = \frac{4(1-\kappa)z^2_{1-\frac{\alpha}{2}}}{w^2}\left[(1-\kappa)(1-2\kappa)+\frac{\kappa(2-\kappa)}{2\pi(1-\pi)}\right]$$

Now, plugging in the values:

$$n = \frac{4(1-0.7)\times 1.96^2}{0.1^2}\left[(1-0.7)(1-2\times 0.7)+\frac{0.7(2-0.7)}{2\times 0.4(1-0.4)}\right]$$

Calculating the expression:

$$n = \frac{1.2\times 3.84}{0.01}\left[-0.12+\frac{0.91}{0.48}\right] = 818.304 \approx 819$$

The required sample size n is approximately 819 when rounded up.

12.9 Sample Size Calculation for Comparing Cohen's Kappa

Cohen's kappa coefficient is a statistical measure used to assess the degree of agreement between two different evaluations of a categorical response variable. The response variable must be categorical, and evaluations can be conducted either by two distinct raters or by the same rater at two different time points. The latter scenario is particularly relevant in test-retest reliability studies. It is essential to note that Cohen's kappa assumes statistical independence of the raters. In the case of repeated measurements by the same rater, the responses at time 2 should be independent of those at time 1 to satisfy this assumption (Bujang & Baharum, 2017a).

Donner and Eliasziw provide a framework for calculating the sample size necessary to ensure adequate power in studies of interobserver agreement involving two raters (Donner & Eliasziw, 1992). They derived the formula for the number of subjects needed to test the null hypothesis $H_0 : \kappa = \kappa_0$ against the alternative hypothesis $H_1 : \kappa = \kappa_1$:

$$n = \frac{\left(z_{1-\frac{\alpha}{2}} + z_{1-\beta}\right)^2}{A+B+C} \tag{12.8}$$

where

$$A = \frac{\left[\pi(1-\pi)(\kappa_1 - \kappa_0)\right]^2}{\pi^2 + \pi(1-\pi)\kappa_0},$$

$$B = \frac{2\left[\pi(1-\pi)(\kappa_1 - \kappa_0)\right]^2}{\pi(1-\pi)(1-\kappa_0)}$$

$$C = \frac{\left[\pi(1-\pi)(\kappa_1 - \kappa_0)\right]^2}{(1-\pi)^2 + \pi(1-\pi)\kappa_0}$$

Example 12.6: Consider a scenario where we wish to test $H_0 : \kappa_0 = 0.60$ versus $H_1 : \kappa \neq 0.60$, with $\kappa_0 = 0.60$ indicating a level of agreement characterised as "substantial". To achieve a power of 80% at a significance level of α = 0.05, assuming π = 0.30 with $\kappa_1 = 0.90$, we need to determine the required sample size.

Solution: The available information includes: π = 0:30, $\kappa_0 = 0.60$, $\kappa_1 = 0.90$, α = 0.05 corresponding to $z_{1-\frac{\alpha}{2}} = 1.96$ and 1-β = 0.80 corresponding to $z_{1-\beta} = 0.84$. Substituting these values into the components of Equation 12.7:

$$A = \frac{\left[\pi(1-\pi)(\kappa_1-\kappa_0)\right]^2}{\pi^2+\pi(1-\pi)\kappa_0} = \frac{\left[0.3(1-0.3)(0.90-0.60)\right]^2}{0.30^2+0.30(1-0.30)\times 0.60} = \frac{[0.063]^2}{0.216} = 0.018375$$

$$B = \frac{2\left[\pi(1-\pi)(\kappa_1-\kappa_0)\right]^2}{\pi(1-\pi)(1-\kappa_0)} = \frac{2\left[0.3(1-0.3)(0.9-0.6)\right]^2}{0.3(1-0.3)(1-0.6)} = \frac{0.007938}{0.084} = 0.0945$$

$$C = \frac{\left[\pi(1-\pi)(\kappa_1-\kappa_0)\right]^2}{(1-\pi)^2+\pi(1-\pi)\kappa_0} = \frac{\left[0.3(1-0.3)(0.9-0.6)\right]^2}{(1-0.3)^2+0.3(1-0.3)\times 0.6} = \frac{[0.063]^2}{0.616} = 0.00644$$

$$\left(z_{1-\frac{\alpha}{2}} + z_{1-\beta}0.00644\right)^2 = (1.96+0.84)^2 = 7.84$$

Finally, substituting A, B, and C into the sample size equation:

$$n = \frac{\left(z_{1-\frac{\alpha}{2}} + z_{1-\beta}\right)^2}{A+B+C} = \frac{7.84}{0.018375+0.0945+0.00644} = \frac{7.84}{0.119315} = 65.71 \approx 66$$

To ensure adequate power for detecting a significant difference in Cohen's kappa, a total of 66 subjects are required.

TABLE 12.4

Number of Required Subjects k at $\alpha = 0.05$ and $\beta = 0.20$

		κ_0				
κ_1	π	**0.4**	**0.6**	**0.7**	**0.8**	**0.9**
0.4	**0.1**	–	334	121	49	17
	0.3	–	148	52	21	7
	0.5	–	126	45	18	6
0.6	**0.1**	404	–	1090	195	46
	0.3	190	–	474	83	20
	0.5	165	–	400	71	17
0.7	**0.1**	179	1339	–	770	103
	0.3	84	595	–	336	44
	0.5	73	502	–	282	37
0.8	**0.1**	101	335	1090	–	413
	0.3	47	148	474	–	177
	0.5	41	125	400	–	149
0.9	**0.1**	64	149	272	779	–
	0.3	30	66	118	336	–
	0.5	26	55	100	282	–

Due to the complexity involved in calculating the sample size for the Kappa coefficient, Table 12.4 presents values for the required number of subjects across various configurations of κ_0, κ_1, and π at significance levels of α = 0.05 and 1-β = 0.80.

This table provides a reference for the required sample sizes across different configurations of κ_0, κ_1, and π at the specified significance levels.

References

Bartko, J. J. (1976). On various intraclass correlation reliability coefficients. *Psychological Bulletin, 83*(5), 762.

Bonett, D. G. (2002a). Sample size requirements for testing and estimating coefficient alpha. *Journal of Educational and Behavioral Statistics, 27*(4), 335–340.

Bonett, D. G. (2002b). Sample size requirements for estimating intraclass correlations with desired precision. *Statistics in Medicine, 21*(9), 1331–1335.

Bonett, D. G. (2003). Sample size requirements for comparing two alpha coefficients. *Applied Psychological Measurement, 27*(1), 72–74.

Bujang, M. A., & Baharum, N. (2017a). Guidelines of the minimum sample size requirements for Kappa agreement test. *Epidemiology, Biostatistics, and Public Health, 14*(2). https://doi.org/10.2427/12267

Bujang, M. A., & Baharum, N. (2017b). A simplified guide to determination of sample size requirements for estimating the value of intraclass correlation coefficient: A review. *Archives of Orofacial Science, 12*(1), 1–11.

Bujang, M. A., Omar, E. D., & Baharum, N. A. (2018). A review on sample size determination for Cronbach's alpha test: A simple guide for researchers. *Malaysian Journal of Medical Sciences, 25*(6), 85.

Donna, S. (2005). *Encyclopedia of biostatistics* (M. H. Gail, P. Armitage, & T. Colton, Eds., Vol. 2, 2nd ed.). Wiley.

Donner, A., & Eliasziw, M. (1992). A goodness-of-fit approach to inference procedures for the kappa statistic: Confidence interval construction, significance-testing and sample size estimation. *Statistics in Medicine, 11*(11), 1511–1519.

Giraudeau, B., & Mary, J. (2001). Planning a reproducibility study: How many subjects and how many replicates per subject for an expected width of the 95 per cent confidence interval of the intraclass correlation coefficient. *Statistics in Medicine, 20*(21), 3205–3214.

Machin, D., Campbell, M. J., Tan, S. B., & Tan, S. H. (2018). *Sample sizes for clinical, laboratory and epidemiology studies.* John Wiley & Sons.

Shoukri, M. M., Asyali, M., & Donner, A. (2004). Sample size requirements for the design of reliability study: Review and new results. *Statistical Methods in Medical Research, 13*(4), 251–271.

Tan, S. M., Loh, S. F., Bujnag, M. A., Haniff, J., Abd Rahman, F. N., Ismail, F., Omar, K., & Mohd Daud, T. I. (2013). Validation of the Malay version of children's depression inventory. *International Medical Journal, 20*(2), 188–191.

Walter, S., Eliasziw, M., & Donner, A. (1998). Sample size and optimal designs for reliability studies. *Statistics in Medicine, 17*(1), 101–110.

Index

For Product Safety Concerns and Information please contact our EU
representative GPSR@taylorandfrancis.com
Taylor & Francis Verlag GmbH, Kaufingerstraße 24, 80331 München, Germany

www.ingramcontent.com/pod-product-compliance
Ingram Content Group UK Ltd.
Pitfield, Milton Keynes, MK11 3LW, UK
UKHW020145200926
475702UK00005B/932
* 9 7 8 1 0 4 1 2 6 2 7 8 7 *